PHENYLPROPANOLAMINE— A REVIEW

LOUIS LASAGNA
Sackler School of Graduate Biomedical Sciences
Tufts University
Boston, Massachusetts

WILEY

A WILEY-INTERSCIENCE PUBLICATION
JOHN WILEY & SONS
NEW YORK / CHICHESTER / BRISBANE / TORONTO / SINGAPORE

Library of Congress Cataloging in Publication Data:

Lasagna, Louis, 1938–
    Phenylpropanolamine—a review.
    "A Wiley-Interscience publication."
    Includes index.
    1. Phenylpropanolamine.   I. Title.
RM666.P57L37   1987   615′.31632   86-28963
ISBN 0-471-81977-8

Printed in the United States of America

10 9 8 7 6 5 4 3 2 1

PREFACE

Phenylpropanolamine has been commercially available for about 65 years. First sold as a mydriatic, phenylpropanolamine has become popular as a cough/cold remedy and for the management of obesity. The population of the United States now consumes about five billion doses of phenylpropanolamine annually. Why, then, should a book be written about it?

In the early 1980s, adverse reaction reports began to appear with increasing frequency. These were usually anecdotal, and, in many instances, described adverse reactions in an individual who had taken several products at the same time. Because case reports often serve as the only signal for unusual drug reactions, careful clinicians were becoming disturbed by the increasing number of such reports. Also disturbing was the observation that most of the adverse experiences occurred with appetite suppressants and very few with cold remedies. This was ironic because, in the United States, the maximum daily dose of phenylpropanolamine is restricted to 75 mg for appetite suppressants, but 150 mg per day can be used in cough/cold remedies. Also, the use of cough/cold remedies containing phenylpropanolamine far exceeds the use of appetite suppressants that contain the drug.

To address the confusion and air the controversy that had developed, a conference on the benefits and risks of phenylpropanolamine was held in New York City in June 1984. At that time, a considerable scientific literature existed, but there had never been a serious attempt to review all of this information. As a followup to the conference, it was decided to assemble a rigorous review of the world literature on phenylpropanolamine.

The book was developed from a comprehensive search of the published literature. Initially, over 2400 articles were identified and considered for inclusion in the book. As the book developed, the literature searches were continued to assure that it would be thorough and up-to-date.

During the initial review, it became apparent that some articles did not report original data, but reiterated the conclusions of earlier reports, thus adding redundancy to the literature and, in some instances, reinforcing inadequate data or incorrect conclusions. Other articles reported the effects of chemical entities termed "phenylpropanolamine" which were not phenylpropanolamine as we know it (*dl*-norephedrine). Because of the confusion, this book was developed not as an annotated bibliography but as a critical review in which, insofar as possible, published information was put into accurate, balanced, scientific perspective. Accordingly, our policy has been to state the consensus view and point out the inadequacy of the supporting evidence, when appropriate, rather than omit a topic because of the absence of information.

This book is not intended to be a handbook for analytical chemists, nor a guide to pharmacologic, behaviorial, or clinical research methods. For these, the reader is referred to the usual channels of information on professional practice. This book is, rather, intended as a general guide to research techniques and their limitations so that the interested reader may be better able to evaluate the published literature. It will also serve as a guidepost for those interested in more specific research information.

Each chapter addresses controversial topics: the relationship of phenylpropanolamine to khat and Ma Huang; isomer nomenclature; national differences in nomenclature conventions; questionable chemical identity and analytical purity of certain products; the chemical and pharmacological relationships of phenylpropanolamine, ephedrine, and amphetamine; the pharmacological effects of phenylpropanolamine in combination with caffeine or ephedrine; tachyphylaxis and phenylpropanolamine activity; therapeutic potency; drug interactions; cardiovascular and central nervous system effects; and abuse potential and use as a "street drug."

This book is intended to inform clinicians and pharmacists regarding the pharmacological actions of phenylpropanolamine and its expected side effects. It will serve as a review of the published literature for pharmacologists, toxicologists, clinical pathologists, and analytical chemists. The book also should be useful to general readers such as public officials and consumers. In short, anyone consulting this book for information on phenylpropanolamine should not go away disappointed.

Finally, I want to thank Nancy J. Chew and her colleagues and staff at NJC Enterprises Ltd. for their thoughtful attention to detail: Roslyn Begun, Norma Colclough, Stephen Gould, Ph.D., James Kittle, Lloyd Weyant, and particularly Donald Hinman, Ph.D. contributed considerably by organizing, assessing, and clarifying a massive amount of disparate information; a special note of appreciation is due to Ann Reilly, who managed the mechanics and scheduling of the book from concept to publication. Thanks also go to Patrice Otani for identifying and locating the source material, to all who have given permission to reprint their original data, and to the editorial staff at John Wiley & Sons.

LOUIS LASAGNA, M.D.

Boston, Massachusetts
January, 1988

CONTENTS

CHAPTER 4. SAFETY

PHENYLPROPANOLAMINE
—A REVIEW

1

HISTORY

Phenylpropanolamine, a component of many over-the-counter (OTC) drug preparations in the United States, has been used both clinically and experimentally for nearly 75 years. The history and development of phenylpropanolamine and its initial synthesis as an analogue of phenylethylamine and the early studies of its pharmacological and therapeutic properties and some recent issues regarding the safety and efficacy of phenylpropanolamine-containing products are reviewed in this chapter. The history of phenylpropanolamine is an interesting example of how the scientific and medical communities have come to appreciate the selective and specific characteristics of this drug. Since phenylpropanolamine is a chemical analogue of sympathomimetic amines, early studies of phenylpropanolamine emphasized the similarities between this drug and pressor amines such as epinephrine or ephedrine, or between phenylpropanolamine and central nervous system (CNS) stimulants such as ephedrine or amphetamine. However, later research efforts emphasized the differences between these related compounds, and it was demonstrated that because of phenylpropanolamine's selectivity of action it could be used therapeutically as a nasal decongestant or an appetite suppressant with a low potency for pressor or stimulant side effects. Unfortunately, this drug selectivity is often ignored and phenylpropanolamine is still often cited as an "amphetaminelike" drug. In addition, this history demonstrates how medical research interacts with social and cultural attitudes regarding pharmacological issues. For example, early pharmacological and clinical studies of phenylpropanolamine were concerned primarily with determining the mechanisms of drug action and the possible therapeutic uses of the drug; issues of drug safety and clinical efficacy were often not specifically investigated. In contemporary clinical pharmacological studies, these latter issues are directly investigated. Finally, in contemporary society, issues such as drug abuse and street drug use are recognized as important medical problems. Phenylpropanolamine has recently come under scrutiny as a component of the so-called amphetamine look-alike and pseudospeed drugs, which often contain phenylpropanolamine combined with caffeine and/or ephedrine. Thus abuse liability of phenylpropanolamine-containing products has become an important issue; the abuse liability of phenylpropanolamine is discussed fully in Chapter 3.

The role of phenylpropanolamine as a therapeutic drug has evolved over a span of 75 years. During the 1920s and 1930s, it was investigated as a member of the class of sympathomimetic pressor amines. Later (1940–1970), it was used extensively as a decongestant and appetite suppressant. More recently, during the 1980s, the efficacy and safety of phenylpropanolamine have been challenged (Bernstein & Diskant, 1982; Dietz, 1981; Horowitz et al., 1980; Mueller, 1983; Mueller et al., 1984). Also, as a component of look-alike drugs and pseudospeed, the drug abuse potential of phenylpropanolamine had become an issue (Griffiths et al., 1978; Chait et al., 1983; Bigelow, 1985). The history of phenylpropanolamine, in terms of the changing attitudes toward this drug, is reviewed in this chapter. In the remaining chapters of this book the scientific literature related to phenylpropanolamine is reviewed and the evidence regarding the safety and efficacy of this drug presented.

EARLY STUDIES OF PHENYLPROPANOLAMINE: SYNTHESIS AND PATENTING

One of the major advances in pharmacology during the first decade of the twentieth century was the investigation of the structure-activity relationships of the β-phenylethylamines. The discovery and synthesis of phenylpropanolamine was part of this effort. β-Phenylethylamine, first isolated from putrid meat by Colombo and Spica in 1875, is the chemical structure from which a large series of sympathomimetic amines was derived. The earliest systematic investigation of these compounds was the study by Barger and Dale (1910), who coined the term "sympathomimetic" to describe the actions of drugs that mimic the sympathetic branch of the autonomic nervous system. These responses include increased arterial blood pressure due to arterial constriction and cardiac acceleration, pupillary dilation, salivation and lacrimation not blocked by atropine, inhibition of gut motility, inhibition of the urinary bladder and contraction of the pregnant uterus. Barger and Dale (1910) described the pharmacological responses to a large series of β-phenylethylamine derivatives and the structural characteristics required for sympathomimetic activity. Although Barger and Dale did not recognize it at the time, the actions of the phenylethylamines were similar to the sympathetic responses because these responses were due to the release of epinephrine and norepinephrine, which are themselves β-phenylethylamines. Nonetheless, these studies provided part of the evidence for the chemical basis of synaptic transmission in the nervous system. Phenylpropanolamine itself was not included in the studies by Barger and Dale.

Another major research effort that led to the development of phenylpropanolamine was the investigation of the pharmacology of the Chinese drug ma huang. Ma huang is an ancient Chinese folk-medicine agent used both therapeutically and as an intoxicant (Emde, 1930). Indeed, Emde (1930) reported that ma huang's "esteem in the old days was such that one had to pay when found riding under the influence." One of the principal alkaloids extracted from ma huang is ephedrine, discovered by the Japanese chemist W. N. Nagai in 1887 (Emde, 1930). Emde also noted that at the time it was believed that "ephedrine only dilates the pupils in Caucasians, not in Mongolians or Negroes. If this is true, the discovery of the mydriatic action will be twice as remarkable because it was made by a Japanese in Europe." The pharmacology of ma huang, ephedrine, and related β-phenylethylamines, including d-norpseudoephedrine and other isomers of ephedrine, was investigated extensively by Chen and co-workers in the 1920s (Chen & Schmidt, 1924, 1930; Chen et al., 1929). In an addendum to their paper, Chen et al. (1929) reported the synthesis of dl-β-phenyl-β-hydroxy-α-methylethylamine HCl (i.e., phenylpropanolamine) by the Sharp and Dohme Company. Phenylpropanolamine produced a pressor activity greater than that of dl-ephedrine, with a potency ratio of 125:105 (phenylpropanolamine:ephedrine). In two humans given 50 mg of phenylpropanolamine (PO), pressor responses of +30 and +16 mm Hg were recorded.

The first synthesis of phenylpropanolamine was reported by Calliess (1912), who referred to the compound as "α-amidopropiophenyl carbinol." He obtained phenylpropanolamine by the reduction of the ketone α-aminopropiophenone with a sodium amalgam and hydrochloric acid. Eberhard (1917) later obtained phenylpropanolamine, which he called "amidoethylphenyl carbinol," in greater yield and purity by the catalytic reduction of the same ketone. Chen et al. (1929) credited Rabe and Hallensleben (1910) with the first synthesis of "racemic C_6H_5-CHOH-CHCH$_3$-NH$_2$," and Kanfer et al. (1983) credited Mannich and Jacobsohn (1910) with the first synthesis of phenylpropanolamine. However, these investigators actually reported synthesis of other phenylethylamine derivatives rather than phenylpropanolamine itself.

The first proprietary phenylpropanolamine preparation was called *Mydriatine,* based on the ability of the drug to produce mydriasis (Nagai, 1920). The synthesis of Mydriatine was described by Nagai (1913), and the first clinical tests were reported by Amatsu and Kubota (1913, 1917) and Hirose (1915). Mydriatine was patented by Nagai (patent application in 1916, approved in 1920).

EARLY BASIC PHARMACOLOGY STUDIES

The earliest studies of the pharmacological responses to phenylpropanolamine demonstrated that it caused dilation of the pupils (Amatsu & Kubota, 1913, 1917; Hirose, 1915; Kanao, 1928). Kanao (1928) described the mydriatic efficacy of various stereoisomers of ephedrine and pseudoephedrine. *dl*-Norephedrine (i.e., phenylpropanolamine) produced mydriasis both in humans *in vivo* and in the isolated eyeballs of frogs. However, phenylpropanolamine has limited clinical usefulness as a mydriatic drug.

Because many sympathomimetic amines are potent pressor agents (Barger & Dale, 1910; Chen et al., 1929), the effects of phenylpropanolamine on blood pressure were measured. Several studies confirmed that IV administration of high doses of phenylpropanolamine increased arterial blood pressure. In anesthetized rabbits, doses of Mydriatine (phenylpropanolamine) greater than 10 mg/kg (IV) produced biphasic effects on blood pressure (Hasama, 1930). An initial depressor response was followed by a pressor response. Both responses were dose-dependent, but neither response was blocked by atropine or ergotamine. In humans as well, administration of IV doses of 20, 25, or 50 mg of Propadrine (phenylpropanolamine) increased blood pressure and decreased heart rate (Loman et al., 1939). The maximum increase in systolic blood pressure was 0 to 28 mm Hg at doses of 20 to 25 mg (IV) and 44 to 82 mm Hg at 50 mg (IV). For diastolic pressure, the maximum increases were 2 to 16 and 14 to 46 mm Hg for 20 to 25 and 50 mg, respectively. The maximum pressor response occurred 1 to 7 min after injection, and the time to recovery was 30 to 95 min. No cardiac arrhythmias were observed after IV Propadrine.

Many sympathomimetic amines are ineffective when given orally because they are metabolically degraded by enzymes in the gut. However, amines with an α-methyl group are effective when given orally (Chen et al., 1929), indicating that phenylpropanolamine might be effective by this route. Indeed, Chen et al. (1929) demonstrated that in two cases, 50 mg of phenylpropanolamine (PO) produced a 16- and 30-mm Hg increase in blood pressure in humans.

The pressor effect of oral phenylpropanolamine was confirmed in dogs, although no quantitative data were presented (Hartung & Munch, 1931). Recent controlled clinical trials using large numbers of subjects taking recommended oral doses of 25-mg immediate-release phenylpropanolamine or 75-mg sustained-release phenylpropanolamine have demonstrated that phenylpropanolamine does not increase blood pressure significantly; these clinical trials are reviewed in Chapter 5.

The sympathomimetic amines have prominent effects on the respiratory and bronchial systems, including constriction of blood vessels in the nasal mucosa and relaxation of bronchial smooth muscle. These effects are the basis for the use of these drugs in symptomatic relief of such conditions as the common cold, hay fever, and asthma. The potential use of phenylpropanolamine as a decongestant was demonstrated by Stockton et al. (1931) who showed that topical application of a 3% solution of phenylpropanolamine in the nostrils produced effective decongestion in humans with acute or chronic sinusitis. No local irritation was noted. This decongestant effect was confirmed experimentally in dogs (Aviado et al., 1959). Anesthetized dogs were prepared for simultaneous recording of blood pressure, carotid blood flow, and intranasal pressure. Phenylpropanolamine (100 μg, intracarotid) decreased both carotid blood flow and intranasal pressure. Presumably the decongestant effect is mediated by constriction of blood vessels in the nasal mucosa.

Two other pharmacological effects may contribute to the efficacy of phenylpropanolamine in cough-cold preparations: relaxation of bronchial smooth muscle and antitussive activity. Early studies demonstrated that phenylpropanolamine decreased bronchial spasm produced by IV injection of choline chloride in anesthetized rabbits (Hasama, 1930). The minimum effective dose for this effect was 4.5 mg/kg IV; the potency of phenylpropanolamine was similar to that of ephedrine and much less than that of epinephrine. In contrast, phenylpropanolamine caused bronchoconstriction in isolated guinea pig trachea-bronchi-lung preparations (Tainter et al., 1934).

The antitussive effects of phenylpropanolamine were demonstrated using experimentally induced coughs in guinea pigs and dogs (Winter & Flataker, 1954). Phenylpropanolamine produced a dose-dependent decrease in coughing in both guinea pigs [0.5–2 mg/kg, subcutaneous (SC)] and dogs (1–8 mg/kg, PO), and was nearly as effective as codeine as an antitussive drug.

Thus most of the phenylpropanolamine research conducted in the 1920s and 1930s focused on the effects on the autonomic nervous and cardiovascular systems. It was not until the 1940s that the CNS effects of phenylpropanolamine were investigated. The prominent CNS stimulating effects of sympathomimetic amines such as ephedrine and amphetamine (Benzedrine) were recognized much earlier (Emde, 1930). In fact, the CNS stimulant effect of ephedrine and its isomers was probably responsible for the popularity of the Chinese drug ma huang as a euphoriant drug.

Since most of the studies of phenylpropanolamine conducted in the 1920s and 1930s were conducted using either anesthetized animals or isolated tissue preparations, possible effects on CNS function could not be investigated. The structure-activity relationships for CNS stimulant activity of a series of 75 sympathomimetic amines were investigated by using locomotor activity in rats as the behavioral model (Schulte et al., 1941). These investigators concluded that there was no relationship between sympathomimetic activity and CNS stimulant effect. The most potent amines in this animal model were amphetamine, ephedrine, epinephrine, and mescaline. Phenylpropanolamine did increase locomotor activity, but only at very high doses. The threshold dose of phenylpropanolamine was 40 mg/kg (SC), and peak effect occurred at 80 mg/kg (SC). By comparison, the minimum lethal dose (MLD) of phenylpropanolamine was 80 mg/kg (SC). In addition, the magnitude of the increase in locomotor activity produced by phenylpropanolamine was much less than that produced by amphetamine or ephedrine.

These results—that phenylpropanolamine has relatively weak CNS stimulant effects and only at near lethal doses—have been confirmed repeatedly in rats (Tainter, 1944; Warren & Werner, 1946) and in mice (Fairchild & Alles, 1967). In addition, phenylpropanolamine given in the diet produced a biphasic effect, with increased motor activity at a dose level of 1.0–1.5 mg/g of food but decreased motor activity at higher doses (Tainter, 1944).

Another major development in the pharmacology of phenylpropanolamine that occurred primarily in the 1940s was the observation of the anorectic effects of the drug. The actual origin of this observation is unclear. Amphetamine (Benzedrine) was used in the mid-1930s as a treatment for narcolepsy (Prinzmetal & Bloomberg, 1935) and later as a treatment for obesity. Recognizing that the CNS stimulant side effects of amphetamine severely limited its usefulness, and recognizing the similarities between Benzedrine and Propadrine, Hirsch (1939) compared the two drugs for treatment of obesity in a series of patients. In this uncontrolled study, Hirsch concluded that phenylpropanolamine was an effective appetite suppressant with no side effects, and particularly no nervousness or insomnia. There appear to be no experimental studies in laboratory animals that antedate the clinical study by Hirsch (1939). In the first reported study in animals, phenylpropanolamine mixed in the diet produced weight loss in rats (Tainter, 1944). The maximum weight loss in the 7-day study was 15% of body weight; the dose level that produced this effect was not reported. Also in this study, phenylpropanolamine decreased weight gain in rats even when control and treated rats were pair-fed; that is, phenylpropanolamine decreased weight gain independent of any effect on food intake. Benzedrine, but not phenylpropanolamine, increased the basal metabolic rate, as measured by an increase in oxygen consumption. Both Benzedrine and phenylpropanolamine decreased the gastric transport time, and Benzedrine decreased food intake. (The effects of phenylpropanolamine on food intake were not reported.) The anorectic effects of phenylpropanolamine in experimental animals has been repeatedly confirmed (Epstein, 1959; Kornblith & Hoebel, 1976; Wellman & Peters, 1980). However, the mechanism of the anorectic effect has not been determined conclusively. Various suggested mechanisms include an effect on feeding and satiety mechanisms in the brain, a peripheral effect on metabolism or glucose utilization, and peripherally mediated conditioned taste aversion. These mechanisms are discussed fully in Chapter 3.

Elucidation of the mechanisms of synthesis, storage, and release of catecholamines by adrenergic neurons has been a major research area during the last 40 years. In addition, two major categories of adrenergic receptors (α- and β-receptors) and several subcategories of receptors (α_1-, α_2-, β_1-, and β_2-receptors) have been identified and characterized. Not surprisingly, the effects of many autonomic drugs, including phenylpropanolamine, have been attributed to effects on these mechanisms. Effects of phenylpropanolamine on these adrenergic mechanisms have not been investigated extensively. Phenylpropanolamine was shown to exert mixed actions on the adrenergic synapse, producing either indirect effects (by release of norepinephrine) or direct effects (by stimulation of adrenergic receptors) depending on the site and dose of the drug (Trendelenburg et al., 1962a,b). More recent studies have demonstrated that phenylpropanolamine binds to α_1-adrenergic receptors, but with low affinity and low intrinsic activity (Minneman et al., 1983). These latter investigators also concluded that phenylpropanolamine acts as a partial agonist at the α_1-receptors.

THERAPEUTIC USES

As mentioned in the previous section, the first proprietary preparation of phenylpropanolamine, Mydriatine, was synthesized (Nagai, 1913) and tested for use as a mydriatic agent (Amatsu & Kubota, 1913, 1917; Hirose, 1915). Whereas this preparation apparently was used clinically as a mydriatic for a time, phenylpropanolamine has never been used extensively for this purpose.

Since phenylpropanolamine was developed as an analogue of the ephedrines, it may be useful to review the therapeutic usages of ephedrines during the period when these compounds were being actively developed. Ephedrine was recommended for "hypotonia, bronchial asthma, hay fever, urticaria, serum exanthem, Quincke edema, chronic bronchitis and emphysema, essential dysmenorrhea, eczema, vasomotor rhinitis, radioscopy effects, Adams-

Stokes disease, choking conditions induced by yellow fever, nerve pains induced by leprosy. Finally, ephedrine is used in ophthalmology as a mydriaticum and in morphine withdrawal to prevent withdrawal symptoms, and for detoxifying scopolamine" (Emde, 1930; translated from German). Thus the decongestant effect of the ephedrine compounds was recognized as early as the 1930s; other important clinical uses of these drugs, such as for appetite suppression or correction of urinary incontinence or retrograde ejaculation, were not discovered until later.

One of the earliest clinical uses of phenylpropanolamine was as a decongestant. The decongestant effects of topically applied sympathomimetic amines (Chen et al., 1929), including phenylpropanolamine (Stockton et al., 1931), was mentioned in the previous section. The therapeutic effects of phenylpropanolamine and ephedrine in treatment of asthma, hay fever, urticaria, and angioneuroedema were compared (Black, 1937). Phenylpropanolamine was given in doses of 24 or 48 mg (PO) every 3 hr (q. 3 hr). Phenylpropanolamine was as effective as ephedrine in symptomatic relief of these conditions. Phenylpropanolamine was considered superior to ephedrine, however, since ephedrine produced side effects of nervousness and insomnia but phenylpropanolamine did not. Single 48-mg doses of phenylpropanolamine (PO) in 41 patients produced a maximum increase in systolic blood pressure of +15 mm Hg and no change in diastolic pressure. In five patients, repeated 48 mg doses (eight doses in 2 days) produced a maximum increase in systolic blood pressure of +10 mm Hg. In one patient with hypertension (170 mm Hg systolic), the systolic pressure decreased 10 mm Hg after a single 24-mg dose of phenylpropanolamine.

Another clinical case study tested the effects of Propadrine (3/8 grain = 24.375 mg phenylpropanolamine, PO) in patients with asthma (Boyer, 1938). The patients were allowed to take the Propadrine *ad libitum,* and the range of doses was one tablet t.i.d. (three times daily) to two tablets q. 2 hr. The patients reported that Propadrine relieved their bronchospasm, rhinitis, and sneezing. Propadrine was rated as better than other drugs by 80% of patients, equal to other drugs by 11%, and less effective than other drugs by 9%.

The decongestant efficacy of phenylpropanolamine was confirmed by Murphy (1939) and Solo (1941). Since that time, the decongestant efficacy of phenylpropanolamine or phenylpropanolamine-containing combination products has been demonstrated in 30 clinical trials published in the clinical literature. These trials are reviewed in Chapter 5. Dozens of phenylpropanolamine-containing cough-cold remedies are marketed over the counter in the United States and throughout the world. Most of these are combination products that combine phenylpropanolamine with an antihistamine, an anticholinergic, a bronchodilator, and/or an expectorant. Indeed, these OTC cough-cold preparations constitute the most common use of phenylpropanolamine today.

Only one report of the clinical use of phenylpropanolamine for its cardiovascular effects was published. The ability of phenylpropanolamine to sustain the arterial blood pressure during spinal anesthesia was tested in a series of 263 patients during 280 operations (Lorhan & Mosser, 1947). Phenylpropanolamine (50 mg, IV or IM) produced a "satisfactory" response in 90% of these operations; "satisfactory" response was defined as maintenance of the blood pressure at not less than 10% below and not more than 25% above the preoperative level. However, undoubtedly because much more effective pressor drugs are available, phenylpropanolamine has not been used clinically for elevation of arterial blood pressure.

The use of phenylpropanolamine for appetite suppression in the treatment of obesity in humans was first reported by Hirsch (1939), who noted that whereas drugs such as amphetamine or ephedrine were successful in curbing the appetite, these drugs produced undesirable side effects, including nervousness and insomnia, in susceptible individuals. Hirsch reported that he had been prescribing Propadrine HCl for appetite suppression in obese patients for 1 year, and that Propadrine was effective as an appetite suppressant without producing these undesirable side effects. Six case reports were presented. The patients were placed on restricted calorie diets (900–1600 cal/day) and ingested one or two Propadrine capsules 20 min before each meal. The phenylpropanolamine content of the Propadrine was not specifically stated, but the preparation in use at that time contained 3/8 grain (24.375 mg) of phenylpropanolamine HCl (Boyer, 1938). All six patients lost weight on this program, with total weight loss ranging from 17 lb in 25 days to 33.5 lb in 2 months. One patient followed the restricted diet-Propadrine regimen for as long as 4 months and lost 24 lb. The greatest rate of weight loss in the six cases was 25 lb in 1 month. Hirsch noted that no patients had complained of side effects due to Propadrine and especially noted no nervousness or insomnia.

Phenylpropanolamine apparently was used for some 20 years as an appetite suppressant without controversy. Although no controlled clinical trials had been published that specifically tested the safety and efficacy of phenylpropanolamine (such trials were not required at that point in history), several case studies (Cutting, 1943; Kalb, 1942) and clinical management opinions (Colton et al., 1943; Reilly, 1950) were published in support of the use of phenylpropanolamine in the treatment of obesity. The first controlled clinical trial of phenylpropanolamine as an appetite suppressant was published in 1959 (Fazekas et al., 1959). In a double-blind, placebo-controlled study, two doses of phenylpropanolamine (25 or 50 mg) and one of d-amphetamine (5 mg) were compared. Drug or placebo was given t.i.d. 1 hr before meals, and the subjects were on a balanced 3000-calorie diet (i.e., not a restricted-calorie diet). The subjects in this study were 81 institutionalized, mentally retarded, obese but physically normal individuals. Both males and females were included, and their IQ levels ranged from "imbecile" to 76. In these individuals, d-amphetamine produced significant weight loss, but neither dose of phenylpropanolamine produced significantly greater weight loss than did placebo.

This study (Fazekas et al., 1959) raised serious questions regarding the efficacy of phenylpropanolamine as an anorectic drug. However, the study was severely criticized as the result of several basic flaws in the experimental design (Federal Trade Commission, 1967; Silverman, 1963). The following criticisms were raised. The study population consisted of mentally retarded individuals, and thus the results may not be directly applicable to a normal population. No dietary restrictions were followed during the study. The "double-blind" conditions were questioned because the overt behavioral effects of amphetamine could be observed by the investigators. Also, drug levels in the blood were not measured, so patient compliance was not determined. There appeared to be an interaction between IQ level and drug effectiveness: in all groups, patients with IQs higher than 33 lost more weight than did patients with lower IQs. In addition, the amount of spontaneous weight loss in this unique population was not estimated. Finally, it was suggested that this patient population was not necessarily motivated to lose weight, and that this motivation may play an important role in the anorectic effect of phenylpropanolamine.

Throughout most of its history, phenylpropanolamine has been available over the counter as an appetite suppressant or as a decongestant. The OTC status of the drug, however, has not been without controversy [see the review by Silverman, (1985)]. A federal Committee on Government Operations conducted a series of hearings regarding "false and misleading" advertising practices in 1957. As a result of these hearings, the efficacy of OTC weight-reducing products was questioned. The Fazekas study was in part a response to the criticisms raised in these committee hearings. In 1965, the Federal Trade Commission (FTC) conducted additional hearings questioning the safety and efficacy of phenylpropanolamine-containing appetite suppressants. As a result of these hearings, the Fazekas study was sharply criticized, and the FTC examiner recommended that phenylpropanolamine (25 mg, t.i.d.) along with dietary restrictions should be considered an effective appetite suppressant. Similar conclusions were reached by the Food and Drug Administration (FDA) advisory review panels in 1978 and 1979.

The efficacy and safety of phenylpropanolamine as an OTC drug was also reviewed by an independent FDA advisory panel (Federal Register, 1976,

1982a, 1982b). As a result of these combined reviews, the FDA approved the continued sale of phenylpropanolamine-containing appetite suppressant and decongestant products.

For a time, combination products containing phenylpropanolamine and caffeine were sold OTC as appetite suppressants. The rationale for including caffeine in the combination is presumably that caffeine would produce mild CNS stimulation and counteract the fatigue that sometimes accompanies dieting. Furthermore, the phenylpropanolamine-caffeine combination may produce greater weight loss than phenylpropanolamine alone, although the difference is not statistically significant (unpublished clinical trial; see Weintraub, 1985). However, to cooperate with the FDA in its effort to control "look-alike" drugs containing phenylpropanolamine and caffeine (see later), manufacturers and marketers of OTC phenylpropanolamine-caffeine combination products voluntarily agreed to cease manufacture and sale of such combinations (Federal Register, 1983). Consequently, all phenylpropanolamine-containing appetite suppressants currently sold in the United States contain no caffeine.

Despite the long history of extensive use of phenylpropanolamine and phenylpropanolamine-containing products for appetite suppression and decongestion with an excellent safety record, and despite the considerable number of clinical trials, the safety of phenylpropanolamine has recently been questioned. The criticisms are based primarily on case reports of hypertensive reactions or CNS stimulation (often labeled "amphetamine-like stimulation" or "psychotic reactions"). In addition, Horowitz et al. (1980) reported a series of severe adverse blood pressure reactions to the commercial preparations Trimolets or Contac marketed in Australia. The pharmaceutical formulation and dosage levels in these products are different from the products available in the United States. These case reports and studies are reviewed in Chapter 4. In assessing this evidence, two considerations are important: (1) extensive clinical trials in published and unpublished studies (reviewed in Chapter 5) have repeatedly confirmed both the safety and efficacy of phenylpropanolamine, and (2) in view of the literally billions of doses of phenylpropanolamine-containing products consumed yearly in the United States, the number of reported adverse reactions is very low. In addition, in several of the case reports there is reason to believe that the reported adverse reaction cannot be attributed to phenylpropanolamine or to a phenylpropanolamine-containing product alone, or that the reported adverse reaction is actually due to an overdose.

Recently, phenylpropanolamine was introduced into therapeutic medicine for two additional indications: correction of urinary incontinence and retrograde ejaculation. At present, these uses of phenylpropanolamine are restricted primarily to Scandinavia and phenylpropanolamine is not approved for these uses in the United States. The rationale for these uses of phenylpropanolamine is its ability to constrict smooth muscles in the urinary bladder.

STREET DRUG ABUSE: AMPHETAMINE LOOK-ALIKES, PSEUDOSPEED, AND COUNTERFEIT CONTROLLED SUBSTANCES

Drug abuse, including abuse of CNS stimulants, is an ancient social and medical phenomenon. Many of the stimulant drugs of abuse are naturally occurring plant alkaloids and have been used and abused since earliest recorded history. These drugs include the ephedrines found in the ancient Chinese drug ma huang (see above), various phenethylamines found in the Khat plant used in Africa and the Middle East, cocaine found in the leaves of the coca plant and used by South American Indians, and caffeine and theophylline found in coffee and teas. More recently, synthetic stimulants, including amphetamine and its various derivatives, have become widely abused.

Phenylpropanolamine has frequently been described in both the scientific and popular literature as an "amphetamine-like" drug or as related to ephedrines or Khat (*Catha edulis*). In fact, whereas phenylpropanolamine, amphetamine, ephedrine, and the components of Khat are chemically related in that they are derivatives of β-phenylethylamine, it is erroneous to assume that these drugs are thus pharmacologically interchangeable. Numerous structure-activity relationship (SAR) studies have demonstrated the marked differences in pharmacological activities of the phenylethylamines; these SAR studies are reviewed in Chapter 3. It has also been mistakenly reported that phenylpropanolamine is a component of the Khat plant. Khat contains various phenylethylamines, including *d*-norpseudoephedrine or cathine (Alles et al., 1961; Wolfes, 1930) and cathinone (Zelger et al., 1980). The chemical relationships between phenylpropanolamine and the isomers of ephedrine are discussed in Chapter 2. Phenylpropanolamine is the racemic *dl*-norephedrine, and this is chemically and pharmacologically distinct from *d*-norpseudoephedrine (cathine).

Legitimate use of amphetamine in clinical medicine began in the 1930s (Prinzmetal & Bloomberg, 1935), when it was used for treatment of narcolepsy or obesity. Since that time amphetamine and its various derivatives have been abused for their ability to produce CNS stimulation and euphoria. During the 1960s, diversion of legally manufactured amphetamines for recreational drug abuse was a major social, legal, and medical problem (Morgan & Kagan, 1978). However, the legal manufacture of amphetamines was severely limited following passage of the Controlled Substances Act of 1970 (Smith,

1983). The production of amphetamines was reduced by approximately 90%, and this reduction had a major impact on illicit as well as licit use of amphetamines. Presumably because the demand for amphetamines continued despite the drastically reduced licit supply, a new source of stimulant drug abuse emerged in the 1970s and continues to the present. This phenomenon is the abuse of the so-called amphetamine look-alikes or pseudospeed (Dougherty, 1982; Halpern, 1983; Morgan & Kagan, 1978; Smith, 1983). These look-alikes are often deliberately manufactured to resemble proprietary amphetamines, but since they contain drugs that can be legally sold OTC, they are often distributed legally by mailorder through popular drug abuse-oriented magazines and newspapers. The look-alikes are also sold "on the street" through conventional drug-abuse channels. In addition, "counterfeit controlled substances" have been identified (Wesson & Morgan, 1982); these drugs are illegally manufactured to look like legal controlled substances but in fact contain other active drugs. The counterfeit drugs are sold illegally "on the street."

Four categories of look-alike drugs and drugs of deception have been described: look-alike stimulants, look-alike cocaine, look-alike depressants, and look-alike opiates (Smith, 1983). Some of the look-alike stimulants and look-alike cocaines contain phenylpropanolamine in combination with other drugs; the specific formulations are described below. Smith (1983) defined look-alike drugs and drugs of deception as follows: "Look-alike drugs contain dosage forms of psychoactive drugs whose names or appearances are designed to associate the characteristics of the emulated psychoactive drug, but in fact contain a completely different substance which is usually neither a controlled nor prescription drug." In the licitly manufactured look-alikes, the contents are usually accurately labeled. The illicitly manufactured look-alikes lack accurate labeling of contents and thus are drugs of deception closely associated with drug culture-derived designations such as "black beauties." A "drug of deception" is "a dosage form of a recreational drug that contains significant amounts of psychoactive substances other than alleged." These drugs of deception necessarily are represented as a desired psychoactive drug such as Quaalude but actually are another drug or combination of drugs.

The abuse of look-alikes and drugs of deception is a relatively recent phenomenon, and it is difficult to estimate the extent of the problem. Between 1975 and 1980, the incidence of poison control case reports involving phenylpropanolamine-containing products increased approximately tenfold (FDA Bulletin, 1981). This is a somewhat misleading estimate, since the incidence of phenylpropanolamine-related poisonings was very low in 1975, not all phenylpropanolamine-related poisonings involved look-alike drugs, and not all look-alike drugs contain phenylpropanolamine. Dougherty (1982) stated that pseudospeed was the third most popular drug of abuse in central New

York (alcohol and marijuana were the most popular), although no data were presented to substantiate this claim. In a retrospective study of toxicologic screening cases in Louisville, Kentucky in 1979–1981, sympathomimetic drugs were identified in 1–12% of cases (Williams et al., 1983). Phenylpropanolamine per se was identified in 0–1.6% of the positive screens, and the incidence increased progressively from 0% in 1979 to 1.6% in 1981. In this study, no distinction was made between licit, illicit, and look-alike drugs.

Look-alike stimulants have received the greatest attention, with considerable emphasis on the toxicity of the substances they contain (Smith, 1983). These are manufactured to resemble amphetamine but do not duplicate the markings of controlled prescription psychoactive drugs. The most "copied" drug is Biphetamine, known primarily as "black mollies" or "black beauties." There are as many as 20 popular controlled stimulant drugs whose look-alikes are known by approximately 25 street names (Jordan, 1981; Newburn, 1981). Many look-alike stimulants contain phenylpropanolamine, caffeine, and ephedrine. The contents of various look-alike stimulants have been analyzed (Stock, 1982a,b).

Stimulant look-alikes contain 37–323 mg of caffeine. Caffeine stimulates the CNS at all levels, as well as the heart and skeletal muscles, and also dilates peripheral blood vessels while constricting cerebral blood flow. About 150–200 mg of caffeine is needed to produce stimulation in the average adult, and doses at this level are considered safe. Excessive amounts may produce headaches, anxiety, sleep disturbances, cardiac arrhythmias, and gastric irritation. Excessively high doses can induce stimulant-induced seizures and psychotic episodes as well as dependence characterized by headaches and depression from withdrawal. The lethal dose of caffeine is estimated to be 10,000 mg. Approximately 30 look-alike stimulants ingested at one time would be a lethal overdose. Many individuals dependent on these look-alike drugs ingest 5–10 doses a day, well within the range of caffeine toxicity.

Ephedrine is also present in many look-alikes. Analyses show that the doses vary between 12.5 and 50 mg. Ephedrine, a sympathomimetic amine, releases endogenous stores of norepinephrine in the brain and stimulates α- and β-adrenergic receptors. It can produce increased blood pressure and heart rate and may induce cardiac arrhythmias. Prolonged high dose abuse can produce a toxic psychosis, and massive overdose can result in seizures, cardiac toxicity, and death.

The dose of phenylpropanolamine in the look-alike drugs typically ranges from 25 to 50 mg, but frequently is higher; thus, the dose of phenylpropanolamine in look-alikes often exceeds the highest dose allowed by law in immediate-release formulations (37.5 mg). At excessive dose levels, phenylpropanolamine can cause anxiety, headache, muscle tremor, palpitations, and elevated blood pressure. Excessively high doses pose a threat of drug-induced psychotic episodes, but relatively little evidence exists of psychotic episodes and seizures associated with phenylpropanolamine alone. Most toxicologic information is associated with the double combination of phenylpropanolamine and caffeine or the triple combination of phenylpropanolamine, caffeine, and ephedrine. The vast majority of cases analyzed involved the triple combination, making it difficult to assess phenylpropanolamine toxicity per se.

Look-alike cocaine has also appeared on the drug scene (Smith, 1983). The look-alike cocaine contains phenylpropanolamine and caffeine, with the addition of local anesthetic agents such as lidocaine, tetracaine, or benzocaine. These cocaine substitute products are topical anesthetics that cause constriction and drying of the nasal mucosa, which can be quite irritating. Look-alike cocaine contains noncontrolled substances and is sold in establishments such as "head shops" and often diverted into the drug culture for recreational use and given a completely different name. There are 12–14 commercial names for cocaine preparations and a similar number of street names for the combinations.

As with all types of drug addiction, abuse of stimulants and look-alikes involves a complex of pharmacological, psychological, social, and cultural factors (Becker, 1967; Smith, 1983). On the basis of observation of patients at the Haight-Ashbury Free Medical Clinic in San Francisco, Smith (1983) described a syndrome of look-alike "dependence" in individuals who used doses of 5–10 look-alike pills per day. Similarly, Dougherty (1982) described stimulant look-alike abuse among teenagers in central New York and estimated the typical daily usage to be five to six doses. Stimulant look-alike abusers claimed that pseudospeed gave a euphoria or "rush" similar to, but not as good as, that from cocaine. They reported that pseudospeed gave an adequate "high," especially when combined with alcohol. Dougherty (1982) also presented three case reports of extreme pseudospeed abuse. These individuals took daily doses of up to 20 pills per day for as long as 18 months. All three individuals combined the pseudospeed with alcohol (one 17-year-old male consumed as much as 12–24 bottles of beer per day); two of them also reported combining pseudospeed, alcohol, and marijuana.

Associated with the increase in abuse of stimulant look-alike drugs, there have been reports of adverse drug reactions (Mueller & Solow, 1982) and overdose cases (Bernstein & Diskant, 1982; Lake et al., 1983; Mueller, 1983; Saxena & Kingston, 1981; Weesner et al., 1982). Paradoxically, perhaps one reason why phenylpropanolamine-containing look-alikes have a liability for overdose is the low potency of phenylpropanolamine for producing CNS stimulation. Since look-alike drug abusers take these drugs for the euphoriant-CNS stimulant effect, the abuser who does not experience the desired effect takes more pills in an attempt to get "high." Since the look-alikes contain phenylpropanolamine plus caffeine and/or ephedrine, and since all of these drugs can produce cardiovascular and CNS toxicity in sufficient doses, adverse or toxic cardiovascular effects are likely to occur when an individual ingests larger doses.

While phenylpropanolamine-containing drugs are undoubtedly involved in the look-alike abuse patterns, several studies in both experimental animals and humans have demonstrated that phenylpropanolamine alone has very low abuse liability. Abuse liability of drugs can be estimated in experimental animals by training them to self-administer drugs in an operant conditioning paradigm. Experimental animals will readily learn to self-administer drugs that show high abuse liability in humans (e.g., opiates, cocaine, amphetamines). On the other hand, animals will not readily self-administer drugs that show low abuse liability in humans (e.g., phenothiazines). Phenylpropanolamine did not reinforce self-administration in baboons (Griffiths et al., 1978), suggesting that phenylpropanolamine has low abuse liability.

Abuse liability can be tested more directly in experiments with human volunteers. In such tests, individuals are given drugs under randomized, double-blind, placebo-controlled conditions and then are questioned regarding their subjective responses to the drugs. Using standardized tests, the individuals are asked to rate the drug responses in terms of "drug liking" or "pleasurableness" [e.g., the Profile of Mood States (POMS)] or to compare the drug responses to other abused drugs that they have experienced [e.g., the Addiction Research Center Inventory (ARCI)]. On the basis of such tests, phenylpropanolamine appears to have low abuse potential in humans (Bigelow, 1985; Bigelow et al., 1984; Chait et al., 1983).

Since the results of animal and human testing have consistently demonstrated that phenylpropanolamine taken alone has a low liability for abuse, the abuse liability of the phenylpropanolamine-containing stimulant look-alikes would seem attributable to the presence of other drugs, such as caffeine and/or ephedrine.

REFERENCES

Alles, G. A., Fairchild, M. D., & Jensen, M. (1961). Chemical pharmacology of *Catha edulis*. *J Med Pharmac Chem, 3,* 323-351.

Amatsu, H., & Kubota, S. (1913). Ueber die pharmakologischen Wirkungen des Ephedrins und Mydriatins. *Kyoto Igaku Zassi, 10,* 301-302.

Amatsu, H., & Kubota, S. (1917). Ueber die pharmakologischen Wirkungen des Ephedrins und Mydriatins. *Kyoto Igaku Zassi, 14,* 77-78.

Aviado, D. M., Wnuck, B. S., & De Beer, E. S. (1959). A comparative study of nasal decongestion by sympathomimetic drugs. *Arch Otolarynogol, 69,* 598-605.

Barger, G., & Dale, H. H. (1910). Chemical structure and sympathomimetic action of amines. *J Physiol* (London), *41*, 19-59.

Becker, H. (1967). History, culture and subjective experience: An exploration of the social bases of drug induced experiences. *J Health Soc Behav, 8,* 163-176.

Bernstein, E., & Diskant, B. M. (1982). Phenylpropanolamine: A potentially hazardous drug. *Ann Emer Med, 11,* 311-315.

Bigelow, G. E., Liebson, I. A., Griffiths, R. R., Trieber, R., & Norowieski, P. (1984). Assessment of phenylpropanolamine (PPA) abuse risk in weight control patients. *Fed Proc, 43,* 571.

Bigelow, G. E. (1985). Quantitative assessments of mood and behavioral reinforcing effect of phenylpropanolamine. In J. P. Morgan, D. V. Kagan, and J. S. Brody (Eds.). *Phenylpropanolamine: Risks, Benefits, and Controversies.* Clinical Pharmacology and Therapeutics Series, Vol. 5. Praeger Scientific, New York (pp. 328-340).

Black, N. J. (1937). The control of allergic manifestations by phenylpropanolamine (Propadrine) HCl. *Lancet, 54,* 101-102.

Boyer, W. E. (1938). The clinical use of phenyl-propanol-amine hydrochloride (Propadrine) in the treatment of allergic conditions. *J Allergy, 9,* 509-513.

Calliess, F. W. (1912). Ueber einige Abkommlinge des Propiophenons. *Arch Pharm,* 141-154.

Chait, L. D., Uhlenhuth, E. H., & Johanson, C. E. (1983). Drug preference and mood in humans: Mazindol and phenylpropanolamine. In L.S. Harris (Ed.), *Problems of Drug Dependence,* NIDA Research Monograph 49: DHHS Publication No. (ADM) 84-1316. Washington, DC (pp. 327-328).

Chen, K. K., & Schmidt, C. G. (1924). The action of ephedrine the active principle of the Chinese drug "ma huang." *J Pharmacol Exp Ther, 24,* 339-357.

Chen, K. K., & Schmidt, C. G. (1930). Ephedrine and related substances. *Medicine, 9,* 1-117.

Chen, K. K., Chang-Keng, W., & Henriksen, E. (1929). Relationship between the pharmacological action and the chemical constitution and configuration of the optical isomers of ephedrine and related compounds. *J Pharmacol Exp Ther, 36,* 363-400.

Colombo, C., & Spica, P. (1875). Sopra alcuni derivati alfatoluici. *Gazz Chim Ital, 5,* 124-125.

Colton, N. H., Segal, H. I., Steinberg, A., Shechter, A., & Pastor, N. (1943). The management of obesity with emphasis on appetite control. *Am J Med Sci, 206,* 75-86.

Cutting, W. C. (1943). The treatment of obesity. *J Clin Endocrinol, 3,* 85-88.

Dietz, A. J., Jr. (1981). Amphetamine-like reactions to phenylpropanolamine. *JAMA, 245,* 601-602.

Dougherty, R. J. (1982). Pseudo-speed. Look-alikes or pea-shooters. *New York State J Med, 82,* 74-75.

Eberhard, A. (1917). Ueber das Amido-athyl-phenyl-carbinol. *Arch Pharmacol, 255,* 140-150.

Emde, H. (1930). Ephedrin. *Arch Pharmacol* (Berlin), *268,* 83-95.

Epstein, A. E. (1959). Suppression of eating and drinking by amphetamine and other drugs in normal and hyperphagic rats. *J Comp Physiol Psychol, 52,* 37-45.

Fairchild, M. D., & Alles, G. A. (1967). The central locomotor stimulatory activity and acute toxicity of the ephedrine and norephedrine isomers in mice. *J Pharmacol Exp Ther, 158,* 135-139.

Fazekas, J. F., Ehrmantrout, W. R., & Campbell, K. D. (1959). Comparative effectiveness of phenylpropanolamine and dextro amphetamine on weight reduction. *JAMA, 170,* 1018-1021.

FDA National Clearinghouse for Poison Control Centers. (1981). Phenylpropanolamine weight control products. *FDA Bulletin, 25,* 16-20.

Federal Register (1976). Establishment of a monograph for OTC cold, cough, allergy, bronchodilator and antiasthmatic drug products. Docket No. 76N-0052.

Federal Register (1982a). Establishment of a monograph for weight control products for over-the-counter human use. Docket No. 81N-0022.

Federal Register (1982b). Establishment of a monograph for oral health care drug products for over-the-counter human use. Docket No. 81N-0022.

Federal Register (1983). Enforcement action under the new drug provisions of the Federal Food, Drug, and Cosmetic Act; Certain OTC drug products; Advisory opinion. Docket No. 83A-0339.

Federal Trade Commission (1967). In the Matter of Alleghany Pharmacal Corp. and Harry Evans, Vincent J. Lynch, and Chester Carity. Docket No. 7176.

Griffiths, R. R., Brady, J. V., & Snell, J. D. (1978). Relationship between anorectic and reinforcing properties of appetite suppressant drugs: Implications for assessment of abuse liability. *Biol Psychol, 13,* 283-290.

Halpern, J. S. (1983). Street speed. *Emerg News, 9,* 224-227.

Hartung, W. H., & Munch, J. C. (1931). Amino alcohols. VI. The preparation and pharmacodynamic activity of four isomeric phenylpropanolamines. *J Am Chem Soc, 53,* 1875-1879.

Hasama, B. (1930). Beitrage zur Erforschung der Bedeutung der chemischen Konfiguration fur die pharmakologischen Wirkungen der adrenalinahnlichen Stoffe. *Arch Exp Pathol Pharmacol, 153,* 161-186.

Hirose, M. (1915). Uber die pharmakologischen Eigenschaften einigen dem Adrenalin nahestehender Substanzen, *o*-Dioxyphenylaethanolamin, Phenylaethanolamin, Ephedrin, Mydriatin. *Mitt med Fak Kais* (Tokyo), *13,* 479-506.

Hirsh, L. S. (1939). Controlling appetite in obesity. *J Med Cinncinati, 20,* 84-85.

Horowitz, J. D., Lang, W. J., Howes, L. G., Fennessy, M. R., Christophidis, N., Rand, M. J., & Louis, W. J. (1980). Hypertensive responses induced by phenylpropanolamine in anorectic and decongestant preparations. *Lancet, 1,* 60-61.

Jordan, P. S. (1981). CNS stimulants sold as amphetamines. *Am J Hosp Pharm, 38,* 29.

Kalb, S. W. (1942). The effect of amphetamine (Benzedrine) sulphate, propadrine hydrochloride and propadrine hydrochloride in combination with sodium delvinal on the appetite of obese patients. *J Med Soc NJ, 39,* 584-586.

Kanao, S. (1928). Uber das Nor- und Nor-ψ-ephedrin. *J Pharm Soc Jpn,* 947-1070.

Kanfer, I., Haigh, J. M., & Dowse, R. (1983). Phenylpropanolamine hydrochloride. *Anal Profiles Drug Subst, 12,* 357-383.

Kornblith, C. L., & Hoebel, B. G. (1976). A dose-response study of anorectic drug effects on food intake, self-stimulation, and stimulation-escape. *Pharmacol Biochem Behav, 5,* 215-218.

Lake, C. R., Tenglin, R., Chernow, B., & Holloway, H. C. (1983). Psychomotor stimulant-induced mania in a genetically predisposed patient: A review of the literature and report of a case. *J Clin Psychopharmacol, 3,* 97-100.

Loman, J., Rinkel, M., & Myerson, A. (1939). Comparative effects of amphetamine sulfate (benzedrine sulfate), paredrine and propadrine on the blood pressure. *Am Heart J, 18,* 89-93.

Lorhan, P., & Mosser, D. (1947). Phenylpropanolamine hydrochloride: A vasopressor drug, for maintaining blood pressure during spinal anesthesia. *Anal Surg, 125,* 171-176.

Mannich, C., & Jacobsohn, W. (1910). Uber Oxyphenyl-alkylamine und Dioxyphenyl-alkyla-mine. *Chem Berichte, 43*, 189-197.

Minneman, K. P., Fox, S. W., & Abel, P. W. (1983). Occupancy of alpha$_1$-adrenergic receptors and contraction of rat vas deferens. *Molec Pharmacol, 23*, 359-368.

Morgan, J., & Kagan, D. (1978). Street amphetamine quality and the controlled substances act of 1970. *J Psychedelic Drugs, 10*, 303-317.

Mueller, S. M., Muller, J., & Asdell, S. M. (1984). Cerebral hemorrhage associated with phenyl-propanolamine in combination with caffeine. *Stroke, 15*, 119-123.

Mueller, S. M., & Solow, E. B. (1982). Seizures associated with a new combination "pick-me-up" pill (letter). *Ann Neurol, 11*, 322.

Mueller, S. M. (1983). Neurologic complications of phenylpropanolamine use. *Neurology, 33*, 650-652.

Murphy, J. A. (1939). Propadrine hydrochloride in the treatment of allergic manifestations. *Pennsylvania Med J, 43*, 65-66.

Nagai, N. (1913). [On the analysis of ephedrine and mydriatine and new alkaloids belonging to the same group.] *Kagaku Kaishi (J Tokyo Chem Soc), 34*, 437-439.

Nagai, W. N. (1920). Mydriatic and process of making same. U.S. Patent 1,356,877.

Newburn, N. (1981). Amphetamine look-alikes. *National Clearinghouse Poison Control Center Bull, 25*, 19.

Prinzmetal, M., & Bloomberg, W. (1935). The use of benzedrine for the treatment of narcolepsy. *JAMA, 105*: 2051-2054.

Rabe, P., & Hallensleben, J. (1910). Uber die bildung eines athylenoxydes aus der quartaren base des phenyl-methyl-oxathyl-amins. *Ber Deut Chem, 43*, 2622.

Reilly, W. A. (1950). The treatment of obesity in childhood. *Am Prac, 1*, 228-234.

Saxena, K., & Kingston, R. (1981). Morbidity of street speed. An update. *Vet Hum Toxicol, 23*, 353.

Schulte, J. W., Reif, E. C., Bacher, J. A., Lawrence, W. S., & Tainter, M. L. (1941). Further study of central stimulation from sympathomimetic amines. *J Pharmacol Exp Ther, 71*, 62-74.

Silverman, H. I. (1985). A history of therapeutic uses of phenylpropanolamine in North Amer-ica. In J. P. Morgan, D. V. Kagan, and J. S. Brody (Eds.). *Phenylpropanolamine: Risks, Benefits, and Controversies*. Clinical Pharmacology and Therapeutics Series, Vol. 5. Praeger Scientific, New York (pp. 11-24).

Silverman, H. I. (1963). Phenylpropanolamine-misused? Or simply abused? *Am J Pharmac, 135*, 45-54.

Smith, D. E. (1983). Look-alike drugs and drugs of deception epidemiological, toxicological and clinical considerations. *Internatl Drug Report*, 4-8.

Solo, D. H. (1941). Phenylpropanolamine hydrochloride as a vasoconstricting agent in otolaryn-gology. *Med Rec, 153*, 101-102.

Stock, S. H. (1982a). The look-alike explosion, part I. *Pharm Chem Newsl, 11*, 3,8,11.

Stock, S. H. (1982b). The look-alike explosion, part II. *Pharm Chem Newsl, 11*, 3-4.

Stockton, A. B., Pace, P. T., & Tainter, M. L. (1931). Some clinical actions and therapeutic uses of racemic synephrine. *J Pharmacol Exp Ther, 41*, 20.

Tainter, M. L. (1944). Actions of benzedrine and propadrine in the control of obesity. *J Nutr, 27*, 89-105.

Tainter, M. L., Pedden, J. R., & James, M. (1934). Comparative actions of sympathomimetic compounds: bronchodilator actions in perfused guinea pig lungs. *J Pharmacol Exp Ther, 51*, 371-386.

Trendelenburg, U., Muskus, A., Fleming, W. W., & Alonso de la Sierra, B. G. (1962a). Modification by reserpine of the action of sympathomimetic amines in spinal cats; a classification of sympathomimetic amines. *J Pharmacol Exp Ther, 138*, 170-180.

Trendelenburg, U., Muskus, A., Fleming, W. W., & Alonso de la Sierra, B. G. (1962b). Effects of cocaine, denervation and decentralization on the response of the nictitating membrane to various sympathomimetic amines. *J Pharmacol Exp Ther, 138*, 181-193.

Warren, M. R., & Werner, H. W. (1946). Acute toxicity of vasopressor amines II. Comparative data. *J Pharmacol Exp Ther, 86*, 284-286.

Weesner, K. M., Denison, M., & Roberts, R. J. (1982). Cardiac arrhythmias in an adolescent following ingestion of an over-the-counter stimulant. *Clin Pediatr, 21*, 700-701.

Weintraub, M. (1985). Phenylpropanolamine as an anorexiant agent in weight control: A review of published and unpublished studies. In J. P. Morgan, D. V. Kagan, and J. S. Brody (Eds.). *Phenylpropanolamine: Risks, Benefits, and Controversies*. Clinical Pharmacology and Therapeutics Series, Vol. 5. Praeger Scientific, New York (pp. 53-79).

Wellman, P. J., & Peters, R. H. (1980). Effects of amphetamine and phenylpropanolamine on food intake in rats with ventromedial hypothalamic or dorsolateral tegmental damage. *Physiol Behav, 25*, 819-827.

Wesson, D., & Morgan, J. (1982). Stimulant look-alikes. *NEWS*, California Society for the Treatment of Alcoholism and Other Drug Dependencies. *9*, 1-3.

Williams, W. M., May, D. C., Hurst, H. E., Jarboe, C. H., & Madden, R. J. (1983). Toxicology screening by gas chromatography mass spectrometry. Three years experience. *J KY Med Assoc, 81*, 24-30.

Winter, C. A., & Flataker, L. (1954). Antitussive compounds: Testing methods and results. *J Pharmacol Exp Ther, 112*, 99-108.

Wolfes, O. (1930). Uber das Vorkommen von D-nor-iso-Ephedrin in *Catha edulis*. *Arch Pharm Berl, 268*, 81-95.

Zelger, J. L., Schorno, H. X., & Carlini, E. A. (1980). Behavioral effects of cathionone, an amine obtained from *Catha edulis* Forsk.: Comparisons with amphetamine, norpseudoephedrine, apomorphine, and nomifensine. *Bull Narc 32*, 67-82.

2

CHEMISTRY

Phenylpropanolamine (see Diagram 2.1) is a member of the extensive class of sympathomimetic amines, the most common of which are derivatives of β-phenylethylamine (see Figure 2.1).

Also called *norephedrine,* and currently indexed by *Chemical Abstracts* under the name α-(1-aminoethyl)-benzenemethanol, phenylpropanolamine is a primary amine with an amino and a hydroxyl group on adjacent carbon atoms. The molecular weight of phenylpropanolamine is 187.67. Its methyl group imparts resistance to degradative metabolic processes that is lacking in members of the phenylethanolamine family such as adrenaline (epinephrine), making possible the oral administration of phenylpropanolamine. Its hydroxyl group confers greater water solubility relative to amphetamine, the de-

PHENYLPROPANOLAMINE

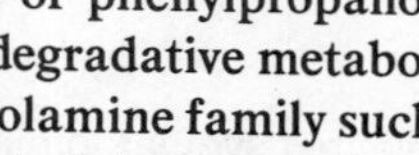

Diagram 2.1

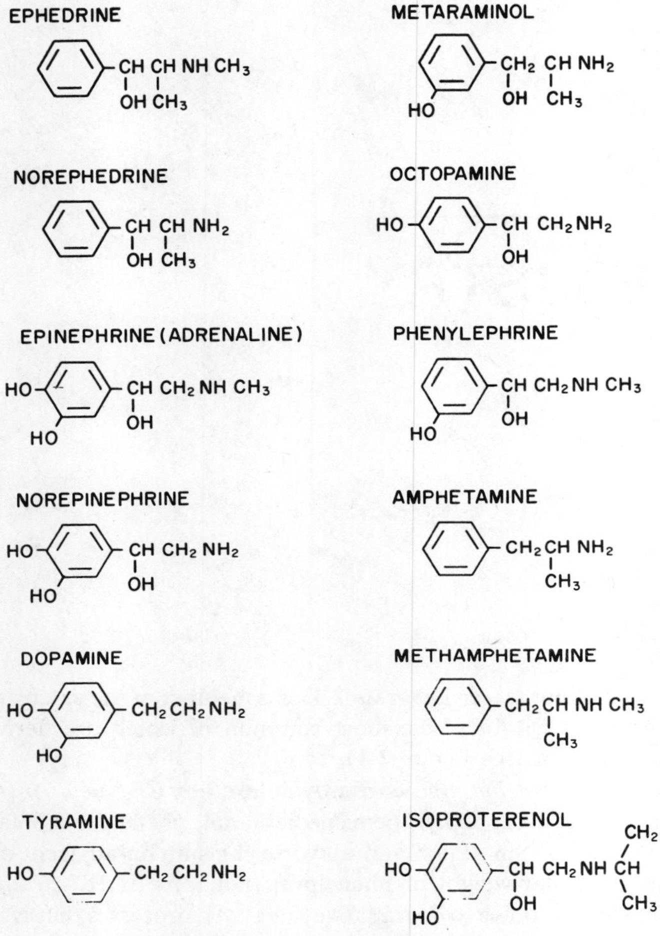

Figure 2.1. Selected sympathomimetic amines

soxy analog, and its partition coefficient (water-heptane) is more than 1000 times greater than that of amphetamine (Vree et al., 1969).

STEREOCHEMISTRY OF PHENYLPROPANOLAMINE

Phenylpropanolamine has two asymmetric or chiral carbon atoms, that is, carbon atoms carrying four different groups. Around each of these two car-

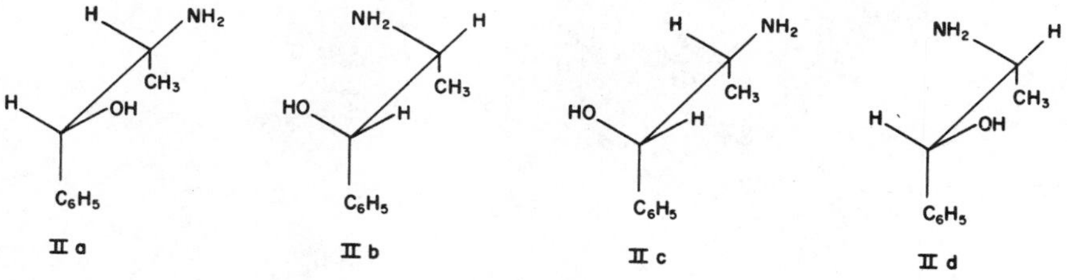

Diagram 2.2

bon atoms, there are two possible configurations of the dissimilar groups and four configurations of the molecule as a whole. Each configuration corresponds to a stereoisomer of phenylpropanolamine and can be depicted by the "sawhorse" drawings (Diagram 2.2). In these drawings the two asymmetric carbon atoms are not shown explicitly but are understood to be at the points where four bonds (lines) meet. Rotation around the bond between the two asymmetric carbons, which causes changes in the positions of the three groups in front with respect to the three groups in back, gives rise to a different conformation of the molecule but not to a different configuration. Provided that groups on an asymmetric carbon atom are not interchanged, the configuration remains the same. None of the stereoisomers represented by IIa–d is superimposable on any of the other three, by virtue of their different configurations, regardless of how one either rotates the molecule as a whole or rotates around single bonds.

Stereoisomer IIb differs from IIa in that the configurations around each asymmetric carbon atom have been inverted (by interchanging the H and OH groups on the carbon atom in front and the H and NH_2 groups on the carbon atom in back). Notice that as a result of this pair of interchanges, IIb is the mirror image of IIa. Stereoisomers such as IIa and IIb that are mirror images of each other are known as *enantiomers*. Similarly, IIc and IId are enantiomers. If the configuration around only one of the two asymmetric carbons is inverted, however, a stereoisomer that is not the mirror image of the original is obtained. Stereoisomers that are not mirror images of each other are known as *diastereoisomers*. Thus IIa and IIc, for example, are diastereoisomers.

Another stereochemical representation of a molecule with asymmetric carbon atoms is the Fisher projection, in which all groups are shown in the plane of the paper, with the understanding that certain groups are in fact projecting above and others below that plane. The Fisher projection corresponding to the four phenylpropanolamine stereoisomers may be written down by viewing the sawhorse projections IIa–d from above, as illustrated by using IIa:

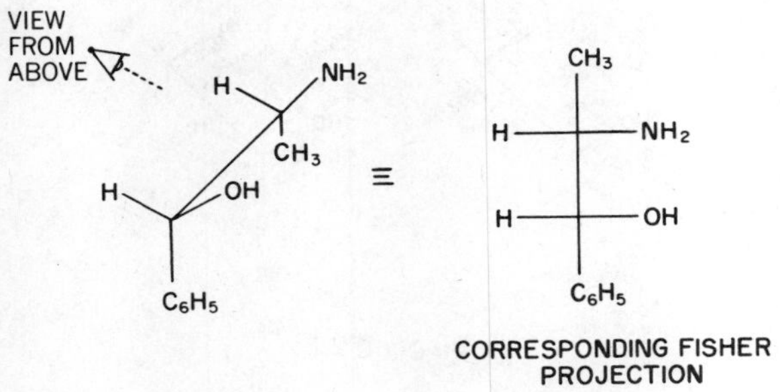

Diagram 2.3

In the Fisher projection, the main carbon chain is drawn vertically and the groups attached to the carbons in that chain are drawn at right angles to it. By convention, the groups on the horizontal lines are understood to be projecting above the plane of the page, while the groups bonded to the terminal carbons of the main chain are understood to project below that plane. The four Fisher projections corresponding to IIa–d are as follows:

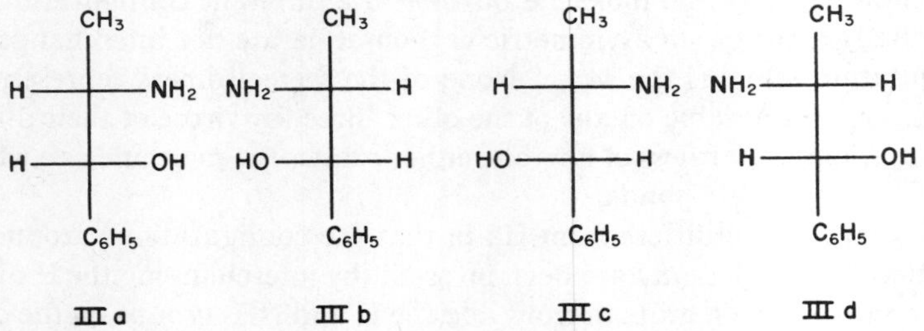

Diagram 2.4

The systematic name 1-phenyl-2-amino-1-propanol for phenylpropanolamine applies equally well to all four of the stereoisomers just described since it refers only to the structure of phenylpropanolamine (i.e., to how the atoms are connected) and not to its configurations. The four stereoisomers have identical structures (the atoms are linked in the same way) but differ in configuration—that is, in the orientation of the atom in space. Additional nomenclature is therefore needed to distinguish among the four stereoisomers.

The pair of stereoisomers represented by formulas IIIa and IIIb (or IIa and IIb) are called *norephedrines;* the second pair of enantiomers (IIIc and IIId) are called *norpseudoephedrines* (or nor-ψ-ephedrines). One member of each pair of enantiomers is dextrorotatory and is denoted by either a lowercase *d* or by a plus (+) sign; the levorotatory forms are denoted by *l* or a minus (−) sign. Experimentally it was found that configurations IIIb and IIIc correspond to the dextrorotatory stereoisomers, so that IIIa and IIId are levorotatory.

Although the foregoing nomenclature provides different labels for each of the phenylpropanolamine stereoisomers, it does not specify their absolute configurations. This can be accomplished by determining whether the configuration around each asymmetric carbon is *R* or *S* according to the Prelog rules, which are outlined in most introductory organic chemistry texts (see Figure 2.2). Numbering the carbon atom carrying the hydroxyl group C-1 and the carbon atom with the amino group C-2, the four stereoisomers, IIa–d, are, respectively, 1*R*, 2*S*; 1*S*, 2*R*; 1*S*, 2*S*; and 1*R*, 2*R*.

Another point of nomenclature that is important to mention because of its widespread use in the literature concerns the prefixes D and L. These prefixes always refer to the configuration around only one asymmetric carbon, selected according to certain rules, regardless of how many other asymmetric carbons are present in the molecule. If the configuration around this carbon is similar to the configuration around the single asymmetric carbon of dextrorotatory glyceraldehyde, in the sense that similar groups are in corresponding positions, then that particular stereoisomer is the D isomer. A D isomer, however, need not be dextrorotatory. In fact, the stereoisomer designated as *D*-norephedrine is levorotatory and is written as D(−)-norephedrine; *L*-norpseudoephedrine happens to be dextrorotatory and is denoted

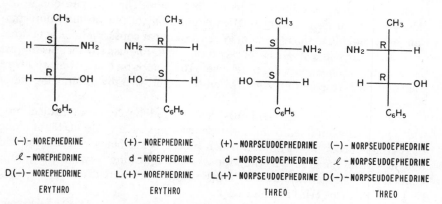

Figure 2.2. Summary of stereochemical nomenclature with reference to the isomeric phenylpropanolamines

$L(+)$-norpseudoephedrine. Do not confuse the lowercase d and l, which do indicate the direction in which the compound rotates polarized light, with the uppercase D and L, which imply nothing about the sign of rotation.

A final point of nomenclature concerns the prefixes *erythro* and *threo*. An *erythro* stereoisomer is one in which similar groups align with each other when the molecule is brought into an eclipsed conformation. Referring to the sawhorse drawings IIa–d, all four conformations have the groups in front eclipsing those in back. However, only the norephedrine stereoisomers, IIa and IIb, have similar groups aligned: the two hydrogens, the OH and NH_2 groups, and the groups containing carbon. Thus, IIa and IIb are *erythro* stereoisomers, whereas IIc and IId are the *threo* forms.

Recently, ^{13}C-NMR spectroscopy has been used to distinguish between the *erythro* and *threo* isomers of phenylpropanolamine and a series of N-substituted derivatives (Engel et al., 1979, 1980). The signal peaks for the methyl- and hydroxyl-bearing and the methyl carbon atoms are shifted upfield by 3–4 ppm in the *erythro* isomer (norephedrine) relative to the *threo* one (norpseudoephedrine).

The absolute configuration of any of the four stereoisomers can, of course, be determined by x-ray crystallography or, determined, in principle, by either optical rotatory dispersion (ORD) or circular dichroism (CD) in conjunction with appropriate model compounds and certain empirical rules (Engel, 1982).

When stereochemistry is not indicated, the term *phenylpropanolamine* usually refers to a racemic mixture of the norephedrine enantiomers, which can be written as either ($\pm$)- or *dl*-norephedrine. The nomenclature discussed previously with respect to phenylpropanolamine is summarized in Figure 2.2.

Now that the configuration of a molecule has been described, the next level of stereochemical description is its conformation. The question one would ideally like to answer is what relative populations of the various conformations are available to the molecule. When looking at conformations generated by rotation around a single carbon-carbon bond, one usually focuses on just three conformations, namely, those where the groups on one carbon atom are staggered with respect to the groups on the other, thereby minimizing steric interactions.

Conformations are conveniently represented by Newman projections, which are easily obtained from sawhorse drawings such as IIa–d. Sight along the carbon-carbon bond around which rotations are being considered, and note in writing the groups as they appear, distinguishing between the groups bonded to the nearer carbon and those bonded to the more distant one. Using ($-$)-norephedrine (IIa) as an example:

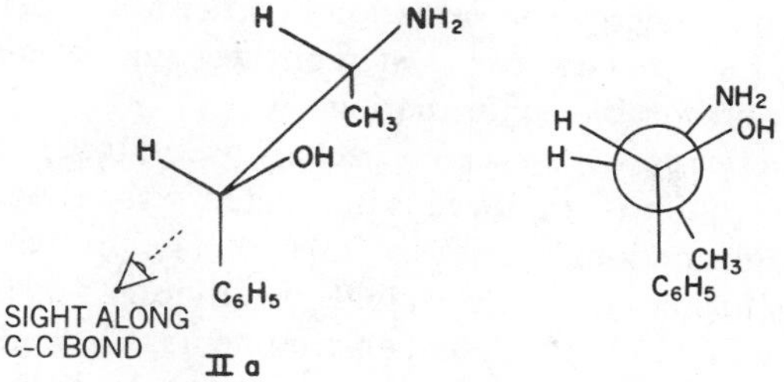

SIGHT ALONG
C–C BOND

II a

Diagram 2.5

Rotating around the carbon-carbon bond in order to reach a fully staggered conformation and writing down the two remaining staggered conformations, one obtains:

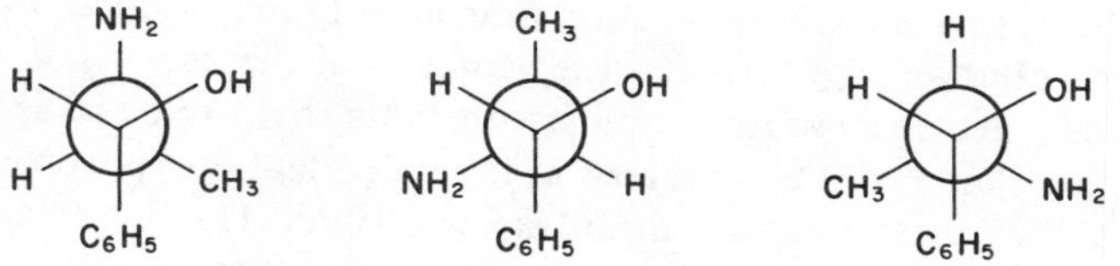

IV a   IV b   IV c

Diagram 2.6

In each conformation, different combinations of groups are brought into proximity. In IVc, for example, but not in IVa or IVb, the phenyl group is (in projection) wedged between the amino and the methyl groups; in IVa and IVc, but not in IVb, the hydroxyl and amino groups are in proximity. Because of differences like these, the three conformations differ in energies. The steric interactions between the phenyl and the nearby methyl and amino groups, for example, tend to destabilize conformation IVc, and to the extent that there is intramolecular hydrogen bonding between the amino and hydroxyl groups in IVa and IVc, those conformations will be stabilized. The relative energies of the three conformations, then, will reflect the sum of a number of interactions, and if the conformations are in equilibrium, the conformation of lowest energy will have the highest population.

The conformational analysis of a series of stereoisomers may help to explain relative activities at a particular type of receptor. A stereoisomer that need not enter a high-energy conformation in order to interact properly with the receptor may have an edge over a stereoisomer that does have to assume an energetically unfavorable conformation.

Nuclear magnetic resonance is an especially useful tool in conformational analysis. One way that it is employed is illustrated with reference to the three norephedrine conformations previously (IVa–c). The protons on each of the two asymmetric carbon atoms give signals in different regions of the NMR spectrum because they are in different environments. They interact with each other, by a process known as *spin coupling,* and their signals consist not of single peaks but of peaks that are "split," that is, slightly separated. The distance between these peaks is called the *coupling constant J_{ab},* where the subscripts identify the interacting protons. The magnitude of the coupling constant varies with the dihedral angle between the hydrogens. When the coupled protons are *anti* to each other (dihedral angle $= 180°$), as in conformation IVb, J_{ab} is a maximum for that particular molecule. When the protons are separated by a dihedral angle of $60°$, that is, *gauche* to each other, as in conformations IVa and IVc, the J_{ab} is much smaller. By examining the NMR spectra of selected model compounds that have groups similar to those in norephedrine but are rigid (so that the geometry of the protons of interest is well defined), one can obtain coupling constants that are close approximations to those that would be observed in the individual norephedrine conformations if they were not rapidly intraconvertible. The J_{ab} measured for norephedrine itself is a weighted average of J_{ab} values corresponding to each conformation. From the observed J_{ab} in the NMR spectrum of norephedrine, it was calculated that conformation IVb is populated only to the extent of about 20%, with the remainder of the molecules at a given instant residing in the other two conformations (Ison et al., 1973).

The importance of stereochemistry in substances that constitute or interact with biological systems cannot be overemphasized. Stereochemistry often makes all the difference. Consider, for example, the near ubiquity of L-amino acids rather than D-amino acids in the proteins and peptides of higher organisms or the presence of D-glucose rather than L-glucose in carbohydrates; proteins and carbohydrates containing the corresponding enantiomers are presumably nonfunctional. As a more concrete example, there are substances (e.g., the terpene carvone) where enantiomers have different odors, presumably because olfactory receptors are chiral and interact differently with each enantiomer (Murov & Pickering, 1973).

Several studies have provided evidence suggesting that enhanced physiological activity is associated with members of the phenylpropanolamine and ephedrine families that have an S configuration around C-2 (the carbon atom carrying the amino group).

For example, the locomotor activity of mice was measured, after the administration of d- and l-amphetamine and the eight stereoisomers in the phenylpropanolamine/ephedrine families, by recording how many times in a given period they interrupted "photoelectric eye" light beams crisscrossing their cages (Fairchild & Alles, 1967). It was found that the isomers having an S configuration around C-2, namely, d-amphetamine, d-norpseudoephedrine, l-norephedrine, d-pseudoephedrine, and l-ephedrine, exhibited greater locomotor stimulatory activity than did their corresponding enantiomers, although two pairs of enantiomers had activity levels so low that the observed differences may not have been statistically significant.

In a study of the effects of essentially the same stereoisomers on appetite suppression and energy expenditure in mice and rats, a similar trend was observed, that is, the association of an S configuration at C-2 with higher activity (Arch et al., 1982).

Still another study measured the relative abilities of a series of sympathomimetic amines to modify the effect of norepinephrine on the isolated vas deferens and atrial tissue of rats (Swamy et al., 1969). Again, the same order of activity was observed in four of the five pairs of enantiomers mentioned previously; the activity of l-norpseudoephedrine was not reported.

It is dangerous to draw sweeping conclusions from studies measuring effects that may reflect quite different modes of action. The caveats that should accompany such interpretations are discussed in more detail in Chapter 3. The important point to make here is that in general stereoisomers show differences in physiological activity, and any full understanding of the mechanism of action of a drug must take stereochemistry into account.

SYNTHESIS OF PHENYLPROPANOLAMINE

Of the four stereoisomers of the phenylpropanolamine family, only two have been found to occur in nature. ($-$)-Norephedrine and ($+$)-norpseudoephedrine have been isolated from various species of the *Ephedra* plant, which is the source of the oriental drug ma huang (Yamasaki et al., 1974). The same two stereoisomers are also present in the plant *Catha edulis* Forsk, commonly known as Khat, and norpseudoephedrine is sometimes called cathine (Schorno et al., 1982). Also isolated from *C. edulis* is ($-$)-α-aminopropiophenone (cathinone), which has the same configuration at the amino-carrying carbon atom as both ($-$)-norephedrine and ($+$)-norpseudoephedrine (Figure 2.3). Phenylpropanolamine itself (i.e., $\pm$ norephedrine) was not isolated from Khat.

The first synthetic phenylpropanolamine was obtained about 1910 by reduction of the ketone carbonyl group in α-aminopropiophenone, using sodium amalgam in the presence of dilute mineral acid. Later syntheses em-

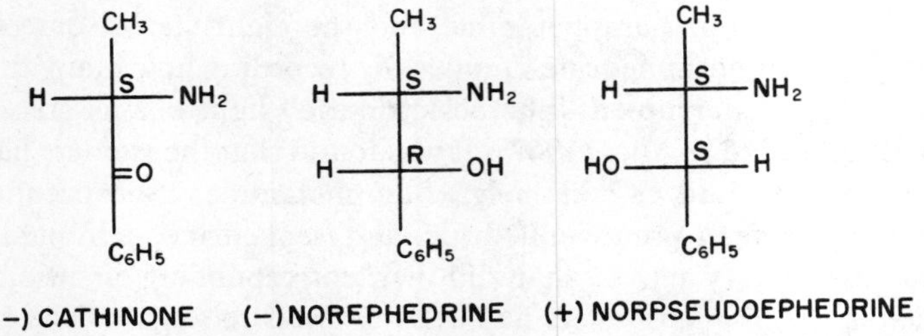

(−) CATHINONE   (−) NOREPHEDRINE   (+) NORPSEUDOEPHEDRINE

Figure 2.3. Stereochemical configurations of cathinone and naturally occurring members of the phenylpropanolamine family

ployed an aldol-type condensation between benzaldehyde and nitroethane, followed by reduction of the resulting nitro compound (Equation 2.1) (Hoover & Hass, 1947; Nagai & Kanao, 1929). The temperature must be controlled during the condensation reaction to avoid side reactions, such as dehydration of the nitroalcohol. Dehydration yields nitroolefins that can subsequently polymerize (Vanderbilt & Hass, 1940) (see Equation 2.1).

The racemic pairs (in the form of either the free bases or the hydrochloride salts) may be separated from each other by fractional crystallization, taking advantage of their different solubilities.

The following melting points (mp) were reported for the purified racemates (Hoover & Hass, 1947):

dl-Norephedrine		*dl*-Norpseudoephedrine
Free base	mp 104°–105°C	mp 71°C
HCl salt	mp 192°C	mp 169°C

Each racemic mixture can be resolved into the corresponding enantiomers by conversion of the amines to salts of optically pure tartaric acid (Kalm, 1960). These salts are diastereoisomers that can be separated by fractional crystalli-

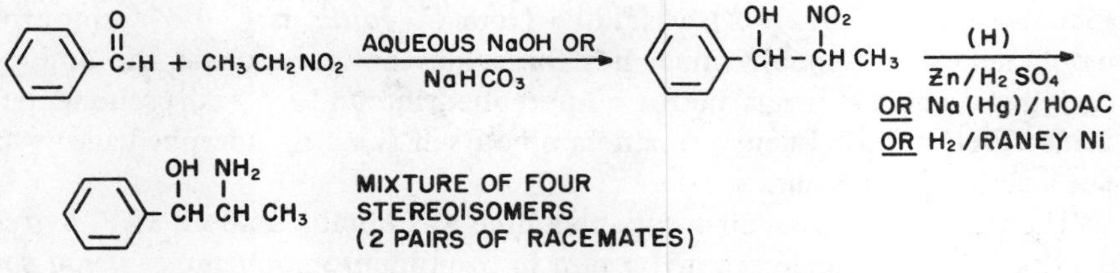

Equation 2.1

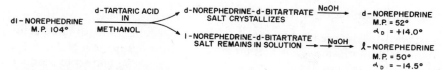

Figure 2.4. Resolution of dl-norephedrine into corresponding enantiomers

zation, and the amines can then be regenerated by treatment with alkali. The scheme shown in Figure 2.4 summarizes the method of resolution, using the *dl*-norephedrine racemate as an example.

To the extent that purification is complete and the physical measurements are precise, the enantiomers have identical melting points and equal but opposite rotations. Notice, though, that the melting point of either enantiomer is different from that of a 50–50 mixture of the two (i.e., the starting racemate), which is not unusual, since a mixture of enantiomers will in general pack into a crystal quite differently than would either of the individual enantiomers.

A benzylic hydroxyl group (an OH group on a carbon atom attached to a benzene ring) is ordinarily quite sensitive to acid. In principle, it can be protonated and lost as water in the course of substitution and dehydration reactions. However, when optically pure isomers of the ephedrine-norephedrine family were kept for 10 days at 100°C in solution at pH 3, no change in rotation was observed, indicating that no reaction occurred (Kisbye, 1959). The observed stability is probably due to the presence of the neighboring amino group, which is protonated first, thereby making it difficult for a second proton to be introduced onto the hydroxyl group. (The second proton must overcome the repulsion of the existing positive charge.) Under more vigorous conditions, though, namely, 5 N HCl, 100°C, reaction does occur. If one starts with either norephedrine or norpseudoephedrine (initially optically pure), an equilibrium mixture of the two diastereoisomers is obtained, with norpseudoephedrine predominating.

PHARMACEUTICAL PREPARATIONS CONTAINING PHENYLPROPANOLAMINE

Accompanying the steadily increasing costs of new-drug development and concern about product liability, there has been a trend in the pharmaceutical industry to recast well-established drugs into new and more effective dosage forms. The cornerstone of this effort has been the development of sustained- or controlled-release drugs (Sanders, 1985).

SUSTAINED RELEASE PREPARATIONS

Sustained-release preparations are designed to avoid the sawtooth-like fluctuations of drug plasma levels that often occur with multiple, equal doses. [A regimen of divided doses of *unequal* size can generally be chosen to produce plasma levels close to those of a sustained-release formulation (Westlake, 1975)]. The object is to maintain the plasma levels of the drug within the so-called therapeutic window, that is, high enough to be therapeutically effective but not to cause undesirable side effects. Since sustained-release drugs can be administered less frequently than traditional dosage forms, they are more convenient to use and tend to increase patient compliance.

The technical details regarding commercially available sustained-release systems for phenylpropanolamine are proprietary, but among the general approaches discussed in the literature are the following:

1. Blends of tiny beads containing a core of phenylpropanolamine wrapped in wax or polymer coats of variable thickness, permeability, and/or digestability have been incorporated into capsules. Such an encapsulated blend of coated beads constituted the Spansules introduced in the 1950s by Smith, Kline & French and which gained popularity as Contac cold relief capsules in the 1960s.

2. Phenylpropanolamine has been uniformly distributed within various polymer matrices. The incorporation of the drug within a matrix may be only a physical occlusion or there may be chemical interaction. An example of the latter is Pennwalt's Pennkinetic system in which protonated phenylpropanolamine is complexed with an ion-exchange resin. The drug-resin complex is coated with a polymer that is permeable to the drug and to inorganic cations. Hydrogen, sodium, and potassium ions penetrate the polymer coat over time and slowly displace the drug from the resin, whereupon it diffuses outward through the coat.

3. Phenylpropanolamine has been packaged inside a semipermeable membrane that contains a tiny, laser-drilled hole. Water slowly migrates inward by osmosis and the resulting osmotic pressure forces the drug solution out through the hole at a constant rate. This device, developed by the Alza Corporation, is termed OROS (for osmotic release oral system) and is used in Ciba-Geigy's appetite suppressant, Acutrim.

An advantage of a sustained-release preparation consisting of many tiny, individually coated particles of the active material is that those particles distribute themselves over the stomach and intestine so that local variations in the composition and pH of the gastric and intestinal fluids are averaged out.

Through delivery of the drug in many small particles, the possibility of significant incomplete release of active material is minimized. Pellets or even crystals of the drug may be coated with different polymers, each with different release characteristics, and then blended together in a capsule or a disintegrating tablet to give a formulation with the overall release pattern desired.

Among the coatings that have been used for these encapsulated pellets are Eudragit series of methacrylic ester copolymers, manufactured by Roehm Pharma (Lehmann et al., 1978; Lehmann, 1984). A certain proportion of pellets, for example, may be coated with copolymers of methacrylic esters and dimethylaminoethylmethacrylate. In the stomach, acid reacts with the tertiary amino groups of the copolymer to form a salt, thereby facilitating dissolution. Another fraction of the pellets is given an enteric coating (i.e., one that dissolves in the intestine rather than in the stomach) of a methacrylic acid-methacrylic ester copolymer. In addition to the two copolymers already mentioned, an acrylic polymer containing a small number of quaternary amino groups is used to coat still other pellets in the blend. This polymer is insoluble throughout the gastrointestinal (GI) tract but swells and permits slow outward diffusion of the drug.

The acrylic-resin coats can be applied to the drug pellets as acetone or isopropyl alcohol solutions or as aqueous latex dispersions obtained by emulsion polymerization. When aqueous dispersions of acrylic polymers are used, the latex particles first agglomerate and then flow together into a smooth, homogenous coat during drying.

Like many latexes, those of the Eudragit series support microbial growth, but 5 ppm active chlorine (from hypochlorite) can check these organisms. Alternatively, aqueous dispersions such as Eudragit E30D can be freeze-dried to give a powder of agglomerated latex particles; before use, the particles can be suspended in water and the carboxylate groups on the polymer are partially neutralized to form a stable, film-forming latex. Slow-release tablets can be produced by coating drug-laden granules with, for example, Eudragit E30D and then compressing them into tablets.

A recent study (Goodhart et al., 1984) compared the in vitro release properties of an Eudragit latex and Aquacoat (FMC Corporation); Aquacoat is an aqueous dispersion of ethylcellulose stabilized with small amounts of sodium lauryl sulfate and cetyl alcohol. Aquacoat requires an added plasticizer (e.g., dibutyl sebacate or triethyl citrate) for satisfactory coalescence of the latex particles into a smooth, even coating; Eudragit requires no plasticizer.

The release of phenylpropanolamine hydrochloride from Aquacoat systems was pH dependent (higher release at higher pH), which was attributed to the influence of sodium lauryl sulfate on the partitioning of the drug into the simulated gastric fluids. Eudragit-coated pellets did not exhibit pH-dependent release. The permeability of Eudragit films could be varied by incorporation of hydrophobic powders such as talc or magnesium stearate; variation in the nature and quantity of plasticizer likewise gave leverage over release rates through the Aquacoat coatings.

Dissolution tests have been described in which coated, spansule-type granules are successively immersed in simulated gastric and intestinal fluids. Excellent correlation was observed between the in vitro dissolution behavior and in vivo gastrointestinal drug release calculated using urinary excretion data (Tomida et al., 1977; Yamakawa et al., 1984).

Another method for altering the rate of dissolution is to formulate tablets containing a mixture of an amine salt and its free base. The release time for a sustained-release tablet or capsule containing phenylpropanolamine hydrochloride and free base was 3–8 hr longer than a preparation containing an equivalent dose of phenylpropanolamine hydrochloride alone (Oshlack & Leslie, 1984). The amine salt-free base mixtures also exhibit superior hardness and are thus less susceptible to fragmentation during tablet formation.

Another type of sustained-release formulation is entrapment of phenylpropanolamine in a polymer matrix; this can be achieved in different ways. In one technique (El Egakey & Speiser, 1982), methylcyanoacrylate monomer is added slowly to a suspension of phenylpropanolamine hydrochloride in acetone while the mixture is sonicated. The amino groups of phenylpropanolamine initiate polymerization of methylcyanoacrylate (a small proportion of free base presumably exists in equilibrium with the protonated amine). Aqueous methanol is added to quench the polymerization reaction and cause flocculation of the polymer particles. As the monomer:drug ratio is increased, a larger percentage of the drug is entrapped; a decrease in that ratio, on the other hand, leads to smaller and more uniform floc particles. Since the rate of release of the drug from the polymer matrix depends on both the initial drug content and the flocculate size (i.e., on the surface area), release rates can be adjusted by selecting the appropriate drug:monomer ratio (as well as by using blends of flocculates).

In another entrapment procedure a solution of a phenylpropanolamine salt is added to an aqueous dispersion of an acrylic copolymer (Rhodes et al., 1970). The salt ions adsorb onto the colloidal polymer particles which alters their surface charges and induces flocculation. The amount of phenylpropanolamine entrapped as the polymer flocculates and the rate of its subsequent release are influenced by the pH as well as by the salt of phenylpropanolamine. For the particular polymer studied, phenylpropanolamine acetate yielded a product with very satisfactory sustained-release characteristics, increasing the half-life for phenylpropanolamine excretion from 4.6 to 8.0 hr in five volunteers.

A long-acting tablet was described that exhibited zero-order release of phenylpropanolamine hydrochloride (i.e., the percentage released increased linearly with time) (Dunn & Haas, 1984). In addition to the active component, the tablet consisted of the dissolution retardants polyethylene glycol 6000, microcrystalline cellulose, and a polyacrylic acid; the diluent dibasic calcium phosphate; the lubricants fumed silicon dioxide (Syloid 244) and magnesium stearate; the plasticizer hydrogenated cottonseed oil; and the disintegrant lactose. These ingredients were dry-blended, then wet-granulated using isopropyl alcohol. The granules were then dried, sieved, and compressed into tablets.

A dosage form that has a two-stage release pattern and is a combination of the two sustained-release formulations discussed so far has been described (Lindahl & Ekman, 1986). This dosage form contains a core of the active drug, but the water-insoluble surrounding coat also contains the drug as randomly distributed tiny particles. Initially, the drug contained in the coating leaches out in a relatively rapid release stage; this process leaves pores in the coating and the core material can diffuse through the pores in a second, slower release stage. A variety of cellulose derivatives and acrylic polymers was suggested as coating material.

In another sustained-release system, the Pennkinetic system, protonated phenylpropanolamine is complexed to a cation exchange resin (a crosslinked divinylbenzenesulfonic acid) (Raghunathan et al., 1981; Robinson, 1986). As the complex travels through the GI tract, cations present in the gastric and intestinal fluids displace the drug from its inert, nonabsorbable carrier. However, in preliminary work, the rate of this ion exchange was found to be too high for acceptable sustained release. The drug-resin complex was thus given a barrier coat through which incoming ions and the outgoing drug would have to diffuse. Ethylcellulose was chosen as the coating material and was applied to the resin-drug complex as a solution in either ethanol or 10:1 methylene chloride:acetone. A refined vegetable oil was used as a coating plasticizer.

One problem with the Pennkinetic system was that water absorbed into the resin, causing it to swell and disrupt the ethylcellulose-barrier coat. Incorporating polyethylene glycol (PEG 4000) into the porous resin prior to coating the drug-resin complex prevented this problem. The PEG 4000 retarded water uptake, preserved the integrity of the outer coat, and slowed release of the drug.

The coated resin particles were mixed with uncoated phenylpropanolamine-resin complex to produce the desired overall release profile. The blend was used either in capsules or a suspension and provided effective plasma concentrations of phenylpropanolamine for 12 hr.

In a similar system, beads of an Amberlite ion-exchange resin carrying phenylpropanolamine were converted to microcapsules having sustained-release properties (Kaser-Liard, 1985). A mixture of n-propanol and n-butanol was added to a suspension of the phenylpropanolamine-resin beads in a

10% aqueous gelatin solution. The gelatin is forced out of solution by the organic solvents but tenaciously retains water of hydration and forms viscous droplets that envelop the phenylpropanolamine-resin beads. The spherical microcapsules, which initially have diameters ranging from 50 to 400 μm, are subsequently "hardened" by crosslinking the gelatin with formaldehyde vapor.

In most of the dosage forms discussed so far, the drug is delivered by outward diffusion from a central core through a semipermeable membrane or other coating. Oral osmotic devices represent a radically different concept. A drug is encapsulated by a semipermeable membrane and a laser is used to drill a hole in the membrane. Gastrointestinal fluids diffuse inward by osmosis; this diffusion increases the internal pressure and forces the drug out through the orifice at a constant rate (Chien, 1985).

Oral osmotic devices (OROS systems) can be classified in terms of structure, content and the rate and extent of drug delivery (Theeuwes, 1985). The most common device, the "elementary osmotic pump", consists of the drug (as a solid or in a saturated solution and sometimes accompanied by effervescent agents or diluents) surrounded by the semipermeable membrane. These devices typically deliver 60–80% of their contents at a constant rate. A "push-pull" osmotic pump is being developed that has an additional compartment with no drug. This unit is designed to deliver more than 80% of its contents at a constant rate.

An OROS device containing phenylpropanolamine is currently on the market. Acutrim is designed to deliver 90% of the active drug over a period of 18 hr and to maintain plasma levels of 60 ng/ml for 16 hr. Acutrim consists of a solid tablet of phenylpropanolamine hydrochloride coated with a cellulose triacetate membrane; the tablet also is coated with a thin layer of an immediate-release formulation of phenylpropanolamine.

The in vitro rates of release of phenylpropanolamine hydrochloride from the appetite suppressants Acutrim and Dexatrim were compared (Liu et al., 1984). As mentioned previously, Acutrim is based on the OROS system, whereas Dexatrim uses the spansule technology of coated granules. Samples were immersed in dissolution cells containing simulated gastric fluid for 2 hr; then the pH was adjusted to 7.5 to simulate intestinal pH. The phenylpropanolamine concentration in the dissolution medium was determined as a function of time. Dexatrim released its entire dose within 7 hr compared with a 16–18 hr release time for Acutrim.

Transdermal devices are patches affixed to intact skin which release a drug directly into the systemic circulation, thus avoiding the GI tract and possibly decreasing GI side effects. Also, metabolism of the drug by the liver can be decreased. One transdermal device that could be used for transdermal administration of phenylpropanolamine consists of two compartments containing the active drug—an adhesive layer in direct contact with the skin and a reservoir layer above it. The layers are separated by an oil-saturated polypropylene membrane that moderates the diffusion of the drug from the reservoir (Enscore & Gale, 1984). The matrix containing the drug is made of polyisobutylene, mineral oil, and fumed silicon dioxide (Cab-O-Sil); the latter component is a thickener that also increases the permeability of the matrix.

Unless the adhesive of the transdermal device is applied only around the edges, the adhesive must be permeable to the drug. The adhesive must also not cause skin sensitization (a problem with some acrylic and natural rubber-based adhesives). Silicone adhesives meet the requirements of permeability and biocompatibility but are subject to another problem: Contact with amino alcohols such as phenylpropanolamine can cause loss of adhesive strength over time. This problem can be solved by chemical modification of existing silicone adhesives (Metevia & Woodard, 1986).

Liposomes are tiny vesicles having walls composed of a lipid bilayer. They have an aqueous interior and have been used to deliver water-soluble drugs parenterally. A recent patent (Muntwyler & Hauser, 1985) described the preparation of liposomes suitable for phenylpropanolamine incorporation. In a typical preparation, equimolar amounts of a phospholipid such as soya lecithin and the hydrochloride salt of the drug of interest are combined in an organic solvent. The solvent is evaporated and water is added to the residual lipid film; high-speed mixing yields an opalescent, aqueous dispersion of the drug-carrying liposomes, which have diameters in the range of 0.02 to 0.06 μm.

FORMULATIONS OF COUGH-COLD PREPARATIONS

Among the medications currently on the U.S. market, those designed for common coughs and colds are probably the most numerous and over 150 of these contain phenylpropanolamine. (This number includes the various dosage forms that may be available under a single brand name.)

Liquid cough-cold preparations include syrups, elixirs, suspensions, and nasal drops or sprays. Phenylpropanolamine hydrochloride is usually present in a concentration of 10–15 mg/5 ml (5 ml = 1 teaspoon); in addition, these formulations contain one or more of the following: antihistamines, antitussives, expectorants, and analgesics. The commonly used drugs are listed here, with typical concentrations (in mg/5 ml) of the more frequently used drugs in parentheses. The structures of the listed compounds are shown in Figure 2.5.

Antihistamines
    Chlorpheniramine maleate (2)
    Pheniramine maleate
    Pyrilamine maleate

Antitussives
   Dextromethorphan hydrobromide (5-10)
   Codeine phosphate (10)
   Hydrocodone bitartrate
Expectorant
   Guaifenesin (100)
Analgesic-antipyretic
   Acetaminophen (150)

Phenylephrine hydrochloride, another sympathomimetic amine, is included in some products at a level of 5 mg/5 ml; like phenylpropanolamine, it acts as a decongestant. In addition, syrups and elixirs may contain flavoring and coloring agents and preservatives; alcohol is often present, usually at 5-10% by volume, but as high as 25% in some products. In formulating a syrup containing phenylpropanolamine, one must pay attention to the sweetener used as it was observed that the drug may very slowly react with aldoses and ketoses. Thus dextrose, fructose, corn syrup, and sucrose are not sweeteners of choice; a polyalcohol like sorbitol is more compatible (Barry et al., 1982).

Immediate-release tablets and capsules generally contain 15-25 mg of phenylpropanolamine, and sustained-release forms contain 50-75 mg. Other active ingredients are essentially the same as those listed for the liquid forms; the expectorant guaifenesin and the antitussive dextromethorphan are much less common in solid dosage forms, and codeine phosphate and hydrocodone bitartrate are not used. When used, acetaminophen is present at a level of 325 mg per tablet or 500 mg in "extra-strength" tablets; some formulations contain aspirin instead of acetaminophen.

Tablets also contain a variety of inert ingredients (excipients) that serve as fillers, binders, disintegrants, and processing aids (Seugling, 1980). Among the common fillers and binders are lactose, sucrose, mannitol, and microcrystalline cellulose; tablet disintegrants include starch, cellulose, alginates, and inorganic material such as bentonite clay; magnesium stearate, talc, and polyethylene glycol are a few of the compounds used as tableting lubricants.

Excipients may strongly influence the bioavailability of the active ingredient. For example, a formulation of phenylpropanolamine capsules containing a surfactant and the hydrophobic ingredients beeswax and peanut oil produced a plasma-level profile that resembled that of a sustained-release formulation (Francois et al., 1982). Optimization methods have been used to establish the excipients levels and processing conditions that produce optimum tablet properties, such as the dissolution/disintegration rate (Gould, 1984).

Tablets may be coated with colored films to aid in identification, provide

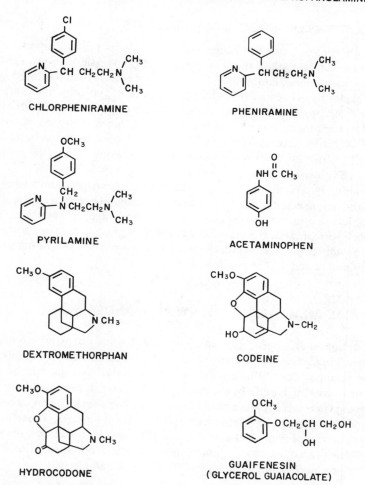

Figure 2.5. Compounds frequently accompanying phenylpropanolamine in commercial cough/cold preparations

requisite mechanical properties, and protect the active ingredients from light and the environment. Hydroxypropyl methylcellulose is often used as a film-forming material; it is water soluble and also soluble in the organic solvent mixtures used in film coating (Stern, 1983). The colorants in films are often "lakes," water-insoluble inorganic solids (e.g., alumina, clay, titanium dioxide, calcium carbonate) on which organic dyes have been adsorbed.

FORMULATIONS OF APPETITE SUPPRESSANTS

The formulations of appetite suppressants containing phenylpropanolamine are far more uniform than those of cough-cold preparations. Since 1984, all phenylpropanolamine-containing appetite suppressants manufactured in the United States have been caffeine-free preparations. Typically, these are sustained-release preparations containing 75 mg phenylpropanolamine or immediate-release preparations containing 25 or 37.5 mg phenylpropanolamine. The OROS tablet Acutrim contains 20 mg phenylpropanolamine in its external coating which dissolves to provide an immediate dose; the tablet core contains an additional 55 mg that is extruded slowly over 16 hr.

Formerly, combination products containing phenylpropanolamine and caffeine were marketed in the United States. Immediate-release capsules consisted of 25 mg phenylpropanolamine hydrochloride accompanied by 100 mg caffeine, approximately the amount of caffeine in a cup of regular, percolated coffee. Sustained-release formulations generally contained 50–75 mg phenylpropanolamine and 200 mg caffeine.

CHEMICAL ANALYSIS OF PHENYLPROPANOLAMINE

The selection of an appropriate analytical method for phenylpropanolamine is governed in part by the problem at hand. The requirements are quite different, for example, depending on whether one is analyzing a spoonful of cough syrup or a drop of blood. In the first case, the sample contains only a few constituents in relatively large amounts; in the second case, the analyst is usually looking at trace quantities in a complex biological matrix. Therefore, the following survey of analytical methods is divided into two sections: the analysis of phenylpropanolamine in pharmaceutical preparations and the analysis of phenylpropanolamine in biological fluids (blood and urine).

ANALYSIS OF PHENYLPROPANOLAMINE IN PHARMACEUTICAL PREPARATIONS

SPECTROPHOTOMETRIC METHODS

Spectrophotometric methods are among the earliest employed in assays of phenylpropanolamine. The methods differ from one another in 1) the means of separation of phenylpropanolamine from other constituents of the sample, and 2) the form in which phenylpropanolamine is measured. To introduce some order into the following discussion of a rather diverse collection of procedures, the methods are arranged according to the final form in which phenylpropanolamine is quantified rather than by the way it is separated from other components of the pharmaceutical product.

UV ABSORPTION OF PHENYLPROPANOLAMINE ITSELF

A method designed primarily for the quantitation of phenylephrine in the presence of other drugs such as phenylpropanolamine hydrochloride, aspirin, acetaminophen, glyceryl guaiacolate, dextromethorphan, and chlorpheniramine used column chromatography to separate the constituents (Levine & Doyle, 1967).

A dilute solution in pH 5.8 buffer was prepared from either an elixir or from ground tablets and was mixed with diatomaceous earth. The resulting agglomerate was transferred to a column containing a diatomaceous earth/pH 5.1 buffer mixture. Constituents other than the phenylephrine and phenylpropanolamine hydrochlorides, including flavoring and coloring matter, were eluted with chloroform and ether.

The two alkanolamine salts were then eluted with an ether solution of the ion pair-forming agent, bis-2-ethylhexylphosphate (DEHP). Phenylpropanolamine was subsequently separated from phenylephrine by passing the eluate through a second column packed with an alkali/diatomaceous earth mixture. Phenylephrine, a phenol, was retained on this column as the phenolate salt while phenylpropanolamine was again eluted as a DEHP ion pair. Finally, the ether solution of the phenylpropanolamine-DEHP ion pair was extracted with dilute sulfuric acid, bringing phenylpropanolamine back into aqueous solution. The UV absorbance of this phenylpropanolamine solution was measured and compared with that of a standard.

In another assay, ion-exchange chromatography was used to separate phenylpropanolamine hydrochloride from other constituents of commercial syrups and tablets (Smith, 1974). The sample was introduced onto a column of Dowex cation exchange resin, and the protonated amines were retained by resin sulfonate groups.

After excipients, coloring matter, and other neutral constituents were eluted, the amines were displaced from the resin—the more weakly basic ones first—by adding hydrochloric acid of increasing concentration. Again, phenylpropanolamine hydrochloride was determined by comparing its UV absorption with that of standards.

UV ABSORPTION OF BENZALDEHYDE DERIVED
FROM PHENYLPROPANOLAMINE

Quantitation of phenylpropanolamine by direct spectrophotometric measurement lacks sensitivity because of the relatively low molar absorptivity of phenylpropanolamine at the wavelength of maximum absorption. However, phenylpropanolamine can be quantitatively oxidized to benzaldehyde which has a 60- to 75-fold greater molar absorptivity (Chafetz, 1971). The oxidative cleavage of phenylpropanolamine is usually carried out by sodium periodate, a reagent used widely in early carbohydrate chemistry for its ability to cleave 1,2-glycols. Periodate reacts with 1,2-hydroxyamines according to equation 2.2, where R may be hydrogen or a not-too-bulky alkyl group but not an acyl group:

$$\underset{\substack{|\quad\; |\\ \\}}{C_6H_5\ CH-CH\ R'} + IO_4^{\ominus} \quad \xrightarrow[\text{PH 7.5}]{\substack{\text{ROOM TEMPERATURE,}\\ \text{15 MINUTES}}} \quad C_6H_5\ CHO + R'\ CHO + RNH_2 + IO_3^{\ominus}$$

with OH and NHR substituents on the first and second carbons respectively.

Equation 2.2

Tertiary amines are unreactive, whereas catecholamines follow a different reaction course, cyclizing to indole derivatives.

Spectrophotometry of the aromatic aldehyde produced on periodate oxidation will not distinguish between compounds such as phenylpropanolamine and ephedrine since both would yield benzaldehyde. However, the reaction affords a convenient method for determining phenylpropanolamine and phenylephrine in combination. Phenylpropanolamine yields benzaldehyde, which is extracted from the aqueous solution with hexane and quantitated by UV absorption measurement at 242 nm (Chafetz, 1971); phenylephrine yields m-hydroxybenzaldehyde, which remains in aqueous solution and is quantitated as the corresponding phenolate. (The phenolate has a higher UV absorption than the phenol.) Alternatively, phenylpropanolamine and phenylephrine can be sequentially extracted into chloroform, with UV measurements made in that solvent (Brown & Portmann, 1971).

Periodate oxidation was used to quantitate phenylpropanolamine in the presence of the antihistamine brompheniramine in sustained-release tablets (Hugosson et al., 1972). An aqueous solution of the tablets was mixed with a buffered solution of picric acid and extracted with chloroform to remove brompheniramine as a picrate ion pair. Phenylpropanolamine was not extracted at the selected pH and remained in the aqueous layer; sodium periodate was added and the benzaldehyde produced was extracted into cyclohexane. Absorbance of the cyclohexane solution was measured to determine the phenylpropanolamine content.

Syrups and other formulations may require preliminary treatment to remove propylene glycol and various sugars that react with periodate. In one example, an initial separation was achieved by column chromatography

(Clark, 1973). A commercial elixir was diluted with water and an aliquot was mixed with potassium hydrogen phosphate (K_2HPO_4) and Celite to provide a slightly alkaline stationary phase. The resulting mass was transferred to a column and methylene chloride was added to elute nonphenolic amines, weak acids, and neutral compounds; sugars, glycols, and phenolic amines such as phenylephrine were retained on the column. The eluate was introduced directly into a second, slightly acidic column that contained K_2HPO_4 and KCl. Weakly basic amines were eluted from this column either as the free bases or as chloride ion pairs, depending on the pK values; the more strongly basic phenylpropanolamine was retained on the column. Finally, ammonium hydroxide was added to elute phenylpropanolamine and to provide the slightly basic pH needed for the periodate oxidation; the eluate was introduced directly into a column containing a Celite/aqueous periodate mixture. Benzaldehyde that formed on this column was eluted with additional methylene chloride and measured spectrophotometrically. Phenylpropanolamine was determined in a series of commercial elixirs containing brompheniramine maleate, pyrilamine maleate, acetaminophen, dextromethorphan, codeine phosphate, phenyltoloxamine citrate, and several other common ingredients in various combinations.

The technique of difference spectrophotometry was used to assay phenylpropanolamine in the presence of either guaifenesin or dextromethorphan, without any preliminary separation (Tan & Salvador, 1985). A difference spectrum was generated using two solutions that were spectrally identical except for the difference brought about by the oxidation of phenylpropanolamine to benzaldehyde. An aliquot of standard (or sample) solution containing phenylpropanolamine hydrochloride was rendered alkaline with disodium hydrogen phosphate and treated with sodium periodate to produce benzaldehyde; the excess periodate was destroyed by adding sodium bisulfite (solution A). In a separate flask, identical quantities of phosphate, periodate, and bisulfite were added, but an identical aliquot of the phenylpropanolamine standard (or sample) solution was added only after the periodate was destroyed (solution B). The absorbance of solution A vs. solution B was measured, after raising the zero point (baseline); the height of the maximum peak vs. concentrations for a series of standards (in the range of 25–100 $\mu g/ml$) was used to construct a linear standard curve from which the amount of phenylpropanolamine in the unknown sample was determined.

Phenylpropanolamine has also been converted to benzaldehyde using ceric sulfate as the oxidant, with subsequent quantitation by UV spectroscopy. Alternatively, ceric sulfate titration can be used to determine milligram quantities of phenylpropanolamine or ephedrine in pharmaceutical dosage forms (Basyoni & Ibrahim, 1984).

COLORIMETRIC DETERMINATION OF PHENYLPROPANOLAMINE AFTER DERIVATIZATION

The reactive triketone ninhydrin (triketohydrindene hydrate) is a popular chromogenic agent for amino acids. Ninhydrin also reacts with phenylpropanolamine (pH 5, 100°C, ca. 30 min) to form a highly colored adduct that can be quantitated colorimetrically at 570 nm (Burke et al., 1974). The absorption is linearly related to concentration in the range of 2–8 μg/ml. This method has been used for the analysis of phenylpropanolamine in tablets and capsules; no interference was observed from aspirin, acetaminophen, tertiary amines such as atropine and chlorpheniramine, or excipients such as lactose, starch, or magnesium stearate.

The reaction between ninhydrin and phenylpropanolamine also was incorporated into an automated procedure for the specific determination of dextromethorphan hydrobromide, glyceryl guaiacolate, and phenylpropanolamine hydrochloride in cough syrups (Weber & Heveran, 1973).

The commercially available reagent 7-chloro-4-nitrobenzo-2-oxa-1,3-diazole reacts with primary, secondary, and tertiary amines to yield derivatives that absorb visible light. The absorbance is measured at 455 nm and is linear for phenylpropanolamine concentrations between 0 and 40 μg/ml. The method is applicable to formulations containing aspirin, acetaminophen, or caffeine but not to those containing pheniramines or other amines (Street & Abrenica, 1986).

COLORIMETRIC DETERMINATION OF PHENYLPROPANOLAMINE AS AN ION PAIR

Phenylpropanolamine was assayed in the presence of phenylephrine by extracting it into chloroform as a complex with bromthymol blue and measuring the absorption of the complex at 420 mm; absorption was linear in the range of 30–50 μg/ml phenylpropanolamine (Shenoy & Das Gupta, 1973). Phenylephrine, which was not extracted into chloroform at the selected pH (6.4), was also determined colorimetrically using 4-aminoantipyrine, a common chromogenic agent for phenols. The antioxidant sodium bisulfite at a level of 0.2% or the preservatives methylparaben (0.02%) or propylparaben (0.01%) produced no interference in the determination of either amine.

FLUOROMETRIC DETERMINATION OF PHENYLPROPANOLAMINE

Fluorescamine (available as Fluram from Roche Diagnostics, Nutley, NJ) reacts specifically with many primary aliphatic and aromatic amines, including phenylpropanolamine, to yield highly fluorescent derivatives (de Silva & Strojny, 1975) (see Equation 2.3).

The reagent and its hydrolysis products are not fluorescent and thus do not interfere with subsequent fluorometric measurements. Optimal reactivity

FLUORESCENCE MAXIMA (for PPA):
EXCITATION: 395 nm
EMISSION: 490 nm

Equation 2.3

with phenylpropanolamine is at pH 9, but the fluorescence of the product is enhanced by adjusting of the pH to 5.0–5.5 and extracting the fluorophor into ethyl acetate. A sensitivity limit of 0.3 $\mu g/ml$ has been reported for phenylpropanolamine, with the linear range having an upper limit of 30 $\mu g/ml$.

Phenylpropanolamine was assayed in a variety of dosage forms containing antitussive, antihistamine, and antipyretic agents but no other primary amines (Shankle, 1978). The sample was diluted in water and buffer, then treated with a 0.3% solution of fluorescamine in acetone to give a solution containing 0–3 $\mu g/ml$ of phenylpropanolamine (in terms of the free base). Fluorescence was determined at 480 nm with excitation at 398 nm. Quenching of the fluorescence occurred at concentrations exceeding about 30 $\mu g/ml$.

GAS CHROMATOGRAPHY

Despite the relatively low volatility of phenylpropanolamine, it can be analyzed by gas chromatography (GC) without derivatization (see Table 2.1). In certain special situations, sample preparation is quite simple. For example, cold tablets containing aspirin, chlorpheniramine maleate, and phenylpropanolamine hydrochloride were partitioned between chloroform and dilute aqueous sodium hydroxide (Madsen & Magin, 1976); the amines were extracted into chloroform, and aspirin remained in the aqueous solution as the sodium salt. After addition of an internal standard, an aliquot of concentrated chloroform solution was injected onto the gas chromatography column.

In another relatively simple sample preparation, a commercial cough-cold syrup containing phenylpropanolamine hydrochloride, glycerol guaiacolate, chlorpheniramine maleate, and dextromethorphan was acidified with hydrochloric acid and extracted with carbon tetrachloride to remove flavor and color additives that might interfere with chromatographic separation (Mario & Meehan, 1970). Glycerol guaiacolate, a glycol, remained in the aqueous phase along with the hydrochloride salts of the three amines. The aqueous

TABLE 2.1. Conditions for Selected Analyses of Phenylpropanolamine (PPA) by Gas Chromatography

Sample Form	Column	Column Temperature (°C)	Retention Time of PPA as Derivative (min)	Reference
Tablets, capsules, syrup	2.0 m × 4 mm (ID) glass, 0.1% silicone oil (DC-710) on 60/80 mesh dimethyl-dichlorosilane-treated glass beads	100–200 at 10°/min	3.0 (silyl derivative)	Hishta & Lauback (1969)
Syrup	2.44 mm × 3.2 mm (OD) Pyrex glass, 2% SE-30 on 80/100 mesh Chromosorb W (HP)	180	1.3	Mario & Meehan (1970)
Tablets	1.8 m × 2.7 mm (ID), 1% SE-30 on Chromosorb G	190	0.5	Gobbeler (1971)
Botanical material	2.0 m × 4 mm (ID) glass, 15% PEG 1000 on 60/80 mesh Celite 545	175	2.7	Yamasaki et al. (1974)
Tablets	1.8 m × 4 mm (ID), 3% OV-17 on 100/120 mesh Gas Chrom Q	230	0.9	Madsen & Magin (1976)
Capsules	1.8 m × 2 mm (ID), glass, 8% OV-101 on 80/100 Chromosorb W (HP)	170–270 at 9°/min	7.0 (as acetylated derivative)	de Fabrizio (1980)
Plasma	30 m × 0.25 mm (ID) fused silica capillary coated with polymethyl(5% phenyl) siloxane (J&W Scientific)	117° for 10 min then 3°/min to 125°	10.8 (tri-fluoro-acetyl derivative)	Crisologo et al. (1984)
Serum, urine	0.32 mm (ID) fused silica capillary, SE-54, 0.52 μm film (Hewlett-Packard)	55° for 1 min then 30°/min to 130° 130° for 0.5 min then 25°/min to 180° for 0.5 min then 16°/min to 225°	5.8	Ehresman et al. (1985)

TABLE 2.1. Continued.

Sample Form	Column	Column Temperature (°C)	Retention Time of PPA as Derivative (min)	Reference
Plasma, urine	15 m × 0.32 mm (ID) Durabond DB-1 fused silica capillary (J&W Scientific)	120–280° at 8°/min	2.4	Perrigo et al. (1985)
Tablets, syrups, elixirs	30 m × 0.32 mm (ID), fused silica capillary, 0.25 mm bonded film of OV-1	200° for 4 min then 5°/min to 235°	2.3	Thompson (1986)
Plasma	12.5 m × 0.32 mm (ID), fused silica capillary, 0.5 μm film of Ultra-1 methyl silicone (Hewlett-Packard)	110° for 1 min then 10°/min to 280°	2.7	Watts & Simonick (1986)

Adapted from Kanfer et al. (1983).

phase was then made alkaline to generate free amines, and was extracted with chloroform. The chloroform extract was concentrated and an internal standard was added before chromatography.

A more complicated extraction scheme was required for the GC analysis of belladonna alkaloids (atropine, scopolamine, and hyoscyamine) from tablets that also contained chlorpheniramine maleate and phenylpropanolamine; quantitation of phenylpropanolamine was not the objective of this method (Santoro et al., 1973). Tablets were triturated with dilute sulfuric acid, an internal standard was added, and the resulting slurry was diluted to known volume. Insoluble residue was separated by centrifugation, and the supernatant liquid was extracted with chloroform to remove wax excipients. The wax-free solution was adjusted to pH 8.0 and extracted with cyclohexane to remove chlorpheniramine, the weakest base among the remaining tablet constituents. A lower pH would have left too much chlorpheniramine behind, while a higher pH would have freed some of the belladonna amines. The aqueous solution was then adjusted to pH 9.0 and belladonna alkaloids were extracted with methylene chloride. Phenylpropanolamine, the strongest base in the formulation, remained in aqueous solution.

The foregoing gas chromatographic separations proceeded satisfactorily without derivatization of the relatively nonvolatile compounds. The retention time for phenylpropanolamine was typically less than 5 min, with columns maintained at temperatures from 180 to 230°C. A number of workers, however, have prepared derivatives of phenylpropanolamine and accompanying drugs before chromatography. One advantage of derivatization is that the highly polar, relatively nonvolatile amines are rendered less polar and more volatile and can be resolved at lower temperatures and/or in less time. Derivatized amines also have less tendency to adsorb to the column packing material or to the column itself, a phenomenon that causes loss of resolution and quantitation errors. (In recent years, the use of glass and fused-silica columns rather than metal ones and the use of more inert column packing material have minimized the problem of adsorption of highly polar compounds.) Derivatization also affects the partitioning of sample components between the mobile and stationary phases and thus may allow separations difficult to obtain with the underivatized compounds.

Phenylpropanolamine derivatization generally replaces hydrogen atoms on hydroxy or amino groups. The classical reaction is acetylation, in which "active" hydrogens (those bonded to oxygen or nitrogen) are replaced by an acetyl ($CH_3C=O$) group. For example, a sample was prepared from capsules containing salicylamide, phenylpropanolamine hydrochloride, caffeine, chlorpheniramine maleate, phenylephrine hydrochloride, and pyrilamine maleate. The sample was mixed with acetic anhydride, pyridine, and 1.2% 4-(dimethylamino) pyridine; the latter catalyzes the acetylation of hydroxyl groups (de Fabrizio, 1980). Of the three compounds that were acetylated—phenylpropanolamine, phenylephrine, and salicylamide—the last was the least reactive and required more vigorous reaction conditions. (A drawback of derivatization in general is the possibility of incomplete reaction, which results in multiple peaks.) The acetylating reagents and solvent gave early-eluting peaks that did not interfere with the separation of the six main components, and the analysis time was 15 min.

A derivatizing agent introduced in the 1960s is N,O-bis(trimethylsilyl) acetamide (BSA), (see Diagram 2.7). This reagent replaces active hydrogens by trimethylsilyl [$-Si(CH_3)_3$] groups. It was used in the analysis of decongestant tablets and syrups containing phenylpropanolamine hydrochloride, phenylephrine hydrochloride, and the two antihistamines phenyltoloxamine dihydrogencitrate and chlorpheniramine maleate (Hishta & Lauback, 1969).

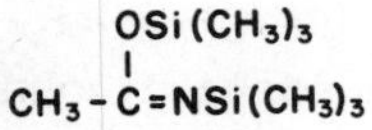

$$OSi(CH_3)_3$$
$$|$$
$$CH_3-C=NSi(CH_3)_3$$

(VI)

Diagram 2.7

The mixture was dissolved in water and sodium carbonate was added to generate the free amines. Additional salts (sodium chloride and sodium sulfate) were added and the mixture was extracted with isopropyl alcohol. (This is an interesting extraction because isopropyl alcohol is normally miscible with water in all proportions but is immiscible with aqueous solutions having high concentrations of dissolved salts.) A small amount of trifluoroacetic acid was added to the isopropyl alcohol fraction, which contained all four amines, and the solution was evaporated to dryness. (Trifluoroacetate salts of the amines tend to be more stable than the corresponding hydrochloride salts.) The residue was redissolved in a pyridine solution containing an internal standard, the silylating agent BSA was added, and an aliquot was chromatographed. Silylated phenylpropanolamine eluted at 3 min after the column temperature had reached about 130°C in a temperature-programmed determination.

As mentioned previously, derivatization sometimes enhances the separation of compounds that are otherwise difficult to resolve. For example, ephedrine and its diastereoisomer pseudoephedrine often elute as a single broad peak. However, when the two isomers were converted to oxazolidines (Equation 2.4) they were well resolved and eluted in about half the time (Yamasaki et al., 1974).

Under the same reaction conditions, phenylpropanolamine formed a Schiff base which also eluted earlier than underivatized phenylpropanolamine (see Equation 2.5).

Compounds may sometimes form unexpected products within the gas chromatograph itself. For example, when a solution of phenylpropanolamine in carbon disulfide was injected into the chromatograph, an unexpected extra peak was observed that was shown to correspond to an addition-cyclization product analogous to the oxazolidines in Equation 2.4 (Santoro et al., 1976).

Quantitation is usually accomplished by the use of an internal standard, a compound that elutes near (but does not overlap with) the chromatographic peaks of interest. The internal standard should be available in high purity, should not react with any of the compounds in the sample, and should not be present in the original sample. A standard solution is prepared containing the

Equation 2.4

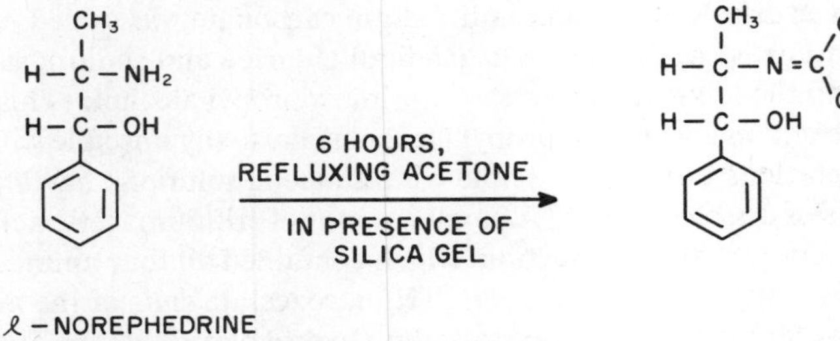

ℓ – NOREPHEDRINE

Equation 2.5

components of interest in concentrations close to those anticipated in the sample. The internal standard is added in identical concentrations to this standard solution and to the sample solution. The concentration of the component of interest is then calculated from the following equation:

$$(C_x)_{sample} = \frac{(H_x/H_s)_{sample}}{(H_x/H_s)_{standard}} (C_x)_{standard}$$

where $(C_x)_{standard}$ is the concentration of the constituent of interest in the standard solution and the H_x/H_s values are the ratios of peak heights (compound of interest:internal standard) determined from the respective chromatograms of the sample and standard solutions. Some of the compounds that have been used as internal standards in the GC analysis of phenylpropanolamine are pramoxine, n-tetracosane, dicyclohexylphthalate, and tribenzylamine.

The GC work described previously was performed on packed rather than capillary columns. Capillary columns have not been quite as widely used as packed columns in the analysis of pharmaceuticals although they are the columns of choice in the analysis of drugs in biological fluids. A recent report, however, gave the relative retention times, on a 0.32 mm id fused silica capillary column, of 39 common drugs (Thompson, 1986). Mixtures of 10–15 drugs, including phenylpropanolamine, were well resolved in either isothermal or temperature-programmed determinations. Because capillary columns are more inert to polar compounds than packed columns, peaks are more symmetrical, which allows better resolution and quantitation; analysis times also may be decreased 50% or more using capillary rather than packed columns.

Gas chromatography using a capillary column gave excellent resolution of a mixture containing 50 ng each of phenylpropanolamine, ephedrine, amphetamine, caffeine, and 14 other drugs. Phenylpropanolamine had the next to the lowest flame-ionization detector response (Trivedi, 1985).

HIGH-PERFORMANCE LIQUID CHROMATOGRAPHY

High-performance liquid chromatography (HPLC) has several advantages over GC that are particularly important in the analysis of phenylpropanolamine. First, separations may be carried out at room temperature rather than at elevated temperatures. Second, separation may be performed on aqueous solutions, so that amine salts can be analyzed directly, without prior liberation of the free amine. Third, HPLC offers the added dimension of a mobile phase that can be "fine-tuned" by the chromotographer to achieve optimal separations. In GC, the mobile phase is the carrier gas which is usually either helium or nitrogen; in HPLC the mobile phase can be varied widely.

High-performance liquid chromatography is usually carried out in either of two modes: normal phase or reverse phase. Normal-phase HPLC resembles traditional column chromatography in that the sample is introduced into a column containing a relatively polar packing material, such as silica, and is eluted with a relatively nonpolar and usually water-insoluble solvent (e.g., hexane, chloroform). In reverse-phase HPLC, the polarities of the mobile and stationary phases are reversed: The stationary phase often consists of silica particles that have been chemically bonded with lipophilic groups, whereas the mobile phase is usually a very polar mixture of water and water-miscible organic solvents (e.g., acetonitrile, methanol, tetrahydrofuran). However, departures from these standard modes are possible, and successful separations of phenylpropanolamine from other drugs have been reported for example, using bare, unbonded silica gel as the stationary phase and polar, aqueous mobile phases (Richardson & Bidlingmeyer, 1984).

Most HPLC separations today are conducted in the reverse-phase mode which has several advantages: Water-soluble solutes such as amine salts can be chromatographed directly without pretreatment with alkali and extraction into an organic solvent; there is more flexibility in choosing a mobile phase since, for example, the pH can be varied by buffers, and other ionic species may be added; furthermore, the overall cost of solvents is generally less in reverse-phase HPLC.

Sample preparation for HPLC analysis of dosage forms containing phenylpropanolamine is usually straightforward. Syrups and elixirs are simply diluted with water to a known volume; tablets are ground into a fine powder (10–20 at a time to give a representative sample), heated briefly with water or dilute hydrochloric acid to bring into solution, then diluted to known volume and filtered. Sonication may also be used to dissolve the tablets, and centrifugation may be employed to obtain a clear solution. Typically, an aliquot of 1–30 μg of phenylpropanolamine hydrochloride in 10–50 μl of solution is injected into the chromatograph. It is important to avoid these errors in using HPLC—overloading the column, which causes loss of resolution, and exceeding the range of linearity of the detector response.

The most commonly used detector for HPLC analysis of phenylpropanolamine is the fixed-wavelength UV detector operating at 254 nm. The 254 nm wavelength rarely coincides with the maximum-absorption wavelength of any given ingredient in a pharmaceutical preparation; therefore, sensitivity is adequate but never optimal. A variable wavelength UV detector operated at 198 nm may offer increased sensitivity without loss of precision (Cox et al., 1977). In analysis of formulations containing acetaminophen, the strong absorption of this drug at 254 nm saturated the detector, but more satisfactory analysis was achieved at 214 nm (Richardson & Bidlingmeyer, 1984).

Although phenylpropanolamine hydrochloride has a UV absorption maximum near 254 nm, its molar absorptivity (extinction coefficient) is low. This can be a problem in analysis of multicomponent formulations if one of the ingredients has a much greater UV absorption than phenylpropanolamine and is also present in severalfold excess. In this situation, it would be necessary to change the detector attenuation during the analysis. In the case of an appetite suppressant containing phenylpropanolamine hydrochloride and caffeine in a 1:4 ratio, the problem was solved by oxidizing phenylpropanolamine with sodium periodate and chromatographing an aliquot of the diluted reaction mixture (Tan & Salvador, 1983). Caffeine is stable toward periodate, but phenylpropanolamine is converted to benzaldehyde which has UV absorptivity 60–75 times that of phenylpropanolamine hydrochloride.

Phenylpropanolamine hydrochloride has a relatively short retention time and its chromatographic peak is sometimes partially obscured by certain early-eluting excipients. Here, too, periodate oxidation of phenylpropanolamine hydrochloride solved the problem (Taylor et al., 1984). In this instance, benzaldehyde was extracted into hexane, and chromatography was carried out on a silica column. This approach, of course, cannot be used if other alkanolamines are present that will yield benzaldehyde on periodate oxidation.

Another strategy that enhances the UV detectability of phenylpropanolamine in HPLC analysis is to form a derivative that contains a strongly absorbing group. For example, both phenylisothiocyanate (Noggle, 1980) and 8-quinolinesulfonyl chloride (Noggle & Clark, 1984) yield derivatives of phenylpropanolamine that give greater UV absorption.

Although it has relatively weak UV absorbance, phenylpropanolamine exhibits natural fluorescence and has been quantitated in two-component mixtures by using a fluorescence detector in series with a variable-wavelength UV detector (Cieri, 1986). Excitation and emission wavelengths for the fluorescence detector were 255 and 285 nm, respectively; the UV detector was set at about 300 nm since aspirin, acetaminophen, and caffeine—the other drugs analyzed—have adequate absorbance at this wavelength but phenylpropanolamine does not.

An important factor in developing an HPLC method is to find a mobile phase that gives good separation of component peaks without unduly long retention times. For example, the separation of phenylpropanolamine from the huge excess of acetaminophen in a commercial cold tablet posed a problem because the leading edge of the large acetaminophen peak crowded the small, earlier-eluting phenylpropanolamine peak. However, by increasing the water content of the mobile phase and decreasing the pH, the retention time of acetaminophen was increased and that of phenylpropanolamine was decreased, resulting in satisfactory resolution (Das Gupta & Heble, 1984).

The retention times of ionic species, such as protonated phenylpropanolamine, can also be varied by the addition of a lipophilic anion, such as an alkyl sulfonate, to the mobile phase. The anionic *counterion* and the protonated amine form an ion pair which has a greater affinity for the nonpolar stationary phase than does either of the unassociated ions. This increases the retention time of the amine. Counterions of increasing alkyl chain lengths generally increase the retention of the (protonated) amine (Koziol et al., 1979). However, in any given solvent system, there is a maximum chain length for the added ion beyond which precipitation occurs (Halstead, 1982). Other variables influence the extent of ion-pair association with the stationary phase: the nature and volume of the stationary phase, the counterion concentration, and the presence of secondary electrolytes that compete with the counterion (Achari & Jacob, 1980). The retention of a nonionic species (e.g., methyl paraben at acidic pH) is generally unaffected by an ion-pairing counterion.

Cough syrups containing phenylpropanolamine, guaifenesin, codeine phosphate, and the preservative sodium benzoate were analyzed successfully by using sodium heptanesulfonate as an ion-pairing agent (Muhammad & Bodnar, 1980). No sample preparation other than a 10-fold dilution was required. Similarly, combination cough-cold tablets containing phenylpropanolamine were analyzed using sodium pentanesulfonate in a mobile phase buffered at pH 1.4 (Greco, 1984). Additional applications of ion-pair HPLC to the analysis of cough syrups and elixirs are illustrated in Figure 2.6.

A method for separating components of cough-cold formulations using a cyano stationary phase was limited by the short column life (Achari & Stillman, 1986). To overcome this limitation, a method was developed using an ordinary nonpolar, C-18 column and sodium hexadecanesulfonate as an ion-pairing agent. A high proportion of organic solvent was required to keep the sulfonate in solution at the customary concentration level, but this mobile phase gave unsuitable retention times. Reducing both the sulfonate concentration and the proportion of organic solvent, however, yielded satisfactory separations of decongestants, antihistamines, and antitussives in several cough-cold formulations.

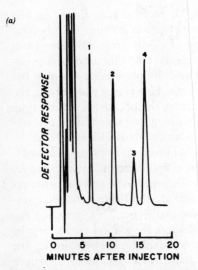

(a)

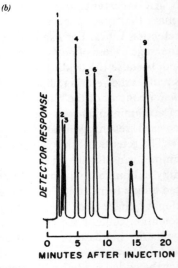

(b)

Figure 2.6.a. Chromatogram of a typical cough-cold syrup (Halstead, 1982)
1) phenylpropanolamine
2) benzphetamine (internal standard)
3) dextromethorphan
4) chlorpheniramine

Figure 2.6.b. Chromatogram of a variety of cough-cold ingredients (Halstead, 1982)
1) maleic acid
2) guaifenesin
3) phenacetin
4) phenylephrine
5) phenylpropanolamine
6) methoxyphenamine
7) benzphetamine (internal standard)
8) dextromethorphan
9) chlorpheniramine

Figure 2.6. Separation of phenylpropanolamine from other drugs by high-performance liquid chromatography

A mixture of ion-pairing reagents (pentanesulfonic and heptanesulfonic acids) was used to optimize the separation of phenylpropanolamine, phenylephrine, and several nonbasic species (Costanzo, 1984). There are many procedures for optimizing the mobile phase for a particular separation (see key references in Costanzo, 1984).

Another group (Lovett et al., 1986) used a cyanopropylsilyl-bonded column with an aqueous buffer/acetonitrile mobile phase (pH 2.3) to separate up to seven drugs often accompanying phenylpropanolamine in cough-cold preparations. The diastereoisomers ephedrine and pseudoephedrine were not separated nor were acetaminophen and caffeine, but these pairs are

(c)

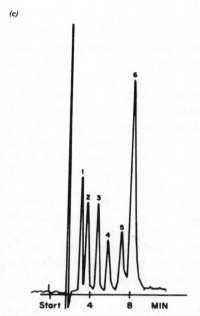

Figure 2.6.c. Chromatogram of a standard mixture of β-phenylethylamines and caffeine (Lurie, 1980)
1) phenylpropanolamine
2) ephedrine
3) amphetamine
4) methamphetamine
5) phentermine
6) caffeine

(d)

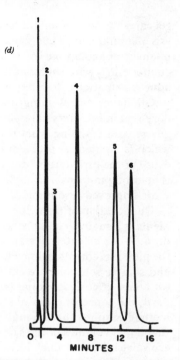

Figure 2.6.d. Chromatogram of a variety of cough-cold ingredients (Koziol et al., 1979)
1) maleic acid
2) phenylephrine
3) pseudoephedrine
4) naphazoline
5) chlorpheniramine
6) brompheniramine

not usually formulated together. Since acetaminophen and aspirin are usually present in far greater amounts than other active ingredients, two sample injections at different recorder attenuations were used to record the heights of all peaks; a lidocaine internal standard was used for quantitation.

Not to be confused with the ion-pair technique is HPLC using an ion-exchange resin. Ion-exchange resins themselves tend to have poor separation efficiencies and tend to swell with changes in ionic strength, but chemists have chemically bonded ion-exchange moieties to a silica gel support. Silica gel carrying surface sulfonate groups, for example, is suitable for HPLC analysis of amine salts. Thus, the components of a commercially available elixir—phenylpropanolamine hydrochloride, phenylephrine hydrochloride, and guaifenesin—were successfully separated on a cation-exchange column with aqueous ethanol buffered at pH 4.8 as the mobile phase (Cox et al., 1977).

Guaifenesin-containing phenylpropanolamine formulations from a half-dozen manufacturers have been found to contain an impurity associated with guaifenesin (ranging from 0.2 to 2.3% of the guaifenesin). The impurity, which is a potential problem in HPLC analysis of phenylpropanolamine because of the proximity of their chromatographic peaks, was identified as an isomer of guaifenesin; a slight modification of the mobile-phase organic solvents improved resolution (Schieffer et al., 1984).

Quantitation of phenylpropanolamine hydrochloride and the other ingredients is usually accomplished by using either an external or internal standard. When an external standard is used, a solution is prepared that contains the pure ingredients in known concentrations. Equal volumes of the standard and sample solutions are chromatographed. From the ratio of peak heights (or areas) of corresponding peaks and the known concentrations in the standard, the concentrations of the sample constituents may be calculated. This method requires that no material is lost during dilution and/or transfer and that equal volumes of the sample and standard solutions are injected. (Modern valve injectors which introduce the sample from a fixed-volume loop have eliminated the variability of syringe injection to a large extent, so the second requirement is generally fulfilled.)

Quantitation employing an internal standard has already been discussed in the preceding section on GC. Among the compounds that have been used as internal standards in the HPLC analysis of phenylpropanolamine hydrochloride are methyl *p*-hydroxybenzoate (methyl paraben) (Tan & Salvador, 1983), 2,5-dihydroxybenzoic acid (Schieffer & Hughes, 1983), amphetamine (Schorno et al., 1982), norpseudoephedrine (Sprieck, 1974), and benzphetamine (Halstead, 1982).

Typical conditions for HPLC analyses of phenylpropanolamine are presented in Table 2.2, and representative chromatograms are shown in Figure 2.6.

Phenylpropanolamine hydrochloride is generally present in pharmaceutical formulations as a racemic mixture, and the enantiomers are not resolved on the columns used in the analyses discussed so far. However, enantiomers can be separated by: 1) preparing diastereoisomeric derivatives and using a standard, achiral stationary phase or 2) using an achiral stationary phase. Both approaches have been used in the separation of phenylpropanolamine enantiomers.

As an example of the first strategy, the enantiomers of phenylpropanol-

TABLE 2.2. Conditions for Selected Analyses of Phenylpropanolamine by HPLC

Sample Form	Column	Mobile Phase	Detector	Flow Rate (ml/min)	Retention Time of PPA (min)	Reference
Elixir, syrup, tablets, capsules	μ-Bondapak phenyl, 30 cm × 4 mm (ID) (Waters)	Water–methanol–acetic acid (55:44:1) 0.005 M sodium heptanesulfonate	UV, 254 nm	2.0	2.6	Koziol et al. (1979)
Syrup	μ-Bondaphenyl, 30 cm × 3.9 mm (ID) (Waters)	Water–methanol (62:36), 0.004 M sodium heptanesulfonate and 1% glacial acetic acid	UV, 254 nm	0.5	16.8	Muhammed & Bodnar (1980)
Tablets	Partisil-10-ODS, 25 cm × 4.6 mm (ID) (Whatman)	2.85×10^{-3} m ethylene–diamine sulfate buffer (pH = 7.44)–acetonitrile (1:1)	UV, 216.5 nm	3.8	4.0	Heidemann (1981)
Syrup	μ-Bondapak C_{18}, 30 cm × 4 mm (ID) (Waters)	5.8 g sodium dioethyl sulfosuccinate in 680 ml methanol 290 ml water, 40 ml tetrahydrofuran, 1 ml 85% phosphoric acid (pH = 3.8)	UV, 254 nm	1.3	7.1	Halstead (1982)
Plant material	Li Chrosorb Si60, 25 cm × 5 mm (ID) (Merck)	Ethylene chloride–methanol–acetic acid–diethylamine–water (800:200:10:5:5) (normal-phase operation)	UV, 257 nm	0.8	16	Schorno et al. (1982)
Syrup, tablets, capsules	Partisil-10 C_8 25 cm × 4.6 mm (ID)	Water–methanol–acetic acid (27:12:1) 0.005 M sodium pentanesulfonate	UV, 254 nm	2.0	6.1	Schieffer & Hughes (1983)
Tablets, elixirs	μ-Bondapak phenyl, 30 cm × 4 mm (ID) (Waters)	0.02 M aq. potassium dihydrogen phosphate adjusted to pH 2.6 with 85% phosphoric acid	UV, 256 nm	2.5	3.5	DasGupta & Heble (1984)

TABLE 2.2. Continued.

Sample Form	Column	Mobile Phase	Detector	Flow Rate (ml/min)	Retention Time of PPA (min)	Reference
Tablets	μ-Bondapak phenyl, 30 cm × 3.9 mm (ID) (Waters)	acetonitrile-acetic acid-water (26.5:1:72.5), 0.005 M sodium pentanesulfonate, pH 2.4	UV, 254 nm	0.75	5.9	Greco (1984)
Urine, plasma	Spherisorb S5W silica, 25 cm × 5 mm (ID) (Phase Separations, UK)	methanol-aqueous ammonium nitrate buffer, adjusted to pH 10.1 with ammonia (9:1)	UV, 254 nm	2.0	2.3	Law et al. (1984)
Tablets, syrup	μ-Porasil silica Radial-PAK, 10 cm × 8 mm (ID) (Waters)	methanol-0.01 M aqueous ammonium hydrogen phosphate, pH 7.8 (3:1)	UV, 214, 254 nm	4.0	2.4	Richardson & Bidling-meyer (1984)
Tablets, capsules, syrup	μ-Bondapak C18 (Waters)	water-methanol (4:1)	UV, 254 nm	1.5	4.5	Schieffer et al. (1984)
Urine, plasma	Spherisorb S5W silica, 12.5 or 25 cm × 4.9 mm (ID) (Phase Separations, UK)	methanolic ammonium perchlorate (10 mM), plus 1 ml/l methanolic sodium hydroxide (0.1 M), pH 6.7	UV, 254 nm electro-chemical, 1.2 v	2.0	1.8	Jane et al. (1985)

	Column	Mobile phase	Detection			Reference
Urine, plasma	5 μ Ultrasphere ODS, 15 or 25 cm × 4.6 mm (ID) (Beckman)	for plasma: 0.8 g sodium heptanesulfonate in 2400 ml of acetonitrile, 1600 ml water, 12 ml acetic acid	fluorescence of post-column derivative	1.0	8.5	Shi et al. (1985)
Tablets, capsules, syrups, elixirs	10 μ-Bondapak C18 30 cm × 3.9 mm (ID) (Waters)	sodium hexadecanesulfonate (0.0015 M); acetic acid-water-acetonitrile (2:48:50)	UV, 265 nm	1.2	7.2	Achari & Stillman (1985)
Tablets	10 μ C18 25 cm × 4.6 mm (ID) (Alltech)	1 g sodium pentanesulfonate in 500 ml water plus 500 ml methanol	fluorescence $\lambda_{ex} = 255$ nm $\lambda_{em} = 285$ nm	1.5	6	Cieri (1986)
Tablets, capsules, syrup	5 μ Ultrasphere cyanopropylsilane, 15 cm × 4.6 mm (ID) (Beckman)	ammonium dihydrogen phosphate, 0.01 M, adjusted to pH 2.3 with phosphoric acid; buffer-acetonitrile (85:15) 40°C	UV, 215 nm	1.5	2.5	Lovett (1986)

Source: Adapted from Kanfer et al. (1983).

59

Equation 2.6

amine (norephedrine), ephedrine, pseudoephedrine, amphetamine, and methamphetamine were resolved on a standard reversed-phase, C_{18} column after conversion to diastereomeric thiourea derivatives using commercially available 2,3,4,6-tetra-O-acetyl-β-D-glucopyranosyl isothiocyanate (Gal, 1984; Noggle & Clark, 1986) (see Equation 2.6).

In an example of the second approach, a chiral stationary phase was prepared by bonding the amino acid L-proline to silica gel; proline was also complexed with copper (II) ions. Several amino alcohol enantiomers including phenylpropanolamine were then resolved by forming a differential (and reversible) complex with the proline-bound copper. To adequately complex the amino alcohols at a pH compatible with the stability of the stationary phase, however, the Schiff-base derivatives (Equation 2.5) rather than the amino alcohols themselves were chromatographed; these derivatives were prepared by reacting the amino alcohols with either salicylaldehyde or ketones of similar structure (Gelber et al., 1984).

Samples generated by in vitro dissolution studies were analyzed by HPLC. A potential problem with such analyses is the mismatch between the sample medium (e.g., simulated gastric fluid at pH 1.2) and the mobile phase (which usually must have a much higher pH for efficient separations). Such a mismatch can cause baseline instability that would interfere with quantitation. The problem of baseline instability was solved, however, by the use of a fluorophosphate buffer in the mobile phase and a silica-alumina column packing (Severin, 1986). The amphoteric nature of the aluminum-oxygen bond tends to modulate the effect of injecting a sample which is several pH units above or below that of the mobile phase. Interestingly, this work employed reversed-phase eluants (i.e., polar, aqueous solvents) with what is usually considered normal-phase column packing (namely, unbonded silica-alumina).

MISCELLANEOUS ANALYTICAL METHODS

ROOM-TEMPERATURE PHOSPHORESCENCE

Phenylpropanolamine can be assayed by room-temperature phosphorescence (RTP) a technique that offers both high selectivity and sensitivity and that permits analysis without prior separations.

Phosphorescence is the light emitted when a molecule in a triplet excited state (electron spins unpaired) returns to the ground state. Triplet states are usually not produced directly by absorption of light; rather, they arise from a singlet excited state (electron spins paired) by a transition called intersystem crossing, which involves flipping an electron spin. Compared to fluorescence (the light emitted when a molecule in a singlet excited state returns to the ground state), phosphorescence has a much longer "lifetime"; that is, it takes much longer—typically milliseconds instead of nanoseconds—for a substantial fraction of molecules to return to the ground state.

Nonradiative relaxation processes compete more effectively with phosphorescent emission than with fluorescent emission. Thus, phosphorescence has traditionally been studied at very low temperature (the boiling point of nitrogen, $77°K$) so that the sample is frozen into a solid matrix and collisions are reduced. However, in the last decade it was discovered that phosphorescence can be detected at room temperature by adsorbing phosphors onto paper, silica gel, or other solids, or incorporating the phosphors into micelles.

Selectivity is achieved in an RTP analysis by choosing the appropriate excitation and emission wavelengths and/or by taking advantage of differences in relaxation times for different phosphors. For example, if a phosphor other than the one of interest has a very short relaxation time, measurements can be made after a predetermined delay time thereby avoiding interference by that phosphor. Making measurements at prearranged times is often referred to as "gated detection" or "time discrimination."

Since phenylpropanolamine itself is not phosphorescent, a fluorescamine derivative was prepared (Long et al., 1985). A quantity of derivative equivalent to 225 ng of phenylpropanolamine was placed on a paper disk, followed by a solution of potassium iodide. (Heavy atoms such as iodine facilitate intersystem crossing and enhance the rate of radiative relaxation.) Spectrofluorometric measurements were made on the dried sample, which was bathed in a stream of dehumidified nitrogen since both water and oxygen strongly quench phosphorescence. The content of phenylpropanolamine was determined from its phosphorescence compared to a standard curve.

NUCLEAR MAGNETIC RESONANCE

Counterfeit drugs of abuse containing combinations of ephedrine, phenylpropanolamine, and caffeine are used within the drug culture to imitate controlled drugs such as amphetamine, phentermine, mephentermine, diethylpropion, phenmetrazine, and phendimetrazine. Nuclear magnetic resonance (NMR) spectroscopy can be used to identify these "look-alike" drugs (Avdovich et al., 1985). The suspect tablet is pulverized, mixed with D_2O, and centrifuged; ^{13}C- and ^{1}H-NMR spectra are obtained on both the supernatant solution and on a deuterated-chloroform extract obtained after addition of potassium carbonate to liberate the free amines. The ^{13}C-NMR chemical shifts of the alkyl side-chain carbon atoms (and the N-methyl carbon atoms of caffeine) are distinctive enough to discriminate among the various drugs of interest.

RAMAN SPECTROSCOPY

A mixture of phenylpropanolamine hydrochloride and acetaminophen was assayed by laser Raman-scattering spectroscopy without any preliminary separation (King et al., 1985). Sharp, well-resolved peaks were obtained from a mixture of phenylpropanolamine, acetaminophen, and potassium nitrate as an internal standard. Sample spectra were measured between 990 and 1220 cm^{-1} and compared with precisely measured spectra of the individual components (plus internal standard); a computer-based technique of cross correlation was used in the analysis. In essence, cross correlation indicates the extent to which each normalized reference spectrum contributes to the sample spectrum.

ANALYSIS OF PHENYLPROPANOLAMINE IN BIOLOGICAL FLUIDS

There are many reasons why rapid, convenient, and reliable analytical methods for the determination of phenylpropanolamine and other drugs in biological fluids are in demand. Analytical capability is needed in emergency situations when a person has ingested one or more potentially toxic agents. A physician may follow the course of treatment when a patient has taken an overdose or monitor drug levels in order to adjust the dose. A pharmaceutical chemist uses these analytical techniques to study the metabolism and excretion of a drug. Officials at an athletic competition may need to determine whether athletes have taken drugs of abuse and employers may need to do the same with their employees.

SPECTROPHOTOMETRIC DETERMINATION

One of the earliest methods for measuring phenylpropanolamine in a biological fluid was described in the report of an evaluation of a sustained-release formulation (Heimlich et al., 1961). Samples consisted of 0.5 ml of urine taken periodically from persons who had received the drug. The samples were diluted, made alkaline to phenolphthalein indicator, and treated with sodium periodate which converted phenylpropanolamine to benzaldehyde. The benzaldehyde was extracted into ether, its UV absorption was measured, and the absorbance was related to phenylpropanolamine concentration by means of a previously constructed standard curve. The sensitivity of the method, which is still used today, is of the order of 10 μg of phenylpropanolamine hydrochloride per ml of urine.

THIN-LAYER CHROMATOGRAPHY

Blood and urine levels of phenylpropanolamine, phenylephrine, chlorpheniramine, and dextromethorphan were determined by a thin-layer chromatography (TLC)-fluorometric technique (Lange et al., 1968). A 0.1 ml sample of capillary blood was treated with aqueous trichloroacetic acid to precipitate plasma proteins before application to the TLC plate. The chromatogram was developed with ammoniacal chloroform : ether (1 : 1), and the area containing the separated drug was extracted with ethanol. The extracted drug was treated with rose bengal, a fluorescein derivative that forms intensely fluorescent complexes with many amines, and the resulting fluorescence was measured. Drug concentrations were determined by comparison to appropriate blanks and standards. The limit of detection was approximately 0.5 μg/ml. Urine samples (0.1 ml) were chromatographed directly.

Much of the TLC work on phenylpropanolamine and other drugs has been in connection with screening programs for drug abuse, and urine has been the biological fluid of choice for these studies. Several different methods have been recommended for the preliminary concentration of the drugs present in the urine. In one procedure, a 40 ml sample of urine was made alkaline and added to a column of XAD-2 resin, a porous, nonpolar copolymer that retains a wide range of neutral organic compounds (Bussey & Backer, 1974). After the column was washed free of excess urine, the adsorbed compounds were eluted with a smaller volume of organic solvent (e.g., ethylene chloride-ethyl acetate). The solvent was evaporated, and the residue was redissolved in a still smaller volume (ca. 50 μl) of solvent. Other workers have suggested a two-stage elution from the XAD-2 column as part of a scheme to separate acidic and basic drugs before chromatography, thereby reducing interferences (Bastos et al., 1973).

Another device for concentrating urine constituents is a 6 cm square piece of paper containing a cation-exchange resin (Kaistha et al., 1975). The ion-exchange paper is immersed for an hour with intermittent agitation, in 20–50 ml of fresh, undiluted urine (at pH 5–6). It is then rinsed with water and extracted with alkaline buffer. The buffer is extracted in turn with chloroform-isopropanol, which is evaporated to yield the drug concentrate.

Still another technique that yields a suitable concentrate for chromatography is the extraction of neutral urine with a chloroform-isopropanol solution of the ion pair-forming surfactant sodium dioctylsulfosuccinate (Hill et al., 1982). The lipophilic anion facilitates the extraction of basic drugs, like phenylpropanolamine, in their protonated form. Neutral and weakly acidic drugs are extracted by the solvent alone. With the use of a slightly smaller volume of urine (ca. 10 ml) than that employed in the other methods, detection limits as low as 1 μg/ml were claimed.

Analytical Systems, Inc. (Laguna Hills, CA) offers a TLC-based drug-screen system called Toxi-Lab (Michaud & Jones, 1980). The system has been used for the detection of phenylpropanolamine and other common drugs, including a series of β-adrenergic blocking agents (Bonicamp & Pryor, 1985) and various drugs of abuse (Bonicamp & Pryor, 1986). Typically, a 5-ml urine sample or a 1-mg drug sample is added to an extraction tube (Toxi-tube) containing organic solvents and an aqueous buffer at pH 9. After mixing and centrifugation, the drug-containing organic solvent layer is separated and concentrated on a small disk of chromatographic media. The disk is then inserted into a circular cavity located at one end of a standardized TLC plate (Toxi-Gram) that may be purchased preimpregnated with sets of commonly occurring drugs. After development of the chromatogram, the plate is treated with a succession of reagents; the various drugs give characteristic color reactions that help reduce the chance of obtaining false positive results.

Selected solvent combinations for TLC are listed in Table 2.3 together with observed R_f values.

GAS CHROMATOGRAPHY

The first GC procedure for routine, quantitative analysis of phenylpropanolamine and other sympathomimetic amines in urine was reported in 1965 (Beckett & Wilkinson, 1965). A 1- to 5-ml sample of urine was combined with 10 μg of (2,6-dimethylphenoxy)ethylamine internal standard and a small amount of hydrochloric acid (to ensure that the amines remained in aqueous solution as their salts). The urine was extracted with ether to remove neutral and acidic constituents, and was then made alkaline with sodium hydroxide. The sample was again extracted with ether, and the amine-containing extracts were concentrated by evaporation; a 3- to 5-μl portion of this concentrate was chromatographed.

The order of elution was methylephedrine, ephedrine, and norephedrine—the order of increasing polarity for these amines which differ from each other by successive removal of a methyl group from the nitrogen. The diastereoisomers ephedrine and pseudoephedrine were not resolved; the diastereoisomers norephedrine (phenylpropanolamine) and norpseudoephedrine were only poorly resolved. These results were duplicated by other workers (Yamasaki et al., 1974).

The concentration of the amines was determined by calculating the ratio of peak heights of the amine to that of the internal standard and comparing this

TABLE 2.3. Selected Solvent Systems for TLC of Phenylpropanolamine and Other Drugs[a]

	Hexane-Ethyl Acetate (50:50) (Shah & Shah, 1976)	Chloroform-ethanol (83:17) (Shah & Shah, 1978)	Methanol-Ammonia (100:1.5) (Hadzija & Mattocks, 1983)	Methanol-Ammonia (100:1.5) (Bussey & Backer 1974)	(See Footnote[b]) (Kaistha et al., 1975)	(See Footnote[c]) (O'Brien et al., 1982)	Chloroform/methanol/ammonia (63:7:2.5) (Wu et al., 1986)	(See Footnote[d]) (Bonicamp & Pryor 1986)
Ephedrine	0.43	0.35	0.22	—	0.36	—	0.15	—
Pseudoephedrine	—	—	0.25	—	0.34	0.15	0.15	—
Phenylpropanolamine	0.76	0.29	0.43	0.56	0.44	0.32	0.32	0.35
Phenylethylamine	—	—	0.39	0.33	0.39	—	—	—
Chlorpheniramine	—	—	—	0.57	0.51	—	—	—
Caffeine	—	—	0.68	—	0.51	0.60	0.60	—
Amphetamine	—	—	—	0.47	0.47	0.37	0.37	0.70
Pyrilamine	—	0.50	—	—	0.59	—	—	—

Data are R_f values.

[a] Silica gel TLC plates from a variety of manufacturers were used.

[b] The chromatogram was partially developed with ethyl acetate–cyclohexane–methanol–ammonia (70:15:10:5). The plate was then removed from the first solvent, dried, and completely developed in ethyl acetate–cyclohexane–ammonia (50:40:0.1).

[c] Ethyl acetate–methanol–water 95:3.5:1.5 + 7.5 μl concentrated ammonia/ml solvent.

[d] Same solvent as c; Toxigrams TLC plates (Analytical Systems, Laguna Hills, CA).

to the standard solutions. (Refer to the earlier discussion of gas chromatography in this chapter.) The lowest concentration of the amines determined in this study was 5 μg/ml.

This foregoing work was later expanded into a screening protocol designed to identify about 100 drugs that might be used to enhance athletic performance (Beckett et al., 1967). In interpreting the results of such drug screens, however, one must realize that the excretion of many drugs is often dependent on the pH of the urine. For example, about 30–40% of an amphetamine dose is excreted in the urine over 48 hr at normal urinary pH. However, if the urine is made more acidic (pH about 5.0), the proportion of drug excreted rises to 60–70%, and if the urine is made alkaline (pH about 8.0), the proportion of amphetamine excreted falls to less than 10%.

In this later work, the preliminary extraction of acidified urine was deleted from the procedure, and the free amines were immediately extracted from urine rendered alkaline with sodium hydroxide. However, to extract conjugated phenolic compounds (i.e., glucuronides), the workers added an hydrolysis step—the acidified urine was heated for 1 hr at 80–100°C. There apparently was no problem of interference by endogenous urine constituents, and it was asserted that as little as 0.1 μg of free base per ml of urine could be detected by using up to 10 ml of urine.

Modern drug-screening programs based on gas chromatography use capillary rather than packed columns. Capillary columns offer superior resolution, inertness, and low column bleed (volatilization of the stationary phase). Drugs and their metabolites are identified by their retention times relative to an internal standard, and confirmed by a mass spectrometer interfaced with a second gas chromatograph operating under conditions identical to the first. With careful attention to experimental details, such as adjusting the carrier flow to achieve the preestablished retention time for the internal standard and not overloading the column (50 ng maximum for each drug), the observed retention times are remarkably constant from one analysis to another, varying no more than 0.02 minutes. To achieve consistent sensitivity, it is important to deactivate the interior surface of the column injection liners by silanation and to replace them at regular intervals. Analyses of urine, serum, or aspirated gastric fluids typically require less than 1 hour. With the flame-ionization detector (FID), a wide variety of drugs can be detected at levels of 1 μg/ml (Ehresman et al., 1985).

In addition to the FID, the nitrogen-phosphorus detector (NPD) has been used in the GC screening of drugs (Dugal et al., 1980; Watts & Simonick, 1986). This detector may exhibit a discrimination effect of about 10^4 between molecules that contain nitrogen, for example, and those that do not; that is, a nitrogen-containing compound might give a signal up to 10^4 times as strong as that of an alkane. The detector response depends on both the number of nitrogens as well as the type of nitrogen in the compound. Chromatograms of plasma or urine are simplified to the extent that peaks corresponding to normal constituents containing no nitrogen (or phosphorus) do not appear.

The resolution of 110 nitrogen-containing drugs on a dual-capillary column system was reported (Watts & Simonick, 1986). The two columns—one polar, the other nonpolar—were inserted into a single injection port so that an injected sample was divided between them; both columns were equipped with NPD detectors. Drugs were thus characterized by their retention times (relative to an internal standard) on two columns rather than one, making assignments of peaks more secure. The main concern in a drug screen, after all, is not quantitation but rather the capability of detecting and unambiguously assigning the peaks (or the spots in TLC) corresponding to a large number of drugs. This method accomplished the goal quite well. Drugs were extracted by n-chlorobutane from 2-ml samples of alkalinized blood and detected at blood levels as low as 0.1 μg/ml, with injection of approximately 2–20 ng of each drug into the dual-column system. In temperature-programmed analyses, the absolute retention times on the nonpolar column for amphetamine, methamphetamine, phenylpropanolamine, and ephedrine were 1.3, 1.7, 2.7, and 3.2 min, respectively.

Another group of investigators (Perrigo et al., 1985) used a dual-capillary column system with identical columns but different detectors—an NPD and an FID. A detector response factor was defined as the ratio of peak areas (NPD/FID) for a compound relative to that for an internal standard. For example, an NPD/FID peak area ratio of 117 for caffeine and a corresponding ratio of 10 for the internal standard would give a detector response factor of 11.7. The combination of retention times and detector response factor provided excellent discriminating power in screening 188 drugs.

By suppressing the solvent peak, the NPD permits better quantitation of constituents eluting in what would ordinarily be the tail of that peak. This feature was used to advantage in analysis of phenylpropanolamine and chlorpheniramine in urine: Phenylpropanolamine eluted after only 0.3 min and would have been obscured by the solvent peak if an FID had been used (Kinsun et al., 1978).

The electron-capture detector (ECD) is more sensitive for selected compounds than the flame-ionization and nitrogen-phosphorus detectors. Basically, the principle of operation of the ECD is that a stream of low-energy electrons (β particles) is emitted by a radioactive source such as Ni^{63} or a tritium compound and is collected by an electrode connected to an electrometer. This background current, which is of the order of 10^{-9} or 10^{-8} As, is reduced when molecules of high electron affinity emerge from the column and "capture" electrons. The reduction in current is converted to an output signal. Compounds containing electron-withdrawing nitro and halogen groups give a strong response; paraffinic hydrocarbons, on the other hand, do not capture electrons and give a weak signal, if any. Thus, the detector combines high sensitivity with high selectivity.

Sympathomimetic amines are converted to fluorine-containing derivatives to increase their detectability by the ECD, as illustrated by the following examples.

In a pharmacokinetics study of pseudoephedrine and norpseudo-ephedrine, 0.2-ml samples of serum and 0.1-ml samples of urine were analyzed (Lin et al., 1977). The samples were rendered alkaline, an internal standard was added, and the free amines were extracted into benzene. An aliquot of the benzene solution was treated with heptafluorobutyric anhydride/pyridine to form the heptafluorobutyrate derivatives of the amines. Pseudoephedrine, ephedrine, and norpseudoephedrine were well resolved, but norpseudoephedrine and norephedrine (phenylpropanolamine) were not. The levels measured were between 0.3 and 1 ng/ml.

Another group of investigators analyzed pseudoephedrine and norpseudoephedrine using essentially the same extraction procedure as described previously except that toluene was substituted for benzene. Trifluoroacetate (TFA) derivatives rather than heptafluorobutyrate derivatives were prepared, and the chromatographic instrumentation and conditions were different (Lo et al., 1981). These workers reported that concentrations as low as 50 ng/ml of either amine could be detected in 0.1 ml of plasma or urine. Interestingly, the order of elution of the TFA derivatives of the amines was the opposite of that observed with the corresponding heptafluorobutyrate derivatives, and the differences in retention times were much greater with the TFA derivatives.

Plasma concentrations of phenylpropanolamine hydrochloride as low as 5 ng/ml were routinely quantitated with a similar extraction and TFA-derivatization procedure but using a capillary GC column (Dye et al., 1984).

Very high sensitivity using electron-capture GC was also achieved by preparing the pentafluorobenzoyl derivative of ephedrine; drug levels were measured from either 1-ml samples of plasma or 0.1-ml samples of urine (Midha et al., 1979). Good resolution of ephedrine and norephedrine (phenylpropanolamine) was obtained. The pentafluorobenzoyl derivative of ephedrine exhibited about 1000 times greater electron-capturing affinity toward the Ni^{63} detector than the corresponding trifluoroacetyl derivative. Ephedrine and norephedrine (phenylpropanolamine) yielded di-acyl derivatives (O- and N-acylation) with either trifluoroacetic anhydride or heptafluorobutyric anhydride but the O-acyl groups were readily cleaved by dilute sodium hydroxide. Pentafluorobenzoyl chloride, on the other hand, yielded only the N-pentafluorobenzoyl derivative under similar reaction conditions. To demonstrate the use of the technique, a volunteer was given 24 mg ephedrine hydrochloride and plasma levels of ephedrine were determined. The peak plasma level was about 100 ng/ml and occurred 1.5 hr after the dose; 12 hr after the dose the plasma level was about 20 ng/ml.

A simplification in sample preparation is afforded by the use of still another heavily fluorinated derivatizing agent, pentafluorobenzaldehyde (Neelakantan & Kostenbauder, 1976). This compound is stored and used as its more stable bisulfite addition salt. Its reaction with phenylpropanolamine, for example, is believed to proceed according to Equation 2.7 (compare this with the reaction of alkanolamines with acetone to yield oxazolidines, Equation 2.4).

The solid adduct, two drops of 10% aqueous potassium hydroxide, and the internal standard 2,4-dinitrophenyl-N,N-diethylamine were added to 3 ml of plasma. (The internal standard has 2 nitro groups which would confer sufficient electron-capture sensitivity to this marker compound, but it is probably derivatized as well, increasing the sensitivity.) As little as 0.4 ng of phenylpropanolamine hydrochloride per ml of plasma was detected. In an application of this method to study the pharmacokinetics of phenylpropanolamine, volunteers were given 50 mg of phenylpropanolamine and blood levels were measured at time intervals after dosing. A peak plasma level of 115 ng/ml occurred 1 hr after dosing; 6 hr after dosing the level was 60 ng/ml. In a study to determine the bioavailability of different phenylpropanolamine formulations, the same analytical procedure was used (Francois et al., 1982). In this study, a peak plasma level of 242 ng/ml occurred 2 hr after a single 50 mg dose of phenylpropanolamine; 6 hr after dosing the level was 115 ng/ml.

The same derivatizing agent was used in a more detailed study of phenylpropanolamine pharmacokinetics (Lonnerholm et al., 1984). The procedure was modified as follows. The bisulfite salt was added in solution rather than as a solid, a phosphate-carbonate buffer was used rather than an alkali hydroxide to impart alkalinity, the reaction time was shorter, isooctane was the extracting solvent, and the isooctane layer was washed with sodium hydrox-

Equation 2.7

ide. The limit of detection for phenylpropanolamine in plasma was 10–15 ng/ml.

A study of amine metabolism in the brain required the determination of amphetamine, phenylpropanolamine, and their corresponding phenolic metabolites (Coutts et al., 1984). The analytical procedure developed is instructive because it illustrates how requirements for efficient extraction and the need to produce derivatives suitable for electron-capture GC may sometimes be in conflict; the procedure also makes use of an ion-pairing agent discussed in a previous section.

A sample from rat brain homogenate was extracted with a chloroform solution of bis-(2-ethylhexyl) phosphoric acid (DEHP), which extracts the desired (protonated) amines as ion pairs. After discarding the aqueous layer, the amines were brought back into an aqueous solution by extracting the chloroform solution with dilute, aqueous hydrochloric acid. The aqueous solution was rendered alkaline and amphetamine and phenylpropanolamine were extracted into ethyl acetate. The ethyl acetate solution was evaporated to dryness, and the residue was reacted with pentafluoropropionic anhydride (PFPA) to yield the N-acylated derivative of amphetamine and the N, O-diacylated derivative of phenylpropanolamine.

To increase the organic solvent extractability of the phenolic metabolites of amphetamine and phenylpropanolamine—p-hydroxyamphetamine and p-hydroxynorephedrine—an alkaline aqueous solution of the phenolics was treated with acetic anhydride (Ac_2O). The amines were acetylated on both the nitrogen and the phenolic oxygen but the β-hydroxyl group of p-hydroxynorephedrine was not acetylated. Although acetylation facilitated extraction into ethyl acetate, subsequent treatment with the pentafluoroacylating agent failed to yield a stable fluorine-containing derivative. The problem was solved by treating the diacetylated compounds with concentrated ammonium hydroxide which hydrolyzed the o-acetyl group and freed the phenolic hydroxyl group for later reaction with PFPA. The reactions are summarized for p-hydroxyamphetamine in Equation 2.8.

Equation 2.8

In the foregoing study, derivatization with PFPA was performed on the free amine, obtained after evaporation of an ethyl acetate solution to dryness. In a modification of this procedure, amines were back-extracted into aqueous acid and derivatized as their corresponding salts, thereby avoiding variable results due to the slight volatility of the free amines (Edwards et al., 1985).

HIGH-PERFORMANCE LIQUID CHROMATOGRAPHY

HPLC has not been as widely used for drug-screening method as GC and TLC. Although HPLC retention data for as many as 84 nitrogen-containing drugs, including phenylpropanolamine and a dozen sympathomimetic amines, have been collected on a single column (Law et al., 1984), the power to distinguish among them is limited by the large number of compounds eluting within a narrow range of retention times. Furthermore, the liquid chromatograph cannot yet be linked routinely with a mass spectrometer or an infrared spectrophotometer, as can a gas chromatograph, to confirm the identity of the compounds.

An alternative to mass spectrometry or infrared spectrophotometry to confirm the identity of the compounds is to measure an identification parameter that is largely independent of retention time. In gas chromatography-based drug screens, for example, parallel detectors—such as the FID and the NPD—can be used to obtain a detector response ratio for individual drugs. Similarly, in the HPLC analysis of 462 basic (i.e., nitrogen-containing) drugs, an electrochemical detector was used in series with the traditional UV detector. The stationary phase in this study was bare, unbonded silica and the mobile phase was methanolic ammonium perchlorate, which is both UV-transparent and resistant to oxidation. The pH of the mobile phase was 6.7—low enough to protonate a wide range of basic drugs (only positively charged species were retained on the column in the system used) but high enough to provide a sufficient equilibrium concentration of free amines, which are more readily oxidized than the corresponding protonated species.

Using relative retention times and eight different ranges of detector response ratios, good discrimination among the drugs was achieved. However, the dependence of the electrochemical response on the composition and the age of the electrode is one problem that may delay the widespread adoption of this method for drug screening.

A quantitative HPLC procedure is based on detection of a fluorescent derivative prepared from phenylpropanolamine and o-phthalaldehyde in the presence of 2-mercaptoethanol. Accurate and precise determinations of as little as 5 ng of phenylpropanolamine per ml of plasma were possible using 0.5 ml of plasma (Mason & Mason, 1983; Mason, 1985). The plasma sample was rendered alkaline and extracted with a mixture of butanol and butyl chloride containing a phenylethanolamine internal standard. The amines were back extracted into aqueous acetic acid and derivatized in that solvent.

The retention times of phenylethanolamine and phenylpropanolamine were typically about 5.6 and 6.4 min, respectively, on an octadecylsilyl (C_{18}) column with an acetonitrile-0.1 M sodium acetate buffer, mobile phase. A variety of drugs (e.g., chlorpheniramine) that often are included in phenylpropanolamine-containing products gave no interfering peaks, whereas acidic drugs such as aspirin and acetaminophen were not extracted from the alkalinized plasma sample.

A post-column, in-line derivatization method was reported for the analysis of phenylpropanolamine in urine using the same o-phthalaldehyde 2-mercaptoethanol chemistry as the precolumn derivatization method for plasma discussed previously. No sample preparation was required other than the addition of an amphetamine internal standard and brief mixing followed by centrifugation; the lower limit of detection claimed for phenylpropanolamine was 100 ng/ml of urine. There are no interferences from secondary and tertiary amines such as epinephrine, salbutamol, terbutaline, phenylephrine, metanephrine, and ephedrine since they are not derivatized and do not have sufficient inherent fluorescence to be detected. Primary amines such as phenylethylamine, norepinephrine, dopamine, and tyramine are detected but are resolved (Dye et al., 1984). In an application of the method, it was found that healthy subjects given a single 25 mg oral dose of phenylpropanolamine excreted 80% of the unchanged drug in the urine within 24 hr.

Another HPLC analysis of phenylpropanolamine—in both urine and plasma—was reported in which post-column derivatization with o-phthalaldehyde was used (Shi et al., 1985). A 0.5-ml sample of plasma was extracted under alkaline conditions with methylene chloride containing an α-methylbenzylamine internal standard; the phenylpropanolamine was then converted back to the hydrochloride salt before concentration and injection onto the column. Urine samples (0.2 ml) were injected directly, after a 10-fold dilution with the mobile phase. The detection limits were 2 ng/ml in plasma and 500 ng/ml in urine.

An alternative HPLC method was proposed that required no derivatization, although its detection limit of 25 ng of phenylpropanolamine per milliliter of plasma was slightly higher than that of the preceding method (Dowse et al., 1983). Sample preparation was basically the same as the foregoing: Alkalinization of a 1-ml sample of plasma, extraction with chloroform, and back extraction of the organic phase with dilute acetic acid. Ephedrine hydrochloride was used as the internal standard, and detection was by UV absorption at 220 nm. Phenylpropanolamine was quantitated in 1-ml urine samples as well, with identical sample preparation. Chromatography was carried out on an octadecylsilane column (Bondapak C_{18}), with an acetonitrile-water mobile phase containing the ion-pairing agent sodium l-heptanesulfonate. As one might have anticipated, the slightly more hydrophobic ephedrine had a slightly longer retention time than did phenylpropanolamine (norephedrine): 5.7 versus 4.8 min.

RADIOCHEMICAL METHOD

A radiochemical method for phenylpropanolamine analysis was recently reported that is based on the enzyme-catalyzed transfer of a tritiated methyl group from S-adenosylmethionine to phenylpropanolamine (norephedrine) to yield labeled ephedrine (Reid et al., 1985). The labeled ephedrine is separated from unreacted reagent and labeled side products by extraction and thin-layer chromatography; the radioactivity is measured and compared with that of standards. The method detects 0.3 to 50 ng/ml of phenylpropanolamine in 1 ml of plasma and 4–1500 ng/ml in 0.1 ml of plasma.

DRUG-SCREENING PROCEDURES

The TLC, GC, and HPLC methods discussed previously are research laboratory techniques capable of separating and discriminating among a wide variety of drugs. In selecting one or more of these methods for a drug-screening program, the following factors need to be considered: 1) sensitivity, 2) selectivity, 3) specificity, 4) analysis time, 5) level of technical skill required, 6) ease of sample tracking and documentation, and 7) cost of operation and maintenance.

Gas chromatography is generally the most sensitive method although nature of the anylate is also important as strategies are available for increasing the detectability of a given compound. As discussed before, HPLC with UV-detection is not a very sensitive method for phenylpropanolamine detection due to the weak UV absorbance of the drug; the preparation of a fluorescent derivative, however, and the use of a fluorescence detector greatly enhance detectability. Of course, the preparation of derivatives would require an increase in the level of technical skill and increase the time required and the cost of the analysis.

The selectivity of a method refers to how well it distinguishes among the sample components. Again, this characteristic depends not only on the technique but also on the sample components. Although one has tremendous flexibility in choosing an HPLC mobile phase for optimum selectivity, the nitrogen-specific detector with GC and the possibility of using selective visualization reagents with TLC may provide a level of selectivity that HPLC cannot; the use of specific detectors and reagents is dictated by the compounds of interest.

The specificity of a method is its capacity to identify a compound unambiguously. TLC, GC, and HPLC are all separation methods that generate spots or peaks representing different sample components, but a match of R_f-value or retention time between an unknown and an authentic sample is not considered compelling proof of identity; the more detailed structural information contained in an infrared or mass spectrum is required for proof of identity. Since the GC is most easily linked to either a mass spectrometer or an infrared spectrophotometer, it is clearly superior to other methods in this regard.

TLC requires less training of personnel and certainly less maintenance than do HPLC and GC. However, TLC can be more labor-intensive than either GC or HPLC; GC and HPLC auto-samplers are well-developed and can work unattended around the clock. The GC-mass spectrometer combination requires the highest level of training for operation, maintenance, and for the interpretation of spectra, although the demands of spectral interpretation have eased somewhat in recent years due to the availability of computer-based libraries of spectra, computer-assisted searches, and spectral matching.

Mislabeling and sample mix-up are common causes of errors in drug-screening laboratories. Because GC and HPLC can be linked to computer-based data stations, there is at least the potential for better recordkeeping than with TLC. Documentation is simpler with GC and HPLC, which yield chromatograms that can be stored in a computer memory as well as in hard copy. TLC plates can be scanned densitometrically to give chromatograms looking much like their GC and HPLC counterparts; however, the spots may undergo a series of color changes when exposed to a series of reagents, and this poses a problem for recordkeeping. (The assignment of color also tends to be somewhat subjective when based on the human eye.)

TLC clearly has the lowest initial cost of the three major separation methods; the cost of the average liquid chromatograph is slightly more than that of an average gas chromatograph. Operating costs for TLC include the cost of TLC plates and relatively small amounts of solvents; HPLC costs include columns and solvents; GC costs include carrier and flame gases and columns. The labor required for sample preparation is the major operating cost for all three methods although laboratory robots may eventually reduce these costs dramatically.

The three methods discussed previously have a major drawback: They are research laboratory techniques not readily adapted to on-site drug screening by untrained personnel. Immunoassay methods may fulfill this need.

An immunoassay is based on the fundamental reaction between an antibody and an antigen to form an antigen-antibody complex; in drug-screening applications, the antigen is the drug or family of drugs of interest. A known quantity of labeled antigen is mixed with the sample and a limited quantity of antibody. The labeled antigen thus competes with unlabeled antigen present in the sample for the limited antibody-binding sites. The greater the amount of unlabeled antigen in the sample, the less labeled antigen will be bound to the antibody at equilibrium. The quantity of unbound, labeled antigen is determined and the amount of unlabeled antigen in the original sample is deduced by reference to an appropriate standard or standard curve.

In radioimmunoassays the antigen is labeled with a radioactive isotope and the amount of either the bound or unbound radiolabeled antigen is measured.

In the more recently developed enzyme immunoassays, which avoid the use of radiochemicals, the labeled antigen is conjugated (chemically bonded) to an enzyme. The enzyme catalytic activity depends on whether the enzyme-antigen conjugate is bound or unbound to the antibody; such activity can be gauged by introducing a substrate that yields easily detected reaction products such as those detected colorimetrically. As with radioimmunoassay, determination of the proportion of bound and unbound labeled species permits the determination of unlabeled antigen—in the present discussion, the drug of interest.

The major producers of drug-screening kits based on immunoassay are Syva Co. (subsidiary of Syntex in Palo Alto, CA), which manufactures kits under its EMIT trademark (EMIT = enzyme-multipled immunoassay technique) and Hoffman-LaRoche (Nutley, NJ), which produces the Abuscreen series based on radioimmunoassay. Among other companies entering the field are Medical Diagnostics, a subsidiary of Keystone Medical Corp. (Columbia, MD), which has introduced its KDI Quik Test kit that takes only minutes to screen for cocaine, morphine, PCP, amphetamines, methadone, and codeine, and costs less than $10; Diagnostics Products Corp of Los Angeles is developing a drug-abuse test that can be used with saliva rather than urine or plasma.

False-positive test results are a recurring problem with drug-screen kits (Morgan, 1984), and most manufacturers recommend confirmation by other methods. For example, a Vicks inhaler contains a component that may give a positive result for amphetamines, and ibuprofen can give a positive test result for marijuana. Improvements in the specificity of the tests will likely decrease the number of false positive results. Syva Company, for example, now offers a kit that can distinguish between amphetamine and phenylpropanolamine on the basis of the latter drug's reaction with periodate to yield benzaldehyde.

REFERENCES

Achari, R. G., & Jacob, J. T. (1980). A study of the retention behavior of some basic drug substances by ion-pair HPLC. *J Liq Chromatogr, 3*, 81-92.

Achari, R. G., & Stillman, R. (1986). An HPLC assay of OTC multisymptom cough-cold preparations. *LC-GC, 4*, 454-456.

Arch, J. R., Ainsworth, A. T., & Cawthorne, M. A. (1982). Thermogenic and anorectic effects of ephedrine and congeners in mice and rats. *Life Sci, 30*, 1817-1826.

Avdovich, H. W., Jin, S. H., & Wilson, W. L. (1985). NMR method for identification of look-alike drugs. *Can Soc Forens Sci J, 18*, 24-31.

Barry, R. H., Weiss, M., Johnson, J. B., & DeRitter, E. (1982). Stability of phenylpropanolamine hydrochloride in liquid formulations containing sugars. *J Pharm Sci, 71*, 116-118.

Bastos, M. L., Jukofsky, D., & Mule, S. J. (1973). Routine identification of drugs of abuse in human urine. 3. Differential elution of the XAD-2 resin. *J Chromatogr, 81*, 93-98.

Basyoni, F., & Ibrahim, M. (1984). Cerimetric determination of ephedrine. *Anal Lett, 17*, 1793-1801.

Beckett, A. H., Tucker, G. T., & Moffat, A. C. (1967). Routine detection and identification in urine of stimulants and other drugs, some of which may be used to modify performance in sport. *J Pharm Pharmacol, 19*, 273-294.

Beckett, A. H., & Wilkinson, G. R. (1965). Identification and determination of ephedrine and its congeners in urine by gas chromatography. *J Pharm Pharmacol, 17*, 104S-106S.

Bonicamp, J. M., & Pryor, L. (1986). Differentiating cocaine from other 'caine drugs and common adulterants by thin-layer chromatography. *J Tenn Acad Sci, 61*, 9-11.

Bonicamp, J. M., & Pryor, L. (1985). Detection of some beta adrenergic blocking drugs and their metabolites in urine by thin layer chromatography. *J Anal Toxicol, 9*, 180-182.

Brown, N. H., & Portmann, G. A. (1971). Analysis of phenylephrine and phenylpropanolamine hydrochlorides in combination. *J Pharm Sci, 60*, 1229-1231.

Burke, D., Venturella, V. S., & Senkowski, B. Z. (1974). Selective determination of phenylpropanolamine hydrochloride in pharmaceutical dosage forms by reaction with ninhydrin. *J Pharm Sci, 63*, 269-273.

Bussey, R. J., & Backer, R. C. (1974). Thin-layer chromatographic differentiation of amphetamine from other primary-amine drugs in urine. *Clin Chem, 20*, 302-304.

Chafetz, L. (1971). Specificity of spectrophotometric determination of ephedrine and other phenalkanolamine drugs as benzaldehydes after periodate oxidation. *J Pharm Sci, 60*, 291-294.

Chien, Y. W. (1985). The use of biocompatible polymers in rate-controlled drug delivery systems. *Pharm Technol, 9*, 50-66.

Cieri, U. R. (1986). Use of serial fluorescence and UV absorption detectors to determine phenylpropanolamine hydrochloride or ephedrine hydrochloride and one additional component by HPLC. *LC-GC, 4*, 908, 910.

Clark, C. C. (1973). Collaborative study of an on-column periodate reaction method for the analysis of phenylpropanolamine hydrochloride in elixirs. *J Assoc Off Anal Chem, 56*, 100-104.

Costanzo, S. J. (1984). Selection of mixed ion-pair modifiers for high-performance liquid chromatographic mobile phases. *J Chromatogr, 314*, 402-407.

Coutts, R. T., Prelusky, D. B., & Baker, G. B. (1984). Determination of amphetamine, norephedrine, and their phenolic metabolites in rat brain by gas chromatography. *J Pharm Sci,* 73, 808-812.

Cox, G. B., Loscombs, C. R., & Sugden, K. (1977). Some applications of bonded-phase high-performance liquid chromatography to the analysis of pharmaceutical formulations. *Anal Chim Acta, 92,* 345-352.

Crisologo, N., Dye, D., & Bayne, W. F. (1984). Electron-capture capillary gas chromatographic determination of phenylpropanolamine in human plasma following derivatization with tri-fluoroacetic anhydride. *J Pharm Sci, 73,* 1313-1315.

Das Gupta, V., & Heble, A. R. (1984). Quantitation of acetaminophen, chlorpheniramine maleate, dextromethorphan hydrobromide, and phenylpropanolamine hydrochloride in combination using high-performance liquid chromatography. *J Pharm Sci, 73,* 1553-1556.

de Fabrizio, F. (1980). Simultaneous GLC analysis of salicylamide, phenylpropanolamine hydrochloride, caffeine, chlorpheniramine maleate, phenylephrine hydrochloride, and pyrilamine maleate in capsule preparations. *J Pharm Sci, 69,* 854-855.

de Silva, J. A. F., & Strojny, N. (1975). Spectrofluorometric determination of pharmaceuticals containing aromatic or aliphatic primary amino groups as their fluorescamine (Fluram) derivatives. *Anal Chem, 47,* 714-718.

Dowse, R., Haigh, J. M., & Kanfer, I. (1983). Determination of phenylpropanolamine in serum and urine by high performance liquid chromatography. *J Pharm Sci, 72,* 1018-1020.

Dugal, R., Masse, R., Sanchez, G., & Bertrand, M. J. (1980). An integrated methodological approach to the computer-assisted gas chromatographic screening of basic drugs in biological fluids using nitrogen selective detection. *J Anal Toxicol, 4,* 1-12.

Dunn J. M., & Haas, R. T. (Verex Laboratories, Inc.). Constant release rate solid oral dosage formulation of pharmaceutical compounds having a high degree of water solubility. European patent no. EP 108218 A2, 16 May 1984, 83108974.3, 12 September 1983; 25 pp.

Dye, D., East, T., & Bayne, W. F. (1984). High-performance liquid chromatographic method for post-column, in-line derivatization with o-phthalaldehyde and fluorometric detection of phenylpropanolamine in human urine. *J Chromatogr, 284,* 457-461.

Edwards, D. J., Mallinger, A. G., Knopf, S., & Himmelhoch, J. M. (1985). Determination of tranylcypromine in plasma using gas chromatography—chemical-ionization mass spectrometry. *J Chromatogr, 344,* 356-361.

Ehresman, D. J., Price, S. M., & Lakatua, D. J. (1985). Screening biological samples for underivatized drugs using a splitless injection technique on fused silica capillary column gas chromatography. *J Anal Toxicol, 9,* 55-62.

El Egakey, M. A., & Speiser, P. P. (1982). In vitro and in vivo release studies of slow-release phenylpropanolamine-poly methylcyanoacrylate entrapment products. *Acta Pharm Technol, 28,* 169-175.

Engel, J. (1982). Chemistry of pharmacodynamically active phenylpropanolamines. *Chem Ztg, 106,* 169-183.

Engel, J., Bork A., Nonnenmacher, G., & Schmidt, I. (1979). Determination of the relative configuration of phenylpropanolamines by carbon-13 NMR spectroscopy. *Chem Ztg, 103,* 283-284.

Engel, J., Klinger, K. H., Nonnenmacher, G., & Schmidt, I. (1980). Determination of the relative configuration of substituted phenylpropanolamine drugs. *Chem Ztg, 104,* 325-326.

Enscore, D. J., & Gale, R. M. (Alza Corp). Matrix composition for transdermal therapeutic system. European patent no. BE 899444 A1, 16 August 1984, US 491490, 4 May 1983; 27 pp.

Fairchild, M. D., & Alles, G. A. (1967). The central locomotor stimulatory activity and acute toxicity of the ephedrine and norephedrine isomers in mice. *J Pharmacol Exp Ther, 158*, 135-139.

Francois, D., Denmat, A., Waugh, A., & Woodage, T. (1982). The in vitro and in vivo availability of phenylpropanolamine from oil/paste formulations in hard gelatin capsules. *Pharm Ind, 44*, 86-89.

Gal, J. (1984). Resolution of the enantiomers of ephedrine, norephedrine and pseudo ephedrine by high-performance liquid chromatography. *J Chromatogr, 307*, 220-223.

Gelber, L. R., Karger, B. L., Neumeyer, J. L., & Feibush, B. (1984). Ligand exchange chromatography of amino alcohols. Use of schiff bases in enantiomer resolution. *J Am Chem Soc, 106*, 7729-7734.

Gobbeler, K. H. (1971). Simultaneous quantitative gas chromatographic determination of dextromethorphan, chlorpheniramine, norephedrine and salicylamide from tablets. *Deutsch Apoth Ztg, 111*, 1291-1292.

Goodhart, F. W., Harris, M. R., Murthy, K. S., & Nesbitt, R. U. (1984). An evaluation of aqueous film-forming dispersions for controlled release. *Pharm Technol, 8*, 64-71.

Gould, P. L. (1984). Optimisation methods for the development of dosage forms. *Int J Pharm Tech Prod Manuf, 5*, 19-24.

Greco, G. T. (1984). Ion-pair high-performance liquid chromatographic determination of chlorpheniramine maleate in cough-cold mixtures. *Drug Dev Ind Pharm, 10*, 19-30.

Hadzija, B. W., & Mattocks, A. M. (1983). Simple techniques to detect and identify pehntermine adulteration. *Forensic Sci Internatl, 23*, 143-147.

Halstead, G. W. (1982). Determination of amine ingredients in cough-cold liquids by reversedphase ion-pair high-performance liquid chromatography. *J Pharm Sci, 71*, 1108-1112.

Heidemann, D. R. (1981). High-pressure liquid chromatographic determination of methscopolamine nitrate, phenylpropanolamine hydrochloride, pyrilamine maleate, and pheniramine maleate in tablets. *J Pharm Sci, 70*, 820-822.

Heimlich, K. R., MacDonnel, D. R., Flanagan, T. L., & O'Brien, P. D. (1961). Evaluation of a sustained release form of phenylpropanolamine hydrochloride by urinary excretion studies. *J Pharm Sci, 50*, 232-237.

Hill, D. W., Kelley, T. R., Matiuck, S. W., Langner, K. J., & Phillips, D. E. (1982). Single extraction for the recovery of basic, neutral and weakly acidic drugs from greyhound dog urine. *Anal Lett, 15*, 193-204.

Hishta, C., & Lauback, R. G. (1969). Gas chromatographic analysis of amine mixtures in drug formulations. *J Pharm Sci, 58*, 745-746.

Hoover, F. W., & Hass, H. B. (1947). Synthesis of 2-amino-1-phenyl-1-propanol and its methylated derivatives. *J Org Chem, 12*, 506-509.

Hugosson, S., Nyberg, L., & Nilsson, L. (1972). Selective methods for the determination of brompheniramine and phenylpropanolamine in a sustained release tablet. *Acta Pharm Suec, 9*, 249-258.

Ison, R. R., Partington, P., & Roberts, G. C. K. (1973). The conformation of catecholamines and related compounds in solution. *Molec Pharmacol, 9*, 756-765.

Jane, I., & McKinnon, A. (1985). High-performance liquid chromatographic analysis of basic drugs on silica columns using non-aqueous ionic eluents. II. Application of UV, fluorescence and electrochemical oxidation detection. *J Chromatogr, 323*, 191-225.

Kaistha, K. K., Tadrus, R., & Janda, R. (1975). Simultaneous detection of a wide variety of commonly abused drugs in a urine screening program using thin-layer identification techniques. *J Chromatogr, 107,* 359-379.

Kalm, M. J. (1960). 3-imidomethyloxazolidines. *J Org Chem, 25,* 1929-1937.

Kanfer, I., Haigh, J. M., & Dowse, R. (1983). Phenylpropanolamine hydrochloride. *Anal Profiles Drug Subst, 12,* 357-383.

Kaser-Liard, B. (1985). Herstellung von gelatine-mikrokapseln unter anwendung der emulsionsinduktions-technik. *Pharm Acta Helv, 60,* 326-333.

King, T. H., Mann, C. K., & Vickers, T.J. (1985). Determination of phenylpropanolamine hydrochloride and acetaminophen in pharmaceutical preparations by raman spectroscopy. *J Pharm Sci, 74,* 443-447.

Kinsun, H., Moulin, M. A., & Savini, E. C. (1978). Simultaneous GLC determination of phenylpropanolamine and chlorpheniramine in urine using a nitrogen selective detector. *J Pharm Sci, 67,* 118-119.

Kisbye, J. (1959). Studies on sympathomimetic amines. III. The racemisation of some benzene derivatives. *Dansk Tidsskr Farm, 33,* 137-151.

Koziol, T. R., Jacob, J. T., & Achari, R. G. (1979). Ion pair liquid chromatographic assay of decongestants and antihistamines. *J Pharm Sci, 68,* 1135-1138.

Lange, W. E., Theodore, J. M., & Pruyn, F. J. (1968). In vivo determination of certain aralkylamines. *J Pharm Sci, 57,* 124-127.

Law, B., Gill, R., & Moffat, A. C. (1984). High-performance liquid chromatography retention data for 84 basic drugs of forensic interest on a silica column using aqueous methanol eluent. *J Chromatogr, 301,* 165-172.

Lehmann, K. (1984). Formulation of controlled release tablets with acrylic resins. *Acta Pharm Fenn, 93,* 55-74.

Lehmann, K. O. R., Bossler, H. M., & Dreher, D. K. (1978). Controlled drug release from small particles encapsulated with acrylic resins. *Midl Macromol Monogr, 5,* 111-119.

Levine, J., & Doyle, T. D. (1967). Determination of phenylephrine in combinations with other drugs. *J Pharm Sci, 56,* 619-622.

Lin, E. T., Brater, D. C., & Benet, L. Z. (1977). Gas-liquid chromatographic determination of pseudoephedrine and norpseudoephedrine in human plasma and urine. *J Chromatogr, 140,* 275-279.

Lindahl, A. R., & Ekman, B. M. (ABLEO). Controlled-release pharmaceutical for oral administration. European patent no. EP 173928, 12 March 1986, 85110631, 23 August 1985; 14 pp.

Liu, J-C, Farber, M., & Chien, Y. W. (1984). Comparative release of phenylpropanolamine HCl from long-acting appetite suppressant products: Acutrim vs Dexatrim. *Drug Dev Ind Pharm, 10,* 1639-1661.

Lo, L. Y., Land, G., & Bye, A. (1981). Sensitive assay for pseudoephedrine and its metabolite, norpseudoephedrine in plasma and urine using gas-liquid chromatography with electron-capture detection. *J Chromatogr, 222,* 297-302.

Long, W. J., Norin, R. C., & Su, S. Y. (1985). Pharmaceutical determination by derivatization-room-temperature phosphorescence. *Anal Chem, 57,* 2873-2877.

Lonnerholm, G., Grahnen, A., & Lindstrom, B. (1984). Steady-state kinetics of sustained-release phenylpropanolamine. *Internatl J Clin Pharmacol Ther Toxicol, 22,* 39-41.

Lovett, L. J., Nygard, G. A., Erdmann, G. R., & Wahba Khalil, S. K. (1986). HPLC analysis of multi-ingredient cold remedies. *LC-GC, 4,* 1125-1128.

Lurie, I. S. (1980). Forensic drug analysis by HPLC. *Am Lab, 12,* 35-42.

Madsen, R. E., & Magin, D. F. (1976). Simultaneous quantitative GLC determination of chlorpheniramine maleate and phenylpropanolamine hydrochloride in a cold tablet preparation. *J Pharm Sci, 65*, 924-925.

Mario, E., & Meehan, L. G. (1970). Simultaneous determination of nonderivatized phenylpropanolamine, glyceryl guaiacolate, chlorpheniramine, and dextromethorphan by gas chromatography. *J Pharm Sci, 59*, 538-540.

Mason, W. D. (1985). Analysis of phenylpropanolamine in plasma by high-pressure liquid chromatography. *Methodol Anal Toxicol, 3*, 151-154.

Mason, W. D., & Mason, J. S. (1983). Improved high pressure liquid chromatographic method for phenylpropanolamine in human plasma. *Anal Lett, 16*, 693-699.

Metevia, V. L., & Woodard, J. T. (Dow Corning Corp). Transdermal drug delivery devices with amine-resistant silicone adhesives. European patent no. EP 180377 A2, 7 May 1986, 85307453, 16 October 1985; 76 pp.

Michaud, J. D., & Jones, D. W. (1980). Thin-layer chromatography for broad-spectrum drug detection. *Amer Lab, 12*, 104-106.

Midha, K. K., Cooper, J. K., & McGilveray, I. J. (1979). Simple and specific electron capture GLC assay for plasma and urine ephedrine concentrations following single doses. *J Pharm Sci, 68*, 557-560.

Morgan, J. P. (1984). Problems of mass urine screening for misused drugs. *J Psychoact Drug, 16*, 305-317.

Muhammad, N., & Bodnar, J. A. (1980). Quantitative determination of guaifenesin, phenylpropanolamine hydrochloride, sodium benzoate and codeine phosphate in cough syrups by high-pressure liquid chromatography. *J Liquid Chromtog, 3*, 113-122.

Muntwyler, R., & Hauser, H. (Ciba-Geigy). Pharmaceutical compositions containing unilamellar liposomes. European patent no. EP 152379 A2, 21 August 1985, 85/810050, 11 February 1985; 65 pp.

Murov, S. L., & Pickering, M. (1973). The odor of optical isomers. *J Chem Ed, 50*, 74-75.

Nagai, W. N., & Kanao, S. (1929). ber die synthese isomeren ephedrine und ihrer homologen. *Justus Liebig's Ann Chem, 470*, 157-182.

Neelakantan, L., & Kostenbauder, H. B. (1976). Electron-capture GLC determination of phenylpropanolamine as a pentafluorophenyloxazolidine derivative. *J Pharm Sci, 65*, 740-742.

Noggle, F. T. (1980). Enhanced detectability and chromatography of some amines by high-pressure liquid chromatography. *J Assoc Anal Chem, 63*, 702-706.

Noggle, F. T., & Clark, C. R. (1984). Liquid chromatographic determination of primary and secondary amines as 8-quinolinesulfonyl chloride derivatives. *J Assoc Off Anal Chem, 67*, 687-691.

Noggle, F. T., & Clark, C. R. (1986). Resolution of some enantiomeric amines of forensic interest by high-performance liquid chromatography. *J Forensic Sci, 31*, 732-742.

O'Brien, B. A., Bonicamp, J. M., & Jones, D. W. (1982). Differentiation of amphetamine and its major hallucinogenic derivatives using thin-layer chromatography. *J Anal Toxicol, 6*, 143-147.

Oshlack, B., & Leslie, S. T. (Euro-Celtique S. A.). Extended action controlled release compositions containing a base and its salt in a matrix. European patent no. EP 97523 A2, 4 January 1984, 83303560, 21 June 1983; 32 pp.

Perrigo, B. J., Peel, H. W., & Ballantyne, D. J. (1985). Use of dual-column fused-silica capillary gas chromatography in combination with detector response factors for analytical toxicology. *J Chromatogr, 341*, 81-88.

Raghunathan, Y., Amsel, L., Hinsvark, O., & Bryant, W. (1981). Sustained-release drug delivery system I: Coated ion-exchange resin system for phenylpropanolamine and other drugs. *J Pharm Sci, 70*, 379-384.

Reid, A. A., Fleming, P. J., & Lake, C. R. (1985). Radioenzymatic determination of phenylpropanolamine in plasma [Abstract]. *Proceedings of the Soc Neurosci, 11*, 51.

Rhodes, C. T., Wai, K., & Banker, G. S. (1970). Molecular scale drug entrapment as a precise method of controlled drug release. 3. In vitro and in vivo studies of drug release. *J Pharm Sci, 59*, 1581-1584.

Richardson, H., & Bidlingmeyer, B. A. (1984). Bare silica as a reverse-phase stationary phase: Liquid chromatographic separation of antihistamines with buffered aqueous organic mobile phases. *J Pharm Sci, 73*, 1480-1482.

Robinson, C. P. (1986). Biphasic control drug delivery system. *Drugs of Today, 22*, 13-16.

Sanders, H. J. (1985). Improved drug delivery. *Chem Eng News, 63*, 30-48.

Santoro, R. S., Progner, P. P., Ambush, E. A., & Guttman, D. E. (1973). Selective determination of belladonna alkaloids by GLC. *J Pharm Sci, 62*, 1346-1349.

Santoro, R., Warren, R., & Roberts, G. (1976). Spontaneous formation of 4-methyl-5-phenyloxazolidine-2-thione from phenylpropanolamine. *J Chromatogr, 117*, 375-382.

Schieffer, G. W., & Hughes, D. E. (1983). Simultaneous stability-indicating determination of phenylephrine hydrochloride, phenylpropanolamine hydrochloride and guaifenesin in dosage forms by reversed-phase paired-ion high-performance liquid chromatography. *J Pharm Sci, 72*, 55-59.

Schieffer, G. W., Smith, W. O., Lubey, G. S., & Newby, D. G. (1984). Determination of the structure of a synthetic impurity in guaifenesin: Modification of a high-performance liquid chromatographic method for phenylephrine hydrochloride, phenylpropanolamine hydrochloride, guaifenesin, and sodium benzoate in dosage forms. *J Pharm Sci, 73*, 1856-1858.

Schorno, X., Brenneisen, R., & Steinegger, E. (1982). Qualitative and quantitative study of CNS active principles and distribution in *Catha edulis* (Celastraceae). *Pharm Acta Helv, 57*, 168-176.

Seugling, E. W. (1980). The contribution of tableting aids to pharmaceutical development. *Pharm Tech, 4*, 27-35.

Severin, G. (1986). A novel column/buffer combination for chromatographic analysis of basic drugs in simulated gastrointestinal fluids. *J Pharm Sci, 75*, 211-214.

Shah, J. J., & Shah, R. J. (1976). Thin layer chromatographic identification of some sympathomimetic amines. *J Assoc Off Anal Chem, 59*, 1416-1418.

Shah, J. J., & Shah, R. J. (1978). Identification of some sympathomimetic amines by thin layer chromatography (TLC). *J Tenn Acad Sci, 53*, 95-97.

Shankle, L. L. (1978). Determination of phenylpropanolamine salts in dosage forms through fluorescent derivative formation. *J Pharm Sci, 67*, 1635-1636.

Shenoy, B. B., & Das Gupta, V. (1973). Quantitative determinations of phenylephrine and phenylpropanolamine hydrochlorides in combination. *J Pharm Sci, 62*, 802-804.

Shi, R. J. Y., Gee, W. L., Williams, R. L., Benet, L. Z., & Lin, E. T. (1985). Ion-pair liquid chromatographic analysis of phenylpropanolamine in plasma and urine by post-column derivatization with o-phthalaldehyde. *J Liq Chromatogr, 8*, 1489-1500.

Smith, D. J. (1974). Collaborative study of an ion exchange method for the chromatographic separation of mixtures containing expectorants, sympathomimetic amines, antihistamines, or phenothiazine in pharmaceuticals. *J Assoc Off Anal Chem, 57*, 741-746.

Sprieck, T. L. (1974). High-pressure liquid chromatographic determination of adrenergic and antihistaminic compounds in pharmaceutical preparations. *J Pharm Sci, 63*, 591-593.

Stern, P. W. (1983). Aqueous-based film coatings grow in popularity. *Drug Cosm Indus, 133*, 50, 54.

Street, K. W., & Abrenica, M. B. (1986). Spectrophotometric determination of phenylpropanolamine hydrochloride in pharmaceuticals after derivatization with NBD-Cl. *Anal Lett, 19*, 597-614.

Swamy, V. C., Tye, A., Lapidus, J. B., & Patil, P. N. (1969). Steric aspects of adrenergic drugs XIII. Norepinephrine potentiating effects of isomers of sympathomimetic amine in rat vas deferens and atria. *Arch Internatl Pharmacodyn, 182*, 24-31.

Tan, H. S. I., & Salvador, G. C. (1985). Difference spectrophotometric assay of mixtures of phenylpropanolamine hydrochloride with guaifenesin or dextromethorphan hydrobromide in solid cough formulations. *Anal Chim Acta, 176*, 71-76.

Tan, H. S. I., & Salvador, G. C. (1983). Assay of mixtures of phenylpropanolamine hydrochloride and caffeine in appetite suppressant formulations by high-performance liquid chromatography. *J Chromatogr, 261*, 111-116.

Taylor, P., Braddock, P. D., & Ross, S. (1984). Determination of phenylpropanolamine hydrochloride as benzaldehyde in pharmaceutical preparations using normal phase high performance liquid chromatography. *Analyst, 109*, 619-621.

Theeuwes, F. (1984). Oral dosage form design: status and goals of oral osmotic systems technology. *Pharm Int, 5*, 293-296.

Thompson, D. W. (1986). Evaluation of capillary gas chromatography for multicomponent drug analysis. *J Assoc Anal Chem, 69*, 811-813.

Tomida, Y., Yokohama, S., Maki, M., Toguchi, H., & Shimamoto, T. (1977). In vitro dissolution test correlating quantitatively with sustained released phenylpropanolamine absorption in man. *J Takeda Res Lab, 36*, 83-89.

Trivedi, D. (1985). Capillary gas chromatographic separation of various stimulants. *J Assoc Anal Chem, 68*, 809-810.

Vanderbilt, B. M., & Hass, H. B. (1940). Aldehyde-nitroparaffin condensation. *Ind Eng Chem, 32*, 34-38.

Vree, T. B., Muskens, A. Th. J. M., & Van Rossum, J. M. (1969). Some physico-chemical properties of amphetamine and related drugs. *J Pharm Pharmacol, 21*, 774-775.

Watts, V. W., & Simonick, T. F. (1986). Screening of basic drugs in biological samples using dual column capillary chromatography and nitrogen-phosphorus detectors. *J Anal Toxicol, 10*, 198-204.

Weintraub, M., Ginsberg, G., Stein, E. C., Sundaresan, P. R., Schuster, B., O'Connor, P., & Byrne, L. M. (1986). Phenylpropanolamine OROS (Acutrim) vs. placebo in combination with caloric restriction and physician-managed behavior modification. *Clin Pharm Ther, 39*, 501-509.

Weber, O. W. A., & Heveran, J. E. (1973). Automated, simultaneous determination of dextromethorphan hydrobromide, glyceryl guaiacolate, and phenylpropanolamine hydrochloride in cough syrups. *J Pharm Sci, 62*, 1174-1177.

Westlake, W. J. (1975). Demonstration of claimed controlled-release properties of a drug formulation. *J Pharm Sci, 64*, 1075-1077.

Wu, A., Bretl, D. D., Pearson, M. L., Wolffe, G. S., & Miller, M. L. (1986). Elimination of labetalol-induced false positives in drug analyses. *Clin Chem, 32*, 407.

Yamakawa, I., Shimomura, M., Hattori, T., Watanabe, S., Tsutsumi, J., Shinoda, A., & Miyake, Y. (1984). An example of pharmaceutical studies on sustained release dosage design. *J Pharm Dyn, 7*, s-38.

Yamasaki, K, Fujita, K., Sakamoto, M., Okada, K., & Yoshida, M. (1974). Separation and quantitative analysis of ephedra alkaloids by gas chromatography and its application to evaluation of some ephedra species collected around Himalaya. *Chem Pharm Bull* (Tokyo), *22*, 2898-2902.

3

BASIC PHARMACOLOGY

The basic pharmacology of phenylpropanolamine is reviewed in this chapter. Most of this chapter is based on information from preclinical studies published in the open literature. In some instances where there is no published information from preclinical studies to illustrate an important aspect of the pharmacology of phenylpropanolamine, information from clinical studies or repository sources is included in the discussion. In some instances, no information is available regarding phenylpropanolamine per se and inferences have been drawn from results with norephedrine or other sympathomimetic amines. Such inferences are clearly identified and should be interpreted with appropriate scientific reservations.

In general, phenylpropanolamine can be characterized as a mixed-acting sympathomimetic amine with predominantly α-adrenergic activity. In many of the studies, phenylpropanolamine was shown to have very low potency and low intrinsic activity at adrenergic sites of action. It has been suggested that phenylpropanolamine is a partial agonist at α_1-adrenergic receptors (Minneman et al., 1983), although this property has not been elucidated definitively.

In reviewing the pharmacological studies of phenylpropanolamine it is important to keep in mind the dose range that produces pharmacological responses. In addition, there may be species differences not only in dose ranges, but also in drug metabolism and pharmacodynamic effects. Probably the most commonly investigated animal species is the rat. The effective dose range for most effects of phenylpropanolamine in rats is 5–40 mg/kg [intraperitoneal (IP)], with side effects and toxicity occurring at doses of 80 mg/kg or more. To put these dose ranges in perspective, the minimum lethal dose (see Table 4.1 in Chapter 4) in rats is 80 mg/kg [subcutaneous (SC); data are not available for IP dosing] and the LD_{50} is 160 mg/kg (IP). In humans, the recommended therapeutic dose range for anorexia is 25–75 mg (total dose, PO; equivalent to approximately 0.4–1.1 mg/kg for a 70-kg person) with an estimated minimum lethal dose of 50 mg/kg (PO). These dose ranges in rats and humans cannot be directly compared because they are based on different routes of administration, and toxicity varies considerably according to the route of administration (e.g., in rats the LD_{50} values for PO and IP administration are 948 and 160 mg/kg, respectively).

To evaluate relative potency and efficacy, phenylpropanolamine has been compared to several standard reference compounds. In *in vitro* studies, norepinephrine, the endogenous neurotransmitter in adrenergic neurons, is often used as the reference compound. In *in vivo* studies, norepinephrine is not necessarily a good choice for a reference standard because *in vivo* responses to exogenously administered norepinephrine are sometimes unreliable because of the short duration of action. Phenylpropanolamine often is compared to the chemically related compounds ephedrine or amphetamine. Structurally, phenylpropanolamine is equivalent to $(\pm)$-demethylephedrine or $(\pm)$-β-hydroxyamphetamine. In addition, phenylpropanolamine is sometimes compared to its metabolite, *p*-hydroxyphenylpropanolamine (α-methyloctopamine), or the structural analog metaraminol (*m*-hydroxyphenylpropanolamine). Metaraminol is of interest because of its relative selectivity for cardiovascular effects and also because it may function as a false transmitter in noradrenergic neurons. Finally, since phenylpropanolamine is a racemic mixture of the isomers of norephedrine [i.e., phenylpropanolamine is $(\pm)$-norephedrine)], phenylpropanolamine often is compared to the isomers of norephedrine: $(+)$-norephedrine, $(-)$-norephedrine, $(+)$-norpseudoephedrine, or $(-)$-norpseudoephedrine.

PHARMACOKINETICS

ABSORPTION

Phenylpropanolamine is well absorbed from the GI tract, and oral dosing is the usual route of administration in therapeutic use. No studies are available in which absorption of phenylpropanolamine by oral or parenteral administration were specifically compared. In animal toxicity studies, the lethality following administration of phenylpropanolamine by PO, SC, IP, and IV routes has been reported (see Chapter 4, section on toxicology). These results demonstrate that phenylpropanolamine is well absorbed by all these routes of administration. However, buccal absorption of phenylpropanolamine in human subjects was limited; in this instance, less than 10% of phenylpropanolamine in test solutions was absorbed (Beckett & Triggs, 1967). Buccal absorption was not affected by altering the pH of the solution. Presumably this limited buccal absorption is due to the low lipid solubility and the high pK_a value of phenylpropanolamine.

One specialized route of administration used to evaluate the absorption of phenylpropanolamine is intracerebroventricular (ICV) administration, which is accomplished by injecting a test substance directly into the cerebral ventricles, thereby bypassing the blood-brain barrier. Whereas many phenethylamines produce neurochemical changes in the CNS when administered by the ICV route (Antunes-Rodrigues & McCann, 1970; Breese et al., 1970), phenylpropanolamine produced no change in brain levels of norepinephrine or dopamine when given ICV (Breese et al., 1970). This negative result may indicate either that phenylpropanolamine was not absorbed into the brain after ICV injection or that it was absorbed but had no effect on the levels of these amines. Local application of phenylpropanolamine to the lateral hypothalamus in rats decreased food intake, but application to the medial hypothalamus had no anorectic effect (Hoebel et al., 1975), indicating a direct effect on the brain that was site specific.

DISTRIBUTION

Phenylpropanolamine is widely and rapidly distributed following IV administration in mice or rats (Thiercelin et al., 1976). Tissue distribution of ^{14}C-phenylpropanolamine was determined by autoradiographic analysis in mice given 267 μg/kg of phenylpropanolamine (IV). Uptake of phenylpropanolamine was most rapid in the lungs, adrenal glands, spleen, and heart. Brain levels of radioactivity were low during the first 2 hr following administration of ^{14}C-phenylpropanolamine. Tissue levels and kinetics of elimination from tissues were determined following administration of 535 μg/kg of phenylpropanolamine (IV) to rats. The rank order of tissue levels was lung $\geq$ adrenal > spleen > heart > brain. At 15 min to 2 hr after administration of phenylpropanolamine, all tissue levels of phenylpropanolamine were higher than plasma levels, confirming the rapid and extensive distribution of phenylpropanolamine. Elimination of phenylpropanolamine occurred at equivalent rates from all tissues except the brain. Distribution of phenylpropanolamine to the brain was delayed, with brain levels steadily increasing during the first

45 min following administration, and elimination of phenylpropanolamine from the brain was slower than elimination from any other tissue.

The delayed distribution of phenylpropanolamine to the brain in rodents is paralleled by the tissue distribution of *l*-ephedrine and its metabolite *l*-norephedrine (phenylpropanolamine is *dl*-norephedrine) in dogs (Axelrod, 1953). *l*-Ephedrine was administered IV to dogs, and tissue levels of *l*-ephedrine and *l*-norephedrine were measured. Both *l*-ephedrine and *l*-norephedrine were widely distributed, but levels of *l*-norephedrine were comparatively lower in cerebrospinal fluid and brain than in other tissues 1 hr after IV administration of *l*-ephedrine.

METABOLISM

Phenylpropanolamine is biotransformed to various metabolites by *p*-hydroxylation or oxidative deamination. Early studies demonstrated considerable species variation in metabolism of phenylethylamines (Axelrod, 1953, 1955), and more recent studies demonstrate such variations in the metabolism of phenylpropanolamine (Table 3.1). In rats the primary route of metabolism of phenylpropanolamine is hydroxylation to *p*-hydroxyphenylpropanolamine (*p*-hydroxynorephedrine; α-methyloctopamine). In contrast, in rabbits very little phenylpropanolamine is excreted unchanged or as *p*-hydroxyphenylpropanolamine, and oxidative deamination and side chain degradation to hippuric acid is the primary metabolic pathway. In both monkeys and humans, there is minimal metabolism, and most of the phenylpropanolamine is excreted unchanged.

α-Methyloctopamine (*p*-hydroxyphenylpropanolamine) is a predominant metabolite of phenylpropanolamine in the rat. Tissue levels of α-methyloctopamine were highest in heart, adrenals, and spleen, tissues that have high innervation by adrenergic nerve terminals (Thiercelin et al., 1976). Since α-methyloctopamine may function as a "false neurotransmitter" in adrenergic neurones (Baldessarini, 1971), this tissue distribution pattern suggests that such a mechanism may be important in the pharmacodynamic responses to phenylpropanolamine. However, α-methyloctopamine levels in the brain were low, even though this tissue has dense innervation by adrenergic nerve terminals.

ELIMINATION

In all four species studied, urinary excretion is the primary route of elimination, with negligible excretion via the feces (Table 3.1). Unchanged phenylpropanolamine in the urine is primarily unconjugated (Thiercelin et al.,

TABLE 3.1. Metabolism and Excretion of Phenylpropanolamine: Comparison of Rats, Rabbits, Monkeys, and Humans

| Species | Route | Sex | Dose (mg/kg) | Duration of Sample Collection (hr) | Total Urinary Excretion (% of Dose) | Urinary Metabolites (%) | | Deamination Products | | | Fecal Excretion (% of Dose) | Reference |
						Unchanged PPA	p-Hydroxy-PPA[a]	Hippuric Acid	Not Specified	Other		
Rat	PO	F	12	24	80	48.1	27.8	—	1.1	—	1.7	Sinsheimer et al. (1973)
	PO	F	12	48	77	48	28	1	—	—	—	Caldwell et al. (1977)
	IV	M	0.535	40	81.6	70–75	24	—	—	1–5	0.54	Thiercelin et al. (1976)
Rabbit	PO	F	12	24	89	8.4	2.9	—	76.0	—	2.3	Sinsheimer et al. (1973)
	PO	F	12	24	96	8	3	85	—	—	—	Caldwell et al. (1977)
Monkey	IM	1M,1F	0.3	24	81	77	0	4	—	—	—	Caldwell et al. (1977)
	IM	M	0.3	96	95.2	76.8	—	3.7	—	—	1.7	Dring et al., 1975
Human	PO	M	25[b]	24	94	89.6	0.6[c]	—	3.4	—	—	Sinsheimer et al. (1973)
	PO	M	0.36	24	96	90	<1	5	—	—	—	Caldwell et al. (1977)

Data are means. Dash (—) indicates not reported (in all tables in this volume).
[a] 4-Hydroxy-norephedrine; α-methyloctopamine.
[b] Total dose (approximately 0.36 mg/kg).
[c] Measurable amounts in only 2 of 3 subjects.

88

1976), whereas the metabolites are both unconjugated and conjugated as glucuronides and sulfonides (Sinsheimer et al., 1973; Thiercelin et al., 1976).

Urinary elimination of phenylpropanolamine is relatively rapid in humans, with an elimination rate constant of 0.18/hr and a half-life of 3.9–4.6 hr (Heimlich et al., 1961; Rhodes et al., 1970). The maximum rate of excretion was 7.1 mg/hr.

The mechanism of the urinary excretion of phenylpropanolamine is not known. Axelrod (1953) reported that the renal clearance of l-norephedrine in dogs was greater than the glomerular filtration rate, suggesting a secretory transport mechanism. The renal clearance of phenylpropanolamine (i.e., $\pm$-norephedrine) was not reported.

The urinary excretion of ephedrine and ephedrine analogues in humans is dependent on the urinary pH (Wilkinson & Beckett, 1968). Urinary excretion of ($-$)-norephedrine was more rapid when the urine was acidified to approximately pH 5.0 by administration of ammonium chloride than when it was alkalinized to approximately pH 8.0 with sodium bicarbonate. However, the magnitude of this pH dependence was different for various ephedrine analogues. The urinary excretion of ($-$)-norephedrine, for instance, was only slightly affected by urinary pH, whereas the excretion of ephedrine and methylephedrine was much more sensitive to urinary pH. The pH dependence of the urinary excretion of phenylpropanolamine has not been investigated.

DISAPPEARANCE FROM BLOOD

Disappearance of phenylpropanolamine from blood has been determined following administration of phenylpropanolamine in immediate-release form (Mason & Amick, 1981; Thiercelin et al., 1976) or in sustained-release form (Dowse et al., 1983; Lonnerholm et al., 1984; Neelakantan & Kostenbauder, 1976; Rhodes et al., 1970).

Following IV administration of 535 μg/kg of phenylpropanolamine in rats, phenylpropanolamine disappeared from the plasma by first-order (exponential) kinetics with an elimination rate constant k of 0.715/hr ($t_{1/2} = 0.693/k = 0.97$ hr) (Thiercelin et al., 1976). The plasma concentration of phenylpropanolamine at 15 min after IV administration was 715 pmol/g. Elimination of phenylpropanolamine from all tissues (lungs, adrenals, spleen, heart) except brain was similar to that from the plasma. However, the elimination of phenylpropanolamine from the brain was slower, with an elimination rate constant of 0.668/hr.

Elimination of phenylpropanolamine from the blood in humans is slower than in rats. In humans the elimination half-life following PO administration was 3–6 hr (El Egakey & Speiser, 1982; Lonnerholm et al., 1984).

The steady-state kinetics of disappearance of phenylpropanolamine from blood was investigated in human volunteers (Lonnerholm et al., 1984). Eight adult volunteers (two females and six males) ingested 50 mg of phenylpropanolamine in sustained-release formulation (Rinexin), twice daily at 12-hr intervals for five doses. Blood samples were collected before each morning dose and at intervals of 0.5–24 hr after the last dose. Urine samples were collected at intervals following the final dose. Blood and urine levels of phenylpropanolamine were determined by gas chromatography with an electron capture detector, with a detection limit of 10 ng/ml.

The results are summarized in Table 3.2. Comparison of blood levels in samples collected prior to the morning doses confirmed that steady-state levels of phenylpropanolamine had been achieved after 1–2 days. The disappearance curves for the eight subjects showed little interindividual variation. The curves showed a flat concentration–time profile for 2–8 hr after the dose, demonstrating the sustained-release characteristics of the formulation. Plasma concentrations of phenylpropanolamine at steady state ranged from 30–200 ng/ml. These relatively low plasma level values are related to the large volume of distribution. Absorption of phenylpropanolamine was nearly complete, and the drug was eliminated primarily unchanged in the urine. Phenylpropanolamine is rapidly cleared from plasma, primarily by renal tubular secretion of the unchanged compound. The relatively short plasma elimination half-life of 4–7 hr is consistent with previous estimates of the half-life in humans (El Egakey & Speiser, 1982).

Peak blood levels of approximately 80 ng/ml of phenylpropanolamine occurred 1 hr following PO administration of 25 mg of phenylpropanolamine in solution to human volunteers (Mason & Amick, 1981). Blood levels declined exponentially to barely detectable levels 24 hr after drug administration.

No published information is available regarding compartmental analysis or determination of terminal elimination half-lives of phenylpropanolamine

TABLE 3.2. Disappearance of Phenylpropanolamine from Plasma at Steady State in Humans[a]

Mean steady-state plasma concentration (ng/ml)	114 ± 20
Maximal plasma concentration (ng/ml)	167 ± 28
Minimal plasma concentration (ng/ml)	59 ± 19
Terminal plasma half-life (hr)	5.6 ± 1.0
Total plasma clearance (liters kg^{-1} hr^{-1})	0.56 ± 0.14
Apparent volume of distribution (liters/kg)	4.4 ± 1.2
Urinary excretion of unchanged drug (%)	86 ± 13
Area under concentration–time curve (ng/ml × hr)	1368 ± 242

Source: Data from Lonnerholm et al. (1984).
[a]Mean ± SD ($n = 8$). Data from samples collected on day 3 of a steady-state study of phenylpropanolamine (50 mg, sustained-release, b.i.d.).

in either animals or humans. Likewise, no information is available comparing the pharmacokinetics of phenylpropanolamine in acute and chronic administration.

PROTEIN BINDING

At a concentration of 10 ng/ml, *l*-norephedrine was 20% bound to plasma proteins (Axelrod, 1953). No specific information regarding protein binding of phenylpropanolamine is available.

BIOAVAILABILITY: COMPARISON OF IMMEDIATE- AND SUSTAINED-RELEASE FORMULATIONS

Since many commercial products contain phenylpropanolamine in sustained-release form, it is important to compare bioavailability in immediate- and sustained-release formulations. The *in vitro* rate of release of phenylpropanolamine from the sustained-release formulation is an important predictor of bioavailability (Heimlich et al., 1961). The *in vitro* rate of release is dependent on the pharmaceutical preparation used (see Chapter 2).

Heimlich et al., (1961) compared the bioavailability of three different formulations of spansules containing a combination of 50 mg of phenylpropanolamine, 8 mg of chlorpheniramine, and 2.5 mg of isopropamide. The formulations were unprocessed drug (immediate-release), slow-release, and slower-release formulations. Urinary excretion of phenylpropanolamine was measured in healthy human volunteers. The total 24-hr urinary excretion of phenylpropanolamine in humans receiving 50 mg of phenylpropanolamine in the immediate-release formulation was 96.5%. In contrast, the urinary excretion in individuals given the slow- and slower-release formulations was 79.7 and 53.4%, respectively. The bioavailability of the immediate-release and slow-release formulations were equivalent, but the slower-release formulation was substantially different. Equivalent bioavailabilities were demonstrated by (1) determining that the overall rate of urinary excretion in the slow-release formulation group (7.6 mg/hr) was comparable to the maximum rate of excretion in the immediate-release formulation group (7.1 mg/hr) and (2) demonstrating that the cumulative urinary excretion was not different in individuals given three 50-mg phenylpropanolamine immediate-release spansules at 4-hr intervals compared to individuals given a single 150-mg slow-release spansule.

Equivalent bioavailabilities of immediate- and sustained-release phenylpropanolamine combination formulations were also demonstrated during a multidose, steady-state, crossover bioavailability study (Barrett et al., 1981). Adult male volunteers were given a single sustained-release tablet containing

75 mg of phenylpropanolamine and 12 mg of chlorpheniramine once a day for 4 days, or an immediate-release tablet containing one-third these doses t.i.d. for 4 days. There were no differences between the two groups with regard to the area under the curve for blood level of phenylpropanolamine versus time, peak phenylpropanolamine concentration, or time to peak, recorded on the fourth day of drug administration.

The bioavailabilities of an oral controlled-release drug delivery system and an immediate-release formulation were compared in a multidose, crossover design clinical trial (Marcus, 1984). This oral controlled-release system (the Pennkinetic system; see Chapter 2) consists of a drug-polymer matrix surrounded by an insoluble semipermeable coating. The drug is released into the gastrointestinal tract when ions from the gastrointestinal fluid diffuse across the semipermeable membrane, initiate an ion-exchange process, and release the drug from the matrix. In this study, the controlled-release formulation, Corsym, contained 75 mg of phenylpropanolamine and 8 mg of chlorpheniramine in a polistirex matrix. This formulation contained both uncoated and coated phenylpropanolamine/polymer particles, providing a loading and maintenance dose, respectively. Chlorpheniramine has a longer half-life than phenylpropanolamine and was not in a controlled-release form. Twelve healthy adult volunteers (age and sex not specified) received either Corsym or an immediate-release formulation daily for seven days. Corsym was administered twice daily at 12-hr intervals. The immediate-release formulation contained half the dose of each drug (i.e., 37.5 mg of phenylpropanolamine and 4 mg of chlorpheniramine) and was given four times daily at 6-hr intervals. The pharmacokinetics profile for phenylpropanolamine was measured on the first day and at steady-state (after 7 days of daily dosing) for each formulation. The two formulations were shown to be bioequivalent because the areas-under-the-curves for plasma concentration versus time were not significantly different for the two formulations.

In addition, the peak plasma level of phenylpropanolamine and the time to reach the peak were compared in the controlled- and immediate-release formulations. The peak plasma levels were not significantly different for the two formulations, but as expected the time to reach the peak was longer for the controlled-release formulation. These results indicate that "dose dumping" (i.e., releasing the entire dose faster in the controlled-release formulation than in the immediate-release formulation) did not occur (Marcus, 1984).

The half-life of urinary elimination of phenylpropanolamine (defined as the time for excretion of 50% of the total dose) was determined for a sustained-release phenylpropanolamine formulation prepared by a facilitated entrapment method and an immediate-release formulation (Rhodes et al., 1970). The half-lives for the immediate- and sustained-release formulations were 4.6 and 8.0 hr, respectively.

Finally, in three studies the blood level-time curves for phenylpropanol-amine in sustained-release preparations were reported. In two patients who took 50 mg of phenylpropanolamine in a sustained-release tablet, peak blood levels of approximately 100 ng/ml occurred 1 hr after ingestion of phenylpro-panolamine, and blood levels decreased to approximately 50–60 ng/ml after 6 hr (Neelakantan & Kostenbauder, 1976). Peak blood levels of approximately 250–300 ng/ml occurred at 2–6 hr in human volunteers given 150-mg sus-tained-release phenylpropanolamine tablets (Dowse et al., 1983). The cumu-lative 24-hr urinary excretion of phenylpropanolamine was 60–70% in the lat-ter study. The peak blood levels of phenylpropanolamine in volunteers given 150 mg of phenylpropanolamine in a controlled-release formulation were ap-proximately 320 ng/ml; the peak blood levels occurred approximately 4 hr after administration of the dose (Westlake, 1975). In comparison, peak blood levels of approximately 80 ng/ml occurred 2 hr after ingestion of 25 mg of phenylpropanolamine in solution in human volunteers (Mason & Amick, 1981). However, the results from these studies cannot be directly compared because different analytical methods were used, and insufficient information is available regarding formulations and drug administration schedules to de-termine whether the procedures were comparable.

PHARMACODYNAMICS

PHARMACOLOGY OF β-PHENYLETHYLAMINES

The β-phenylethylamines are a class of drugs that have as a common chemical structure a phenyl ring attached by a two-carbon link to an amino nitrogen. In a classic pharmacological study of the structure-activity relationships of β-phenylethylamine analogues, Barger and Dale (1910) noted that IV admin-istration of these compounds tended to reproduce many of the physiologic responses produced by stimulation of the sympathetic branch of the auto-nomic nervous system. Barger and Dale (1910) thus proposed the term "sym-pathomimetic amines" to describe these drugs. The responses of the β-phen-ylethylamines so closely mimic the sympathetic responses because two of the most potent of the β-phenylethylamines, epinephrine and norepinephrine, are neurotransmitters released from the adrenergic nerve terminals.

Anatomically and functionally, the sympathetic nervous system is com-plex. Postganglionic sympathetic neurons innervate most of the major vis-ceral organs (see Table 3.3). A review of the physiologic functioning of the sympathetic nervous system is beyond the scope of this book [see the review by Mayer (1980)]. In general, stimulation of the sympathetic nervous system produces a cluster of physiologic responses often referred to as the "flight or

TABLE 3.3. Location and Classification of Adrenergic Receptors

Location	Receptor	Response
Eye		
Radial muscle, iris	α	Mydriasis
Ciliary muscle	β	Relaxation
Heart	β_1	Increased heart rate; increased force of contraction
Arteries	α	Constriction
	β_2	Dilation
Veins	α	Constriction
	β_2	Dilation
Lung	β_2	Bronchodilation
Gastrointestinal tract		
Motility and tone	α_2, β_2	Decreased motility and tone
Sphincters	α	Contraction
Kidney	β_2	Renin secretion
Urinary bladder		
Detrusor	β	Relaxation
Trigone, sphincter	α	Contraction
Ureter	α, β_2	Increased tone and motility
Uterus	α	Contraction (pregnant)
	β	Relaxation (nonpregnant)
Male sex organs	α	Ejaculation
Splenic capsule	α, β_2	Contraction
Liver	α, β_2	Glycogenolysis, gluconeogenesis
Pancreas	α	Decreased glucagon secretion
	α	Decreased insulin secretion
	β_2	Increased insulin secretion
Adipose tissue	α, β_1	Lipolysis
Salivary glands	α	Potassium and water secretion
	β	Amylase secretion

Source: Adapted from Mayer (1980).

fright" syndrome. By a combination of cardiac stimulation, inhibition and contraction of various smooth muscles, stimulation of secretion from certain glands, and activation of metabolic processes, the sympathetic nervous system prepares the individual to attack, defend itself, or flee from an aggressor.

The β-phenylethylamines, and particularly the catecholamines norepinephrine and epinephrine, are capable of either stimulating or inhibiting contraction of smooth muscles. Whether a particular drug causes stimulation or inhibition depends on both the pharmacodynamic characteristics of that particular drug and the receptor population of the particular smooth muscle. Ahlquist (1948) introduced the concept of two categories of adrenergic receptors, α- and β-receptors, which mediate primarily excitatory and inhibitory responses, respectively. There are two major exceptions to this pattern of responses: inhibitory responses in the gut are mediated by both α- and β-receptors, and excitatory responses in the heart are mediated primarily by β-receptor activity.

The differentiation between α- and β-receptor activity is based on two lines of evidence. The first line, the rank order of potency of sympathomimetic amines, varies in different tissues. For example, the rank order of potency for producing vasoconstriction is norepinephrine > epinephrine > isoproterenol, whereas the rank order of potency for increasing heart rate is the reverse. The second line of evidence is that certain drugs specifically block effects of sympathomimetic amines at α-adrenergic sites, whereas other drugs specifically block effects at β-adrenergic sites. For example, phenoxybenzamine is a specific α-adrenergic antagonist and propranolol is a specific β-adrenergic antagonist. The classification of various sympathetic activities as α- or β-adrenergic is indicated in Table 3.3.

More recently, it has been demonstrated that the α- and β-adrenergic receptors can be subdivided according to variations in the rank order of potency of the respective agonists, and the development of more specific antagonists. β-Adrenergic receptors can be subdivided into β_1-receptors that are predominantly excitatory in the heart and β_2-receptors located elsewhere in the body, especially in the lungs (Lands et al., 1967). Likewise, α-adrenergic receptors can be subdivided into α_1-receptors, which are primarily postsynaptic receptors, especially in the peripheral nervous system, and α_2-receptors, which are primarily presynaptic receptors in the peripheral nervous system and may also be postsynaptic receptors in the central nervous system (CNS) (Mayer, 1980). The locations of the α_1-, α_2-, β_1-, and β_2-adrenergic receptors in the body are indicated in Table 3.3.

DIRECT, INDIRECT, AND MIXED ACTIVITY OF PHENYLPROPANOLAMINE AT SYMPATHETIC SITES

The classic studies of Liebman (1961) and Trendelenburg et al. (1962a,b) established that the sympathomimetic amines can be categorized into three classes: direct-acting, indirect-acting, and mixed-acting drugs. Direct-acting drugs exert their pharmacodynamic effects at postsynaptic receptor sites on the effector organs and do not require the presence of intact, functional adrenergic neuron terminals for their effects. Examples of direct-acting drugs are epinephrine, phenylephrine, and synephrine. Indirect-acting sympathomimetic amines, in contrast, produce their pharmacodynamic effects by causing release of neurotransmitter, predominantly norepinephrine, from adrenergic nerve endings in the tissues. Consequently, the actions of the indirect-acting amines are reduced or abolished when the adrenergic neuron terminals are nonfunctional as a result of pharmacological or other experimental manipulations. The standard example of an indirect-acting amine is tyramine. Mixed-acting sympathomimetic amines, as the name implies, exert their actions by a combination of direct and indirect actions. The reference standards for mixed-acting amines are ephedrine and p-hydroxyephedrine, although as shown by Trendelenburg et al. (1962a), most sympathomimetic amines are mixed-acting drugs. Indeed, the classification of amines as three distinct categories—direct, indirect and mixed—is somewhat misleading. Rather, the activity of the sympathomimetic drugs is represented by a continuum ranging from predominantly direct-acting to predominantly indirect-acting drugs, with most drugs falling somewhere between the two extremes. In fact, as shown by Trendelenburg et al. (1962a), the ratio of direct to indirect activity of any given drug may vary according to the site of action under investigation.

The direct and indirect activities of a large number of sympathomimetic amines were elucidated in classic pharmacological studies using cats (Trendelenburg et al., 1962a,b). The study design is summarized in Table 3.4. Drug effects on three physiologic responses were measured. The three responses were blood pressure, heart rate, and contraction of the nictitating membrane. To fully elucidate the spectrum of drug actions, the following manipulations were used [reviewed by Trendelenburg et al. (1962a)]. Chronic denervation of the postganglionic nerves to the nictitating membrane or pretreatment with cocaine increased the responses to direct-acting amines, decreased the responses to indirect-acting amines, but had variable effects on responses to mixed-acting amines. To better differentiate between indirect- and mixed-acting amines, two regimens for pretreatment with reserpine were used. Long-term reserpine pretreatment, which caused depletion of norepinephrine

TABLE 3.4. Effects of Direct-, Indirect-, and Mixed-Acting Sympathomimetic Amines in Cats with Spinal Transections

Experimental manipulation	Effect of Experimental Manipulation on Drug Response[a]		
	Direct	Indirect	Mixed
Postganglionic denervation	+ +	−	+/−
Cocaine	+	−	+/−
Reserpine			
Long term	+ +	−	−
Short term	+/−	−	−
		(nonparallel)	(parallel)

[a]Symbols: (+) response increased (dose–response curve shifted to the left); (+ +) response greatly increased; (+/−) variable effect; (−) response decreased (dose–response curve shifted to the right).

and supersensitivity, increased the responses to direct-acting amines and decreased responses to both indirect- and mixed-acting amines. Short-term pretreatment with reserpine, which caused depletion of norepinephrine but not supersensitivity, decreased responses to both indirect- and mixed-acting amines. After short-term reserpine pretreatment, the dose-response curves for indirect-acting amines were shifted to the right with a lower maximum response, whereas the dose-response curves for mixed-acting amines were shifted to the right with no change in the maximum response.

Using this experimental design, Trendelenburg et al. (1962a,b) demonstrated that phenylpropanolamine exerted its effects by mixed actions (see Table 3.5). Moreover, the ratio of direct to indirect actions was different for the three different responses. Thus the effects of phenylpropanolamine on the nictitating membrane were due predominantly to direct actions, whereas the cardiac effects, especially the effects on heart rate, were due predominantly to indirect actions.

Although these results demonstrate that phenylpropanolamine had a combination of direct and indirect effects on smooth muscle and the cardiovascular system, it should be noted that phenylpropanolamine had very low potency for these effects. Phenylpropanolamine was 100–200 times less potent than either epinephrine or norepinephrine in increasing blood pressure and heart rate. In fact, phenylpropanolamine was among the least potent of the 16 sympathomimetic amines tested. In addition, it should be noted that these results were based on IV administration of the test drugs.

Liebman (1961) also demonstrated that phenylpropanolamine (0.01–10 mg/liter) increased the heart rate by a mixture of direct and indirect actions in the isolated heart-lung preparation of the dog. The maximum increase in heart rate of approximately 80 bpm occurred at a concentration of 3.0 mg/liter. Reserpine pretreatment shifted the dose-response curve for phenylpropanolamine to the right, with only a slight decrease in the maximum response.

These studies by Liebman (1961) and Trendelenburg et al. (1962a,b), published more than 20 years ago, established that phenylpropanolamine exerted sympathomimetic effects due to a combination of direct and indirect actions, and that phenylpropanolamine had low potency for these effects. These conclusions were based on indirect measurements in whole animals *in vivo*. More direct measurements of the effects of phenylpropanolamine on adrenergic neurons using more specific techniques are surprisingly limited. Phenylpropanolamine (0.8–125 mg/kg, SC, in mice) was not effective in stimulating release of ^{3}H-norepinephrine in heart tissue but was relatively more effective in preventing uptake of ^{3}H-norepinephrine (Levitt et al., 1974). Phenylpropanolamine was effective in causing constriction of human arteries and veins *in vitro* (Stevens & Moulds, 1981) and in inhibition of smooth-muscle activity

TABLE 3.5. ED$_{50}$'s for Phenylpropanolamine on Nictitating Membrane, Blood Pressure, and Heart Rate in Cats with Spinal Cord Transections

Response	ED$_{50}$ (95% Confidence Limits) (μg/kg, IV)			
	Control	Reserpine Pretreatment[a]	Cocaine	Denervation
Nictitating membrane contraction	1160 (547–2470)	2430 (1200–4930)	2200 (1700–2840)	910 (280–2950)
Increased blood pressure	184 (50–676)	385 (289–514)	—	—
Increased heart rate	145 (61–345)	925 (527–1620)	—	—

Source: Data from Trendelenburg et al. (1962a,b).
[a]Short-term treatment, judged to produce depletion of norepinephrine without inducing supersensitivity.

in the gut and in contracting the uterus *in vitro* (Ghouri & Haley, 1969). However, in the latter two studies, phenylpropanolamine had very low potency, and because of the experimental designs used it is not possible to determine whether the effects were due to direct or indirect actions of phenylpropanolamine. The dose-response curves for contraction of isolated aortic strips by phenylpropanolamine did not differ between untreated and reserpine-pretreated rabbits (Figure 3.1) (Persson et al., 1973), indicating that at least in this tissue phenylpropanolamine acts mainly by direct action. Studies directly measuring the release of norepinephrine from adrenergic neurons *in vitro* or *in vivo* and measuring binding of phenylpropanolamine to adrenergic receptors would be required to definitively determine the direct and indirect actions of phenylpropanolamine on adrenergic neurons. Phenylpropanolamine does bind directly to α-adrenergic receptors from vas deferens, but with very low affinity (Minneman et al., 1983). Additional studies will be required to confirm the indirect actions of phenylpropanolamine on adrenergic nerve terminals, however.

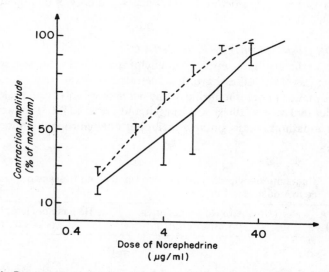

Figure 3.1. Dose response curves for contraction of aortic strips by norephedrine. Abscissa: concentration of (±)-norephedrine (μg/ml). Ordinate: contraction amplitude (% of maximum). Solid line: control. Dashed line: reserpine pretreatment. Mean ± s.d. From *Persson et al. (1973).*

EFFECTS OF PHENYLPROPANOLAMINE ON ADRENERGIC NEURONS

RELEASE OF NOREPINEPHRINE

If the effects of phenylpropanolamine at sympathetic sites of action are mediated in part by release of endogenous norepinephrine from the adrenergic
nerve terminals, it should be possible to demonstrate that administration of
phenylpropanolamine causes an increase in norepinephrine release either *in
vitro* or *in vivo*. Only one report has been published in which the effects of
phenylpropanolamine on release of norepinephrine were directly investigated. Phenylpropanolamine (0.8–125 mg/kg, SC) was administered to mice
either 15 min before or 15 min after administration of radiolabeled norepinephrine (^{3}H-norepinephrine), and uptake and release of radioactivity by
the heart was measured (Levitt et al., 1974). Presumably the ^{3}H-nor-
epinephrine was taken up and released from the readily available pool of
neurotransmitter in the adrenergic nerve terminals in the heart. Phenylpropanolamine, administered 15 min after the dose of ^{3}H-norepinephrine, did
not significantly increase the release of norepinephrine (Table 3.6); even at
the very high dose of 125 mg/kg (SC), release of norepinephrine was marginally decreased. It should be noted that the effective dose range for anorexia in
rats is 5–40 mg/kg (IP) (Epstein, 1959; Kornblith & Hoebel, 1976; Wellman
& Peters, 1980), and significant toxicity occurs at a dose of 80 mg/kg (Davis
& Pinkerton, 1972).

INHIBITION OF NOREPINEPHRINE UPTAKE

In contrast to the negligible effect of phenylpropanolamine on release of norepinephrine, several studies have demonstrated that phenylpropanolamine
inhibits reuptake of norepinephrine by the nerve terminal (i.e., uptake$_1$). The
early studies by Iversen (1964) and Burgen and Iversen (1965) showed that a
series of sympathomimetic amines, including phenylpropanolamine, inhib-

TABLE 3.6. Effects of Phenylpropanolamine on Uptake and Release of
Norepinephrine in Mouse Heart in vitro

Dose of PPA (mg/kg, SC)	Uptake of Norepinephrine (% of Control)	Release of Norepinephrine (% of Control)
0.8	79	—
4	50	—
5	—	113
20	19	—
25	—	74
125	—	68

Source: Data from Levitt et al. (1974).

ited reuptake of norepinephrine in the isolated perfused rat heart. These results have been confirmed in rat vas deferens and heart (Swamy et al., 1969) and in mouse heart (Levitt et al., 1974).

An extensive series of sympathomimetic amines, including phenylpropanolamine, was tested for inhibition of uptake of norepinephrine using the isolated perfused rat heart preparation (Burgen & Iversen, 1965; Iversen, 1964). Inhibition of uptake of radiolabeled norepinephrine by uptake$_1$ (high-affinity uptake) and uptake$_2$ (low-affinity uptake) was measured. Phenylpropanolamine inhibited uptake$_1$ with an IC_{50} (drug concentration required to produce 50% inhibition of uptake) of 2.0×10^{-6} M. The affinity of phenylpropanolamine for uptake inhibition was very low relative to other sympathomimetic amines such as metaraminol, (+)-amphetamine, and (−)-norepinephrine. Effects of phenylpropanolamine on uptake$_2$ were not investigated.

Phenylpropanolamine (0.8–20 mg/kg, SC) effectively inhibited uptake of ^{3}H-norepinephrine in the mouse heart (Levitt et al., 1974) (Table 3.6). Uptake inhibition was measured by administering phenylpropanolamine 15 min before the loading dose of ^{3}H-norepinephrine and measuring uptake of radioactivity by the heart tissue. Note that phenylpropanolamine inhibited uptake of norepinephrine at doses that are within the behaviorally effective range.

Inhibition of norepinephrine uptake by phenylpropanolamine was confirmed by measuring the uptake of I^{125}-metaiodobenzylguanidine (I^{125}-MIBG) into the heart and parotid glands *in vivo* (Sherman et al., 1985; Sisson et al., 1985). I^{125}-MIBG was used as an indirect measure of adrenergic neuron function; it is taken up into neurons, stored in catecholamine-containing storage vesicles, and released in response to acetylcholine. Phenylpropanolamine inhibited uptake of I^{125}-MIBG in the heart and parotid glands in rats (Sherman et al., 1985) and humans (Sisson et al., 1985). In both species, phenylpropanolamine produced a more marked effect in the heart than in the parotid glands.

Inhibition of norepinephrine uptake would produce sympathomimetic effects by prolonging the duration of action of norepinephrine released from the nerve terminals by either physiologic stimuli or pharmacological agents. One experimental method for measuring functional inhibition of norepinephrine uptake is to measure the dose-response curve for exogenously administered norepinephrine in the absence and presence of the uptake inhibitor. Although no report has been published using such a paradigm to test for uptake inhibition by phenylpropanolamine per se, various isomers of norephedrine have been shown to potentiate the effects of exogenously applied norepinephrine (Swamy et al., 1969). In the study by Swamy et al., (1969), $D(−)$- and $L(+)$-norephedrine and $L(+)$-norpseudoephedrine potentiated the effects of norepinephrine on both the isolated rat vas deferens and the isolated rat heart preparations. In both preparations, the (−)-norephedrine isomer was more potent than the (+)-isomer.

EFFECTS OF PHENYLPROPANOLAMINE ON STORAGE OF NOREPINEPHRINE IN NERVE TERMINALS

No studies have been published to determine by either histochemical or neurochemical methods whether phenylpropanolamine has any effect on the storage of norepinephrine in adrenergic nerve terminals. However, indirect evidence from several studies indicates that phenylpropanolamine is not likely to have any significant effect on norepinephrine storage. Structure-activity studies of norepinephrine depletion by sympathomimetic amines indicate that one of the structural requirements for norepinephrine depletion is the presence of either a mono- or dihydroxy substitution on the phenyl ring (Shore, 1966). Since phenylpropanolamine has no substitutions on the phenyl ring, it is not likely to cause norepinephrine depletion. Indeed, phenylpropanolamine (2 mg/kg, IP) caused no change in the level of norepinephrine in rat heart (Shore, 1966); however, insufficient information regarding the methods and results of this investigation were presented to allow a full analysis of these results. In addition, only a single dose of phenylpropanolamine was investigated, and this was a relatively low dose.

Two other lines of evidence indicate that phenylpropanolamine probably does not alter storage of norepinephrine in the nerve terminals. Phenylpropanolamine (40 μg) administered directly into the cerebrospinal fluid by intracerebroventricular injection did not cause a change in the brain levels of either norepinephrine or dopamine (Breese et al., 1970). However, interpretation of this negative result is limited because only a single dose of phenylpropanolamine was administered, and this may have been a subthreshold dose. The other line of evidence comes from a structure-activity study of the thermodynamic stability of complexes formed between various sympathomimetic amines and Cu^{2+}-ATP (Rajan et al., 1974). The rationale for this study was that the norepinephrine stored in the storage granules in the nerve terminal is complexed with Cu^{2+} and ATP. Thus any drug that interferes with this norepinephrine-Cu^{2+}-ATP complex may interfere with storage of norepinephrine. Phenylpropanolamine was not investigated in this study. However, norephedrine (the isomer was not specified) had very low affinity for the Cu^{2+}-ATP complex, in fact the lowest affinity of any of the amines tested. The structural requirements for binding of the amines to the Cu^{2+}-ATP complex included the presence of a mono- or dihydroxy substitution on the phenyl ring, suggesting that phenylpropanolamine would have low affinity for binding to the complex.

FALSE TRANSMITTER

There are no studies available that have specifically tested the hypothesis that phenylpropanolamine could be taken up into the amine storage granules and released as a false transmitter. To demonstrate that a drug acts as a false transmitter, it is necessary to demonstrate that (1) the drug is taken up into the nerve terminal, (2) the drug displaces the endogenous transmitter from its storage sites, (3) the false transmitter is released by physiologic stimuli, and (4) the postsynaptic response to the false transmitter is less than the response to the natural transmitter. No studies are available to demonstrate whether phenylpropanolamine is taken up into the nerve terminals or released by physiologic stimuli. As discussed in the previous section, it is unlikely that phenylpropanolamine displaces norepinephrine from the nerve terminal storage pools. The fourth criterion, low potency relative to norepinephrine, has been demonstrated repeatedly at many sites of action, including most smooth muscles and cardiac tissue. In summary, there is insufficient evidence available to determine whether phenylpropanolamine acts as a false transmitter at noradrenergic neurons. However, indirect evidence and structure-activity studies of false transmitters indicate that it is unlikely that phenylpropanolamine acts as a false transmitter.

It should be noted that one derivative of phenylpropanolamine, m-hydroxyphenylpropanolamine (metaraminol), is a potent depletor of norepinephrine stores (Berti & Shore, 1967; Bhagat et al., 1965; Kopin, 1972; Shore, 1966).

In summary, the effects of phenylpropanolamine on adrenergic mechanisms are as follows. The studies by Trendelenburg et al. (1962a,b) showed that phenylpropanolamine is a mixed-acting sympathomimetic amine and that the ratio of direct to indirect activity depends in part on the site of action. However, there is a paucity of direct evidence to support these original observations. The effects of phenylpropanolamine on norepinephrine release were investigated in only one study, which showed negligible effects of phenylpropanolamine even at near-toxic doses. In contrast, several studies have demonstrated that phenylpropanolamine inhibits reuptake of norepinephrine via uptake$_1$. There is no direct evidence that phenylpropanolamine causes depletion of norepinephrine or that phenylpropanolamine itself acts as a false neurotransmitter at the adrenergic nerve terminal.

EFFECTS OF PHENYLPROPANOLAMINE ON SMOOTH MUSCLE

Most of the studies of effects of phenylpropanolamine on smooth muscle have utilized *in vitro* isolated smooth muscle preparations. These preparations present several advantages over *in vivo* studies of drug actions. In isolated tissue preparations many of the indirect effects of the test drugs, such as effects on blood pressure or blood flow and reflex activities, can be eliminated, and the effects observed can more reliably be attributed to direct effects of the drug at the tissue level. In addition, the concentration of the drug in the tissue bath can be carefully controlled and manipulated, making dose-response (or more properly, concentration-response) determinations more reliable. Dose-response studies conducted in whole animals are in general more susceptible to bias introduced by such factors as variations in absorption, distribution, and elimination kinetics, which all too often are not fully considered in the experimental design. However, there are certain limitations inherent in the isolated tissue preparations that must be considered in interpreting the results. The results from isolated tissue studies cannot always be directly extrapolated to predict effects of the drug in whole animals. For example, direct effects of the drug at the tissue level may be masked or prevented in the whole animal as the result of reflex or indirect effects on neural or cardiovascular functions. Moreover, many drugs are metabolized *in vivo,* and the metabolites may have pharmacological properties different from those of the parent compound. These differences will not be reflected in the isolated tissue preparations unless the various metabolites have been identified and can be systematically investigated. Finally, it is not easy to extrapolate from the concentrations used *in vitro* to either the blood levels or dose levels used *in vivo.* Thus it is necessary to investigate the pharmacodynamic effects of a test drug both *in vivo* and *in vitro* to fully understand the actions of the drug.

EFFECTS ON SMOOTH MUSCLE IN THE VAS DEFERENS

The isolated vas deferens of the rat is often used to investigate effects of α-adrenergic drugs on smooth muscles because this particular tissue contains a very homogeneous population of adrenergic receptors (Minneman et al., 1983). Several reports have confirmed that phenylpropanolamine or norephedrine causes contraction of the rat vas deferens.

Only one study reported the effects of phenylpropanolamine on contraction of the rat vas deferens (Minneman et al., 1983). In this study, the rats were pretreated with reserpine to deplete the endogenous stores of norepinephrine. In addition, the contractions of the vas deferens were measured in the presence of desmethylimipramine to block uptake$_1$, normetanephrine to block uptake$_2$, and propranolol to block β-adrenergic receptors. Phenylpropanolamine had very low potency and low intrinsic activity for contraction of the vas deferens. Phenylpropanolamine had 1/2000 the potency of norepiniphrine or epinephrine, and the intrinsic activity of phenylpropanolamine was less than 50% of the maximum.

Norephedrine also produced contractions of the isolated human vas deferens (Ratnasooriya et al., 1979b). In this study, specimens of the vas deferens were collected from patients undergoing elective vasectomy. Norephedrine produced a dose-dependent increase in contraction strength and in the frequency of spontaneous contractions. The effective concentrations of norephedrine ranged from approximately 1 to 100 μg/ml.

In addition, two isomers of norephedrine, $D(-)$-norephedrine and $L(+)$-norpseudoephedrine, were shown to produce contraction of the rat vas deferens *in vitro* (Patil et al., 1967a,b). Both isomers had low potency and low intrinsic activity for producing contraction; however, $D(-)$-norephedrine was more potent than $L(+)$-norpseudoephedrine.

To determine whether norephedrine-induced contractions of the vas deferens influence fertility and reproduction, norephedrine was applied locally to the vas deferens *in vivo* (Ratnasooriya et al., 1979a, 1981) or to the epididymis (Ratnasooriya et al., 1980), and the effects of drug treatment on fertility and reproduction were measured. Silastic collars containing norephedrine (the isomer was not specified) were implanted around the vas deferens in rats (Ratnasooriya et al., 1979a) and rabbits (Ratnasooriya et al., 1981). Local application of norephedrine to the vas deferens produced infertility, which was associated with reduced semen volume, reduced sperm counts and sperm motility, and abnormalities in sperm morphology. Mating behavior was not affected by such local administration. However, local application of norephedrine to another portion of the male reproductive tract, the epididymis, did not produce infertility (Ratnasooriya et al., 1980), suggesting that the decrease in fertility is due to a selective effect of norephedrine on the vas deferens.

EFFECTS ON GASTROINTESTINAL SMOOTH MUSCLE

The early studies by Chen et al. (1929) demonstrated that sympathomimetic amines caused inhibition of the spontaneous contractions of the isolated rabbit intestine. Effects of phenylpropanolamine on the isolated intestine were not investigated; however, it was noted that while most of the sympathomimetic amines tested inhibited the spontaneous contractions, d-norpseudoephedrine showed a tendency to increase the tone of the contractions.

Phenylpropanolamine increased the gastric transport time in rats *in vivo* (Tainter, 1944). No details regarding the dose, route of administration, or magnitude of the effects of phenylpropanolamine were presented.

The observation that phenylpropanolamine increased gastric transport time was confirmed by studies showing that phenylpropanolamine increased gastric retention in rats (Wellman et al., 1986). Phenylpropanolamine (5 to 40 mg/kg, IP), administered immediately after a test meal, produced a dose-dependent increase in gastric retention compared to saline treatment. The gastric retention was measured 3 hr after administration of phenylpropanolamine.

The effects of a series of α-adrenergic drugs on the spontaneous contractions of the rabbit ileum were investigated (Ghouri & Haley, 1969). Inhibition of the spontaneous contractions by sympathomimetic amines was studied in the presence of blocking concentrations of phentolamine. Phenylpropanolamine had very low potency for inhibition of contractions in this smooth muscle preparation (Table 3.7). Phenylpropanolamine was approximately 1/1000 as potent as l-norepinephrine, the most potent α-agonist studied.

These effects of phenylpropanolamine on gastrointestinal smooth muscle were confirmed by Innes and Kohli (1969). In this study, the effects of 22 sympathomimetic amines on GI smooth muscle were investigated using three different smooth muscle preparations, the isolated rat stomach, the rabbit jejunum, and the guinea pig ileum. Phenylpropanolamine (10^{-8}–10^{-5} g/ml) inhibited spontaneous contractions in all three preparations. The amines were classified into three categories according to whether they produced inhibition or excitation of the GI smooth muscle. One group of drugs, including phenylpropanolamine, inhibited the contractions of all three preparations. The second group, which included β-phenylethylamine and $(-)$-amphetamine, produced excitatory effects in all preparations. This excitatory effect was shown to be due to effects on serotonin receptors. However, the excitatory activity was demonstrated only at relatively high concentrations of the drugs ($\geq 10^{-6}$ g/ml), and the intrinsic activity of the amines was less than 50%, compared to the maximum excitatory response produced by serotonin. The third group of amines produced inhibition in some preparations and excitation in other preparations. Phenylpropanolamine did not produce excitatory effects on GI smooth muscle preparations, suggesting that it does not stimulate serotonin receptors in the gut.

TABLE 3.7. α-Adrenergic Activity of Drugs in Rabbit Ileum and Uterus[a]

	Ileum		Uterus	
Agonist	EC_{50} (μM)	Potency[b]	EC_{50} (μM)	Potency[b]
l-Phenylephrine	0.024	1.0	0.036	1.0
l-Norepinephrine	0.005	5.2	0.004	8.5
dl-Nordefrin[c]	0.040	0.6	0.082	0.45
Metaraminol[d]	0.15	0.16	0.21	0.17
Phenylpropanolamine	5.32	0.0045	5.80	0.006

Source: Data from Ghouri and Haley (1969).
[a]Tissues from estrogen-pretreated rabbits; EC_{50}, concentration required to produce 50% response.
[b]Relative to phenylephrine.
[c]3,4-dihydroxyphenylpropanolamine.
[d]3-hydroxyphenylpropanolamine.

EFFECTS ON VASCULAR SMOOTH MUSCLE

In light of the controversy regarding whether phenylpropanolamine produces hypertensive crisis and cerebrovascular hemorrhage, there is surprisingly little information available regarding the vasoconstrictor activity of phenylpropanolamine.

In isolated aortic strips from the rabbit, phenylpropanolamine produced a dose-dependent contraction of the vascular smooth muscle (Persson et al., 1973); in this article, ($\pm$)-norephedrine was referred to as "norephedrine" and not as "phenylpropanolamine." The threshold and maximum concentrations of phenylpropanolamine for producing contractions were 0.005 and 1.6 μg/ml, respectively. Phenylpropanolamine was 1/50 to 1/80 times as potent as norepinephrine in this preparation.

The vasoconstriction produced by a series of α-adrenergic agonists was studied in postmortem samples of arteries and veins from humans (Stevens & Moulds, 1981; Stevens et al., 1981). In these dose-response studies, phenylpropanolamine was shown to have very low potency for vasoconstriction. Phenylpropanolamine was approximately 1/100 as potent as norepinephrine, but the efficacy of the two drugs was similar. There was no difference in the potency of phenylpropanolamine in arteries and veins, and although the efficacy of phenylpropanolamine was less in veins than in arteries, the difference was not significant.

EFFECTS ON THE URINARY TRACT

The effects of norephedrine on urinary tract smooth muscle in humans were studied both *in vitro* and *in vivo* (Ek, 1977, 1978). The effects of phenylpropanolamine itself have not been reported.

Samples of human urethras were collected from patients undergoing surgery for bladder malignancy. Tissue segments from various portions of the urethra were suspended in an isolated tissue bath to measure spontaneous contractions and determine dose-response curves for several adrenergic and cholinergic drugs. The smooth muscle preparations showed spontaneous contractions. In addition, norephedrine (the isomer was not specified) produced dose-dependent contractions of the isolated urethra that were blocked by phenoxybenzamine, indicating that the effects were mediated by α-adrenergic activity. Unfortunately, no quantitative data were reported in these studies, and it is not possible to assess the potency and intrinsic activity of norephedrine. Segments of smooth muscle taken from various portions of the urethra responded similarly to norephedrine, indicating that there was no anatomic specificity in the drug response. Several other α-adrenergic agonists also produced contractions of the isolated urethra that were blocked by phenoxybenzamine. The β-adrenergic agonist isoproterenol caused inhibition of the spontaneous contractions, and this effect was blocked by propranolol. Finally, acetylcholine produced contraction of the smooth muscle from the urethrovesical junction, but not smooth muscle taken from other portions of the urethra. The effects of acetylcholine were blocked by atropine.

In vivo studies in humans confirmed the effects of norephedrine on the smooth muscles of the urinary tract (Ek, 1977, 1978). The urinary closure pressure profile was measured before and after oral administration of 75–100 mg of norephedrine to female patients with stress incontinence. Norephedrine increased both the maximum urethral pressure and the maximum urethral closure pressure. These effects were blocked by phentolamine and were not influenced by bladder volume or body position.

EFFECTS ON THE ESTROGEN-PRIMED UTERUS

Sympathomimetic amines produce qualitatively different effects on uterine smooth muscle depending on whether the animal is pregnant. In general, adrenergic agonists produce inhibition of uterine tone in nonpregnant animals and contractions of the uterus in pregnant animals (Barger & Dale, 1910). Most experimental studies of the effects of drugs on uterine smooth muscle utilize estrogen-primed animals rather than pregnant animals to more carefully control the endocrine status of the animal.

Phenylpropanolamine, in the presence of a blocking concentration of phentolamine, produced a dose-dependent contraction of the estrogen-primed uterus of the rabbit (Ghouri & Haley, 1969), but with a very low potency (Table 3.7). Furthermore, the potency of phenylpropanolamine for inhibition of spontaneous contractions in the ileum and that for contraction of the estrogen-primed uterus were similar, and the rank order of potency for selected phenylpropanolamine analogues (nordefrin and metaraminol) was similar in the two tissues.

EFFECTS ON THE PUPIL

Topical application of a 2% solution of phenylpropanolamine in saline directly into the eyes of awake, restrained rabbits produced mydriasis, with the maximum effect occurring approximately 40 min after drug administration (Leaders et al., 1970). Furthermore, topical application of phenylpropanolamine to the eye in anesthetized rabbits produced no change in the intraocular pressure as measured by applanation tonometry. By comparing the effects of a series of 20 phenylethylamines on pupil diameter and intraocular pressure, the authors concluded that pressor amines (i.e., α-agonists) generally produce mydriasis without decreasing intraocular pressure, whereas amines with depressor and cardiac stimulating properties (i.e., β-agonists) decrease intraocular pressure without producing mydriasis.

EFFECTS ON THE NICTITATING MEMBRANE OF THE CAT

The nictitating membrane of the cat is a specialized smooth muscle that has been utilized in many classic investigations of drug effects on autonomic sympathetic ganglia and on adrenergically innervated smooth muscles. The nictitating membrane is located underneath the eyelid in the cat; it is absent in most other mammals. The membrane is innervated by postganglionic adrenergic neurons from the cervical sympathetic ganglia. Thus drug effects at three sites of action in the autonomic nervous system can be investigated. Drug effects at the ganglion can be investigated by stimulating the preganglionic nerve trunk and recording drug effects on the contraction of the nictitating membrane. Drug effects on the postganglionic neurons can be investigated by stimulating the postganglionic nerve, bypassing the preganglionic and ganglionic sites of action. Finally, effects on the sympathetic neuroeffector sites can be investigated by measuring contraction of the membrane in the absence of any nerve stimulation. This is possible because adrenergic agonists produce contraction of the nictitating membrane by direct action on the adrenergic receptors in the smooth muscles of the membrane. Therefore, drugs that modulate postsynaptic adrenergic responses can be investigated by determining the effects of the test drug on the dose-response curve for exogenously applied norepinephrine, since IV administered norepinephrine produces a dose-dependent contraction of the nictitating membrane.

Phenylpropanolamine produced a dose-dependent contraction of the nictitating membrane of the cat (Trendelenburg et al., 1962a,b), with a relatively low potency (Table 3.5). The actions of phenylpropanolamine were due primarily to direct effects on the adrenergic receptor sites, and short-term pretreatment with reserpine did not significantly alter the dose-response curve for phenylpropanolamine (Figure 3.2). However, phenylpropanolamine was considerably different from other direct-acting amines in one important aspect. The dose-response curves for most direct-acting amines were shifted to the left by pretreatment with cocaine, since cocaine causes supersensitivity to direct-acting amines. However, the dose-response curve for phenylpropanolamine was not affected by pretreatment with cocaine. These results indicate that phenylpropanolamine is not taken up into the neuron by the amine uptake mechanism. The reason for this unusual response is not known.

EFFECTS ON BRONCHIAL SMOOTH MUSCLE

Although phenylpropanolamine is used clinically in cough-cold preparations, only two studies have been published testing the effects of phenylpropanolamine on bronchial smooth muscle.

In one early study of the pharmacological effects of sympathomimetic amines, the isolated trachea-bronchi-lung preparation of the guinea pig was

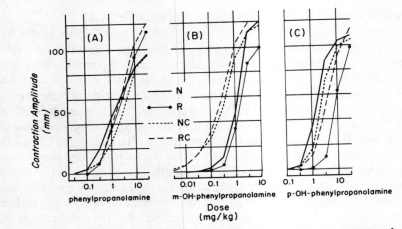

Figure 3.2. Dose-response curves for phenylpropanolamine and analogues for contraction of the nictitating membrane in cats with spinal cord transections. Abscissa: dose (mg/kg, IV). Ordinate: contraction amplitude (mm). N—normal (control). R—reserpine pretreatment. NC—normal, with cocaine. RC—reserpine pretreatment, with cocaine. From *Trendelenburg et al. (1962b)*.

used to test for the bronchodilator-bronchoconstrictor effects of phenylpropanolamine (Tainter et al., 1934). In this study, the preparation was perfused with saline and the rate of flow of saline through it was measured to show bronchoconstriction (decreased flow) or bronchodilation (increased flow). Control bronchoconstrictions were induced by pilocarpine, histamine, and barium chloride. Effects of various sympathomimetic amines on the bronchoconstriction produced by these test compounds were measured. Epinephrine, neosynephrine, and ephedrine were shown to be effective bronchodilators. In contrast, "propadrine" [sic] produced bronchoconstriction, whether administered alone or in combination with pilocarpine or histamine. It is not entirely clear whether these results can be extrapolated to phenylpropanolamine. The investigators stated in the text that they used "phenyl-1-amino-2-propanol-1, which is also known as 'propadrin,' 'mydriatin,' and 'norephedrine.' " However, there is reason to doubt the chemical identity of the actual isomer used because the structure of phenyl-1-amino-2-propanol-1 shown in the article is actually norpseudoephedrine.

More recently, Maitai (1975) reported that khat chewers who are also asthmatics claim that chewing khat relieves their asthma. Since *d*-norpseudoephedrine is a component of khat, the bronchodilator properties of several ephedrine derivatives were tested. Bronchodilation was measured in the isolated guinea pig whole trachea; tracheal volume was measured by manometric techniques. d-Norpseudoephedrine (0.25–1.00 mg/ml) produced weak but dose-dependent bronchoconstriction, whereas d-pseudoephedrine and l-ephedrine produced bronchodilation. Phenylpropanolamine was not investigated in this study.

Thus the bronchodilator-bronchoconstrictor activity of phenylpropanolamine is uncertain. Since bronchodilation is a β_2-adrenergic effect, and since phenylpropanolamine is predominantly an α-adrenergic agonist, it is unlikely that phenylpropanolamine produces significant bronchodilation.

SUMMARY OF EFFECTS OF PHENYLPROPANOLAMINE ON SMOOTH MUSCLE

Effects of phenylpropanolamine on smooth muscle activity have been investigated in a wide variety of smooth muscle preparations both *in vivo* and *in vitro*. Phenylpropanolamine causes contraction of vascular smooth muscle, the urethra, the vas deferens, the radial smooth muscles of the eye, and the estrogen-primed uterus. In the GI tract phenylpropanolamine inhibits spontaneous contractions of smooth muscles. However, phenylpropanolamine has very low potency at all these sites of action as well as low intrinsic activity at most sites. Phenylpropanolamine had no effect at excitatory serotonergic sites in the gut. Effects of phenylpropanolamine on the bronchial smooth muscle have not been demonstrated conclusively. Finally, cocaine pretreatment did not produce supersensitivity to phenylpropanolamine.

This spectrum of pharmacological activity suggests that phenylpropanolamine exerts these pharmacodynamic effects via action on α-adrenergic receptors, since adrenergic vasoconstriction, contraction of the urethra, contraction of the vas deferens, and inhibition of GI motility are generally mediated by α-receptors. However, quantitative studies of antagonism of phenylpropanolamine by selective α- and β-antagonists have not been reported. The effects of norephedrine on the isolated human urethra were blocked by an α-antagonist.

RECEPTOR BINDING STUDIES

Several of the studies discussed in the foregoing sections indicate that phenylpropanolamine exerts at least part of its pharmacodynamic effects through actions on adrenergic receptors, and more specifically through effects on α-adrenergic receptors. One of the most important advances in pharmacology in recent years is the development of techniques to directly measure binding of drugs to specific receptors.

Ideally, binding studies can contribute meaningfully to the understanding of drug action *in vivo* if the results of such studies are correlated with some functional response(s) in isolated tissues or whole animals. In addition, to determine whether the drug effect is due to specific and selective binding to particular receptors, the binding of the test drug to a variety of receptor types and in a number of tissues should be tested. In other words, lack of specific binding to various receptors is as important in determining selectivity of effect as is specific binding to one particular receptor.

α-ADRENERGIC RECEPTORS

The binding of phenylpropanolamine to α_1-adrenergic receptors from rat vas deferens tissue has been reported (Minneman et al., 1983). In addition, effects of phenylpropanolamine on contraction of the isolated vas deferens were also investigated, and thus the results of the receptor binding studies could be correlated with the results of the pharmacodynamic studies in isolated tissue preparations.

Binding of phenylpropanolamine, as well as a series of other sympathomimetic amines, to receptors in homogenates from rat vas deferens tissue was investigated using ^{125}I-labeled BE 2254 [2(β-(4-hydroxyphenyl)-ethylaminomethyl)-tetralone], abbreviated [125]IBE, as the binding ligand. The [125]IBE compound has been shown to be selective and specific for α_1-adrenergic binding sites in rat brain. In the rat vas deferens as well, binding of [125]IBE was shown to be specific, high affinity, and saturable. The K_D for binding of [125]IBE to vas deferens receptors was 105 ± 15 pM as determined by equilibrium analysis, and the B_{max} was 215 ± 30 fmol/mg of protein. Binding of [125]IBE was specifically displaced by α_1-adrenergic antagonists. These results indicate that [125]IBE can be used as a specific binding ligand for measurement of binding to α_1-adrenergic receptor sites in tissue other than brain.

In addition, the ability of these sympathomimetic amines to produce contractions of the isolated rat vas deferens was measured. The rats were pretreated with reserpine 16–20 hr prior to the experiments to deplete the tissues of endogenous stores of biogenic amines. The contraction of the vas deferens was measured in the presence of desmethylimipramine to block uptake of amines by uptake$_1$, normetanephrine to block uptake$_2$, and propranolol to block β-adrenergic receptors. Thus the indirect and nonspecific effects of the adrenergic agonists were eliminated by these multiple pharmacological manipulations, and drug effects could be attributed to direct effects mediated via α_1-adrenergic receptor activity. To determine whether the effects of the adrenergic agonists in the contractile responses were mediated by effects on α_1-receptors, the antagonism of norepinephrine by a series of α_1- and α_2-selective antagonists was investigated. The pA_2 values for the various antagonists were determined from the Schild plots. These results indicated that, indeed, the effects were mediated by specific effects on α_1-receptors.

Twelve sympathomimetic amines were tested in this study. The results of selected amines are shown in Table 3.8. The effects on binding of ^{125}IBE (K_D values) and contraction of the vas deferens are compared. The drugs varied considerably with regard to potency and intrinsic activity. Two major classes were identified: full agonists, which produced maximum contractions equivalent to the maximum contraction produced by norepinephrine; and partial agonists, which produced less than maximum contractions. These differences between full and partial agonists are shown graphically in Figure 3.3. As can be seen in Table 3.8, phenylpropanolamine was classified as a partial agonist with very low potency and low intrinsic activity. In the presence of the specific α_1-antagonist, prazosin, there was a ten- to twentyfold shift to the right of the dose-response curve for phenylpropanolamine. Scatchard plot analysis of the inhibition of binding of ^{125}IBE by phenylpropanolamine indicated a simple mass-action interaction between phenylpropanolamine and the ligand for binding to the receptors, since the Hill coefficient was not significantly different from 1.0.

In summary, this thorough investigation of interactions between phenylpropanolamine and α_1-adrenergic receptors demonstrates that phenylpropanolamine does, indeed, interact with the receptors, but with low affinity and low intrinsic activity. These results are consistent with those of many *in vivo* and *in vitro* studies that indicate that phenylpropanolamine has low potency and low intrinsic activity at adrenergic sites of action. However, these authors indicate that phenylpropanolamine is a "partial agonist" at the α_1-adrenergic receptors. Clearly, phenylpropanolamine is a weak agonist, producing less than maximum response, as indicated by its low intrinsic activity. To prove that phenylpropanolamine is a true partial agonist, it would be nec-

TABLE 3.8. Comparison of K_D for Binding to Receptors and EC_{50} for Contraction of Vas Deferens

Drug	EC_{50}[a] (μM)	K_D[b] (μM)	Ratio (K_D/EC_{50})[c] or Intrinsic Activity[d]
Full agonists			
Norepinephrine	0.12 ± 0.013	11.2 ± 0.76	93.3
Epinephrine	0.09 ± 0.014	7.4 ± 0.51	82.2
Phenylephrine	1.4 ± 0.28	13.1 ± 1.1	9.2
Partial agonists			
Oxymetazoline	0.14 ± 0.018	0.19 ± 0.020	72 ± 1.2
Ephedrine	78.0 ± 7.0	36.0 ± 1.0	52 ± 6.3
Phenylpropanolamine	181.0 ± 45.0	220.0 ± 41.0	47 ± 3.3

Source: Data from Minneman et al. (1983).
[a]For contractile responses.
[b]For inhibition of 125IBE binding.
[c]For full agonists.
[d]For partial agonists.

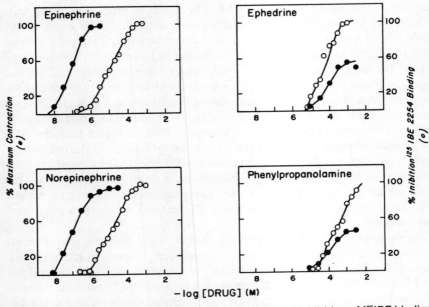

Figure 3.3. Dose-response curves for contraction (●) and inhibition of ^{125}IBE binding (○) in isolated rat vas deferens. Dose-response curves for full agonists on the left, for partial agonists on the right. From *Minneman et al. (1983)*.

essary to show that low doses of phenylpropanolamine and a full agonist were additive in their pharmacodynamic responses, but that at high doses phenyl-propanolamine and the full agonist were antagonistic toward each other. This type of interaction cannot be demonstrated by the data presented. If, indeed, phenylpropanolamine is a partial agonist, much of the existing information regarding effects of phenylpropanolamine would need to be reanalyzed to determine the full spectrum of action of this drug. First, however, it will be essential to test whether phenylpropanolamine is a partial agonist according to the strict pharmacologic definition of the term.

EFFECTS OF PHENYLPROPANOLAMINE ON β-ADRENERGIC RECEPTORS

As mentioned previously, the spectrum of activity of phenylpropanolamine both *in vivo* and in isolated tissues would indicate that phenylpropanolamine acts at α-adrenergic receptors but not at β-adrenergic receptors. The lack of significant effect on bronchial smooth muscle and the apparent lack of effect on cardiac muscle suggest that phenylpropanolamine probably does not affect β-adrenergic sites. However, studies actually demonstrating that effects of phenylpropanolamine are not antagonized by β-blockers, and that phenyl-propanolamine does not bind to β-receptors, have not been published. Perhaps, as is all too often the case, such negative results are available in unpublished studies. As mentioned in the introduction to this section, lack of specific binding to multiple sites is as important in determining the effects of a drug as is the demonstration of specific binding to a particular receptor type. Thus it would be important to investigate the binding of phenylpropanolamine to β-adrenergic receptors.

MECHANISM OF ACTION

Recent studies have investigated the cellular and subcellular mechanisms of action of α-agonist drugs. These studies have demonstrated that binding of α-agonists to adrenergic receptors stimulates the breakdown of polyphosphoinositides to inositol-triphosphates; these inositol-triphosphates are involved in the mobilization of intracelluar Ca^{+2}.

α_1-Agonists stimulated the metabolism of ^{3}H-inositol in the rat vas deferens (Fox et al., 1985). In this study, rats were pretreated with reserpine to deplete endogenous biogenic amines; the vas deferens was removed and incubated in a Krebs-Ringer solution containing ^{3}H-inositol. The accumulation of ^{3}H-inositol phosphates was measured. Phenylpropanolamine increased the accumulation of ^{3}H-inositol phosphates, with an EC_{50} (concentration required to produce 50% of the maximal response) of 34.4 ± 10.0 μM and an intrinsic activity of 98% (compared to norepinephrine $= 100\%$).

Further analysis of the results revealed that, for full agonists, there was a large receptor reserve for stimulation of inositol phosphate turnover; that is, the agonist had to bind to a large proportion of the total receptor population before there was a measurable increase in inositol metabolism. The mechanism was different for partial agonists such as phenylpropanolamine. Partial agonists were equally effective in stimulating inositol metabolism and in causing muscle contraction (i.e., there was no receptor reserve for the partial agonists). These results suggest that there is no linear relationship between the effects of the drugs on inositol metabolism and their effects on smooth muscle contraction (Fox et al., 1985).

In the cerebral cortex as well, α_1-adrenergic agonists increase ^{3}H-inositol metabolism (Minneman & Johnson, 1984). In these studies, slices of rat brain were incubated in a buffer solution containing lithuim chloride and ^{3}H-inositol and the accumulation of ^{3}H-inositol phosphates was measured. Furthermore, the binding of the drugs to α_1-receptors was evaluated by measuring displacement of ^{125}IBE-binding from the particulate fraction of the cortex. (As discussed in a previous section, ^{125}IBE is a radioligand that specifically binds to α_1-adrenergic receptors.)

Full α_1-agonists such as norepinephrine produced dose-related increases in ^{3}H-inositol metabolism; the effects were blocked by prazosin and not by yohimbine, demonstrating that the effects were mediated specifically by stimulation of α_1-receptors (Minneman & Johnson, 1984). Partial agonists such as phenylephrine or methoxamine produced less than maximal stimulation of ^{3}H-inositol metabolism. Even in concentrations as high as 3000 μM, phenylpropanolamine produced no measurable increase in ^{3}H-inositol metabolism in the cerebral cortex. Comparison of receptor occupancy and stimulation of inositol metabolism indicated there was no reserve pool of α_1-adrenergic receptors in the cerebral cortex.

Thus, there are important differences between the mechanism of action of α-agonists in smooth muscle (Fox et al., 1985) and in the CNS (Minneman & Johnson, 1984). Full α-agonists stimulate inositol metabolism and cause pharmacologic responses in both tissues. Phenylpropanolamine, a partial agonist, causes pharmacologic responses in tissues that have spare receptors (e.g., vas deferens) but produces no measurable response in tissues that have no spare receptors (e.g., cerebral cortex).

EFFECTS OF PHENYLPROPANOLAMINE ON THE CARDIOVASCULAR SYSTEM

Despite the controversy regarding whether phenylpropanolamine causes hypertensive crisis and stroke in humans taking phenylpropanolamine in OTC products, there is surprisingly little well-documented information from preclinical studies regarding the effects of phenylpropanolamine on the cardiovascular system. Many of the pharmacological studies in whole animals are early studies from 1930–1960, using primarily the IV route of administration in anesthetized animals. Carefully controlled dose-response studies in conscious animals using oral or parenteral administration of phenylpropanolamine are not available. The lack of information regarding effects of oral doses of phenylpropanolamine on the cardiovascular system is a major limitation in evaluating effects of the drug on cardiovascular parameters, since oral administration is the usual therapeutic route. Also, data regarding the effects of chronic administration of phenylpropanolamine on the cardiovascular system in experimental animals are virtually nonexistent.

In a classic study of structure-activity relationships for pressor effects in a series of sympathomimetic amines, Barger and Dale (1910) noted the following structural requirements for pressor effects. Maximum activity was observed when a two-carbon chain separated the phenyl ring and the amino nitrogen. Primary and secondary amines were more potent than tertiary amines. Whereas the catechol nucleus was not absolutely required for activity, activity was markedly increased by the 3,4-dihydroxy substitution on the phenyl ring. Finally, the β-OH substitution increased activity only when the 3,4-dihydroxy substitution was present. Thus while phenylpropanolamine was not specifically tested in this study, it is not unreasonable to predict that phenylpropanolamine would have pressor activity, but with relatively weak potency compared to other β-phenylethylamines.

The earliest report of the cardiovascular effects of phenylpropanolamine (simply identified as dl-β-phenyl-β-hydroxy-α-methylethylamine · HCl) was that by Chen et al. (1929). In cats with spinal transections, "0.2 cc. of a M/20 solution" (1.88 mg) IV produced an increase in arterial blood pressure equivalent to 0.0125 mg of epinephrine; the effect lasted 45 min. Phenylpropanolamine was 1/150 as potent as epinephrine in this study. Chen et al. (1929) also reported the synthesis and pressor activity of the phenylpropanolamine analog, 3-hydroxy-phenylpropanolamine (α-methyloctopamine). α-Methyloctopamine was more potent than phenylpropanolamine, with a potency ratio of 187:125. In contrast, Trendelenburg et al. (1962a) reported that phenylpropanolamine and α-methyloctopamine were equipotent for pressor effects. These latter authors reported that in two volunteers taking 50 mg of phenylpropanolamine, maximum increases in systolic blood pressure were 30 and 16 mm Hg.

Hartung & Munch (1931) reported the synthesis of four isomeric phenylpropylamines, one of which was phenylpropanolamine. The pressor effects of these drugs were of interest for two reasons: (1) previous studies had shown that while β-phenylethylamine decreased blood pressure and increased force of contraction of the heart, α-phenylethylamine had opposite effects (increased blood pressure, decreased force of contraction); and (2) Barger & Dale (1910) had proposed that the maximum pressor effect occurred when a two-carbon link separated the phenyl ring and the amino nitrogen. These observations were confirmed by demonstrating that phenylpropanolamine (IV, in dogs) had pressor activity that was equivalent to ephedrine. No quantitative results were presented, however.

In one of the earliest clinical studies of its cardiovascular effects, phenylpropanolamine (IV) was shown to increase blood pressure and decrease heart rate (Loman et al., 1939). In eight subjects, 50 mg of Propadrine (IV) increased systolic blood pressure by 44–82 mm Hg, and in four subjects 20–25 mg Propadrine (IV) increased systolic blood pressure by 0–28 mm Hg. The maximum increase in blood pressure occurred at 1–7 min, and the time to recovery was 30–95 min. In the combined dose groups, the decrease in heart rate ranged from 16 to 36 bpm. No cardiac arrhythmias were observed.

Phenylpropanolamine (50 mg, IV) was effective in sustaining blood pressure in patients undergoing spinal anesthesia (Lorhan & Mosser, 1947). This dose produced consistent and reproducible effects, either IM or IV, while a lower dose (15 mg, IV) was ineffective. The mean duration of action of phenylpropanolamine was 45 min, with a range of less than 15 min to 75 min. Phenylpropanolamine produced no change in heart rate. However, it should be noted that the effective response in this study was maintenance of blood pressure at preanesthetic levels (i.e., prevention of spinal anesthesia-induced hypotension), and the relevance of these results to conscious, unrestrained subjects is not known.

The effects of 25 mg of phenylpropanolamine (PO)—alone or in combination with 100 mg of caffeine—on blood pressure and heart rate were measured as part of a clinical safety study (Silverman et al., 1980). Phenylpropanolamine alone did not significantly increase blood pressure or heart rate. As part of a study investigating interactions between phenylpropanolamine and belladonna alkaloids, phenylpropanolamine (50 mg, sustained-release tablet, twice daily for 4 weeks) had no effect on blood pressure or pulse rate compared to placebo in 32 normotensive volunteers (Mitchell, 1968). Noble (1982) presented evidence that phenylpropanolamine (50 mg, PO, t.i.d. for 12 weeks) did not increase the blood pressure in obese patients, compared to placebo (Figure 3.4).

In summary, these studies suggest that phenylpropanolamine produces an

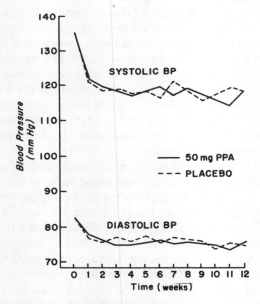

Figure 3.4. Mean systolic and diastolic blood pressure in obese patients taking PPA (50 mg, t.i.d.) or placebo for 12 weeks. Abscissa: time (weeks). Ordinate: blood pressure (mmHg). From *Noble (1982)*.

increase in blood pressure and a decrease or no change in heart rate when administered IV, but no change in either blood pressure or heart rate when given orally. However, certain factors limit the interpretation based on these results. First, in the IV studies the doses of phenylpropanolamine were 20–50 mg (Loman et al., 1939; Lorhan & Mosser, 1947), whereas in the PO studies the doses were 50 mg (Mitchell, 1968; Noble, 1982). Blood levels of phenylpropanolamine following 50 mg (IV) would be considerably higher than following 50 mg (PO), so that a greater pharmacodynamic effect would be expected following IV dosing. Second, the IV studies involved acute administration of phenylpropanolamine, whereas the PO studies were chronic administration.

However, the limited data available from preclinical studies seem to parallel this difference between IV and PO dosing with regard to effects on the cardiovascular system. The comparisons are limited because IV administration of phenylpropanolamine was investigated in anesthetized cats or dogs and PO administration was investigated in unanesthetized rats. Thus species differences and level of anesthesia may confound the comparisons.

In anesthetized cats with intact vagi, IV administration of phenylpropanolamine (±-norephedrine, referred to as "norephedrine" in the article) produced a dose-dependent increase in systolic blood pressure and heart rate (Table 3.9) (Persson et al., 1973). The high dose of phenylpropanolamine (200 μg/kg, IV) was investigated in only one experiment. The increased heart rate in the presence of an increase in blood pressure is difficult to interpret, since the vagi were intact and presumably the baroreceptor mechanism was functioning. However, the time courses of the two responses were not reported, and it is possible that a transient tachycardia occurred prior to the baroreceptor reflex effects. Pressor responses to 100–250 μg/kg of phenylpro-

TABLE 3.9. Effects of Phenylpropanolamine on Blood Pressure and Heart Rate in Anesthetized Cats[a]

Dose (μg/kg, IV)	n	Systolic Blood Pressure (Δ mm Hg)	Heart Rate (Δ bpm)
10	5	12 ± 2	6 ± 3
20	5	25 ± 8	13 ± 3
25	1	20	5
40	3	33 ± 14	18 ± 2
50	4	50 ± 15	14 ± 5
200	1	120	58

Source: Data adapted from Persson et al. (1973).
[a] Mean ± SD; n = total of 9 cats (1–3 doses per cat).

panolamine (IV) were also reported in cats with spinal transections (D'Mello, 1969).

In contrast, phenylpropanolamine (0.5–1.0 mg/kg, IV) produced no consistent effect on systemic blood pressure in anesthetized dogs (Aviado & Schmidt, 1957). The reason for the difference between the responses in cats and dogs is unclear. The cats were anesthetized with pentobarbital, whereas the dogs were anesthetized with morphine and chloralose. In the cat study, relatively lower doses were used (0.01–0.2 mg/kg, IV), whereas in the dog study higher doses (0.5–1.0 mg/kg, IV) were used. Persson et al. (1973) did note that dose-response curves were not reliably produced at doses greater than 0.1 mg/kg in the cat. Thus it is possible that the doses in the dog study were too high to produce reliable responses from IV administration.

However, phenylpropanolamine (20 mg/kg, PO) produced no significant effect on blood pressure in unanesthetized, unrestrained rats (Figure 3.5) (McIlreath et al., 1965). These studies were conducted in adult male rats with intraarterial catheters chronically implanted in the abdominal aorta; blood pressure was monitored continuously following PO drug administration. The maximum increase in blood pressure (6.4%) was not significant, but was as-

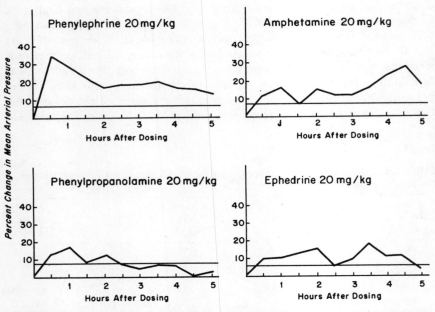

Figure 3.5. Blood pressure in unrestrained, unanesthetized rats following PO administration of sympathomimetic amines. Abscissa: time (hr). Ordinate: mean arterial pressure (% change). From *McIlreath et al. (1965)*.

sociated with a significant decrease in heart rate. The magnitude of the heart rate change was not reported. The rats were monitored for overt side effects, but phenylpropanolamine produced no observable side effects. Even though only a single dose of phenylpropanolamine was tested, this dose is within the behaviorally effective dose range in rats. In comparison, phenylephrine (20 mg/kg, PO) produced a significant increase in arterial blood pressure and decrease in heart rate.

Intravenous phenylpropanolamine [i.e., ($\pm$)-norephedrine] produced a dose-dependent increase in the mean arterial pressure in anesthetized rats (Moya-Huff et al., 1987). In this study, cumulative doses of phenylpropanolamine ranging from 0.3125 to 10 mg/kg were administered IV. The highest dose of phenylpropanolamine (10 mg/kg) increased the mean arterial pressure by 45 $\pm$ 11 mm Hg. Pretreatment of the rats with reserpine to deplete endogenous catecholamines failed to abolish the phenylpropanolamine-induced increase in arterial pressure, indicating this was a direct action of phenylpropanolamine. Comparison of the pressor effects of phenylpropanolamine isomers indicated that *l*-norephedrine and phenylpropanolamine were the most potent, while *d*-norephedrine, *d*-norpseudoephedrine, and *l*-norpseudoephedrine were relatively inactive.

The effects of norephedrine isomers on adrenergic-receptor subtypes were investigated in anesthetized pithed rats (Moya-Huff & Maher, 1987). The receptor-subtype activity was inferred by measuring effects on arterial blood pressure. For all the receptor subtypes, *l*-norephedrine was most potent, *d,l*-norephedrine was intermediate, and *d*-norephedrine was least potent. The cardiovascular effects of *l*-norephedrine were mediated primarily by α_1-adrenergic receptors, with less activity mediated by α_2- and β_1-adrenergic receptors; *l*-norephedrine had very low potency for β_2-receptor activity.

In the rat but not in other species, phenylpropanolamine is metabolized to *p*-hydroxynorephedrine. Since *p*-hydroxynorephedrine is a vasopressor, this metabolite might be involved in the cardiovascular effects of phenylpropanolamine in this species. To investigate this possibility, rats were pretreated with either iprindole or SKF-525A to inhibit *p*-hydroxylation, then given 6 mg/kg of phenylpropanolamine (the route of administration was not specified; Snoddy et al., 1985). Pretreatment with the hydroxylation inhibitors did not alter the cardiovascular effects of phenylpropanolamine, indicating that the metabolite *p*-hydroxynorephedrine was not responsible for the effects.

Phenylpropanolamine (0.01–10.0 mg/liter) produced marked increases in heart rate in the isolated heart-lung preparation of the dog (Liebman, 1961). The maximum increase in heart rate was approximately 80 bpm and occurred at a concentration of 3.0 mg/liter. These results contrast sharply with those from *in vivo* studies demonstrating that phenylpropanolamine did not alter heart rate. Two factors contribute to this difference: (1) 3.0 mg/liter is a very high dose level for phenylpropanolamine [in clinical usage, blood levels of phenylpropanolamine are approximately 50–200 ng/ml (Dowse et al., 1983; Mason & Amick, 1981)]; and (2) in intact animals the baroreceptor reflex mechanism tends to prevent such large fluctuations in basal heart rate. Finally, it should be noted that positive chronotropic effects of sympathomimetic amines are mediated via β_2-adrenergic receptors, whereas phenylpropanolamine has predominantly α-adrenergic activity. The cardioaccelerator effects of high doses of phenylpropanolamine in the isolated heart preparation may represent nonspecific effects of phenylpropanolamine.

Phenylpropanolamine also increased the rate of contraction in the isolated guinea pig atrium (Trendelenburg et al., 1963). The maximum increase in rate was 35/min and occurred at a relatively high concentration of 10 μg/ml phenylpropanolamine. Even higher concentrations of phenylpropanolamine (greater than 100 μg/ml) decreased the rate of contraction. Reserpine pretreatment shifted the phenylpropanolamine dose-response curve to the right (i.e., inhibited the response) but did not completely abolish the response. These results indicate that phenylpropanolamine increased the heart rate primarily by a direct action on the heart and not by releasing endogenous catecholamines.

Sympathomimetic drugs increase the irritability and automaticity of heart muscle (Greiner & Garb, 1950). The isolated cat papillary muscle was used in a bioassay of drug effects on the heart; irritability was measured by determining the minimum electric current required to produce muscle contraction. Eight sympathomimetic amines, including Propadrine, increased the heart irritability. Propadrine was effective at concentrations ranging from 0.54 to 54 μM. Propadrine (5.4 μM; approximately 1.0 mg/ml) induced spontaneous rhythmicity in only one of six papillary muscles; this concentration is considerably higher than the blood levels of phenylpropanolamine in clinical usage (see foregoing).

In isolated tissue studies, phenylpropanolamine produced dose-dependent contractions of smooth muscle from both arteries and veins (Persson et al., 1973; Stevens & Moulds, 1981; Stevens et al., 1981), which would contribute to the increase in arterial blood pressure seen in whole animals. However, phenylpropanolamine had very low potency for vasoconstriction in all the studies. Effects of phenylpropanolamine on force of contraction in isolated heart preparations (e.g., Langendorff heart preparation) have not been reported. Thus the effects of phenylpropanolamine on force of contraction *in vitro* are not known. Since adrenergic receptors in the heart are primarily β_1-receptors, and since phenylpropanolamine exerts its effect primarily via action on α-receptors, it is unlikely that phenylpropanolamine would affect the force of contraction of the heart. Nonetheless, it would be important to test for direct cardiac effects of phenylpropanolamine *in vitro*.

Two studies have tested phenylpropanolamine for effects on specialized cardiovascular responses, both with negative results. Phenylpropanolamine (0.5–1.0 mg/kg, IV, in anesthetized dogs) produced no consistent change in systemic blood pressure, pulmonary blood pressure, pulmonary venous outflow or pulmonary vascular resistance (Aviado & Schmidt, 1957). Levy and Ahlquist (1957) studied a series of drugs with respect to effects on the "epinephrine reversal" phenomenon in anesthetized dogs. The epinephrine reversal refers to the fact that in an untreated animal, epinephrine produces pressor effects, whereas in an animal pretreated with an α-blocker, epinephrine produces depressor effects. Ephedrine was shown to reverse the "epinephrine reversal" in anesthetized dogs, but phenylpropanolamine (20 mg/kg, IV) had no such effect. The significance of these findings is obscure.

One clinically important aspect of the cardiovascular effects of sympathomimetic amines is the phenomenon of tachyphylaxis or acute tolerance. When certain sympathomimetic amines, especially amines with pronounced indirect effects, are given repeatedly at short intervals, the pharmacodynamic effect soon decreases. This phenomenon is known as tachyphylaxis. In the case of indirect-acting amines, tachyphylaxis is thought to be due to acute depletion of norepinephrine, since coadministration of an exogenous dose of norepinephrine reestablishes the full response to the test amine. Tachyphylaxis has been well demonstrated for several sympathomimetic amines and is often assumed to occur with phenylpropanolamine. Tachyphylaxis to the pressor effects of a series of sympathomimetic amines was tested in anesthetized, vagotomized cats (Huidobro & Croxatto, 1951). Tachyphylaxis to Propadrine (0.5 mg of the base, in distilled water, IV; equivalent to approximately 0.125–0.33 mg/kg) was demonstrated in one experiment, although the actual results were not presented. Tachyphylaxis was reversed by administration of epinephrine (IV) 1–3 min before the test dose of Propadrine.

In contrast, there was no tachyphylaxis to the pressor effect of IV phenylpropanolamine in rats (Moya-Huff et al., 1987). In this study, anesthetized rats were given 1 mg/kg of phenylpropanolamine IV once every 5 min for a total of four doses. The first dose of phenylpropanolamine increased the blood pressure by 59 ± 8 mm Hg. Subsequent doses produced increases in the blood pressure that were not significantly different from the effect of the first dose. Similarly, there was no tachyphylaxis to the phenylpropanolamine isomer *l*-norephedrine; on the other hand, there was tachyphylaxis to the pressor effect of *d*-norephedrine. These results indicate that phenylpropanolamine and *l*-norephedrine are direct-acting drugs, whereas *d*-norephedrine is an indirect-acting drug.

One other aspect of chronic administration of sympathomimetic amines, which has not been investigated for phenylpropanolamine, is the paradoxical antihypertensive effect. Although acute systemic administration of norepinephrine produces an increase in systemic arterial blood pressure, local application of norepinephrine to the baroreceptor area produces a paradoxical hypotensive response, presumably as a result of local vasoconstriction causing increased discharge from the baroreceptor. In addition, when pressor amines were chronically administered to hypertensive animals, a paradoxical antihypertensive response to the amines developed (Vidrio & Pardo, 1973). Unfortunately, the effects of phenylpropanolamine in such a paradigm were not investigated.

In summary, the information available suggests that phenylpropanolamine has negligible effects on blood pressure when administered PO but increases blood pressure when administered IV. Phenylpropanolamine may either increase heart rate or reflexly decrease heart rate. No tachyphylaxis developed to the pressor effect of phenylpropanolamine. Well-controlled dose-response studies of the effects of phenylpropanolamine on cardiovascular parameters in unanesthetized unrestrained experimental animals have not been reported, nor have the effects of classical adrenergic antagonists on cardiovascular responses to phenylpropanolamine in intact animals. Evidence from isolated tissue studies indicates that phenylpropanolamine is a weak vasoconstrictor in arteries and veins, an effect mediated via α-receptors. In isolated tissue preparations, phenylpropanolamine increased the heart rate and irritability of the papillary muscle.

PHENYLPROPANOLAMINE: DIRECT- OR INDIRECT-ACTING AMINE?

Phenylpropanolamine has sympathomimetic activity at several sites of action. As detailed above, experimental results indicate that phenylpropanolamine is an α-adrenergic agonist with low potency and low intrinsic activity. However, whether phenylpropanolamine is a direct-, mixed-, or indirect-acting amine is an issue that has not been clearly resolved. In this section, various lines of evidence are reviewed in an attempt to determine whether phenylpropanolamine exerts its pharmacological effects by direct, indirect, or mixed activity.

The criteria for determining whether a sympathomimetic agent is a direct-, indirect- or mixed-acting drug are summarized in Table 3.10. Direct-acting drugs bind to specific receptors to produce either α- or β-adrenergic effects. Indirect-acting drugs, in contrast, do not bind to adrenergic receptors but rather produce sympathomimetic effects by increasing neurotransmission at noradrenergic synapses. Indirect-acting sympathomimetic drugs act via several mechanisms, including stimulating release of norepinephrine, inhibiting reuptake of norepinephrine, and inhibiting the metabolism of released norepinephrine. Most of the sympathomimetic drugs are mixed-acting agents and act via a mixture of direct and indirect actions.

Although sympathomimetic drugs are often classified into these three categories, Trendelenburg et al. (1962a,b) showed that most of the drugs actually demonstrate a spectrum of activity along the direct-mixed-indirect activity continuum. In addition, they pointed out that a given drug can exert direct activity in one physiologic system (e.g., smooth muscle) and indirect activity in another (e.g., the cardiovascular system). These authors concluded, on the basis of an extensive series of *in vivo* experiments, that the effects of phenylpropanolamine on the nictitating membrane (a model for effects on smooth muscle) were due predominantly to direct actions, whereas the cardiovascular effects, and especially the effects on heart rate, were due predominantly to indirect actions.

The indirect activity of phenylpropanolamine on the cardiovascular system was demonstrated both *in vivo* (Trendelenburg et al., 1962a,b) and *in vitro* (Liebman, 1961). In these studies, pretreatment of experimental animals with reserpine, which depleted neuronal stores of norepinephrine, diminished the cardioaccelerator and pressor responses produced by phenylpropanolamine, suggesting that phenylpropanolamine increased heart rate and blood pressure by releasing norepinephrine.

Data suggesting indirect actions of phenylpropanolamine on the cardiovascular system are corroborated by several studies showing that phenylpropanolamine inhibits reuptake of norepinephrine in isolated heart preparations (Burgen & Iversen, 1965; Iversen, 1964; Levitt et al., 1974; Swamy et al., 1969). However, phenylpropanolamine did not stimulate release of norepinephrine (Levitt et al., 1974) and had no effect on norepinephrine levels (Shore, 1966) in isolated heart preparations. The results of Shore (1966) are difficult to interpret because only a single dose level of phenylpropanolamine was investigated, and possible effects of phenylpropanolamine on norepinephrine metabolism, uptake, and release were not investigated.

Further evidence supporting the view that phenylpropanolamine acts indirectly on the cardiovascular system is suggested by the results of studies employing monoamine oxidase (MAO) inhibitors. The effects of phenylpropanolamine on blood pressure were potentiated by MAO inhibitors in humans (Cuthbert et al., 1969; Cuthbert & Vere, 1971) and cats (D'Mello, 1969), suggesting an effect on norepinephrine or phenylpropanolamine metabolism. However, the cardiovascular effects of phenylpropanolamine were not potentiated by MAO inhibitors in dogs (Gatgounis, 1965). This difference in response cannot be attributed to simple species differences in metabolism of phenylpropanolamine, because phenylpropanolamine is not metabolized in humans. (It is excreted primarily unchanged in the urine.) Thus potentiation of phenylpropanolamine by MAO inhibitors cannot be due to inhibition of the metabolism of phenylpropanolamine itself. Studies on the metabolism of phenylpropanolamine in cats and dogs have not been reported. It is possible

TABLE 3.10. Direct Versus Indirect Actions of Sympathomimetic Amines[a]

Tests	Sympathomimetic Amines			Phenylpropanolamine			
	Direct Acting	Mixed Acting	Indirect Acting	Effect	Tissue	Classification	Reference
Receptor binding	+	+	O	(+)[b]	Smooth muscle α-adrenergic	Direct	Minneman et al. (1983)
Reserpine	O(I)[c]	I/O	D	D	Cardiovascular	Indirect	Trendelenburg et al. (1962a, b) Liebman (1961)
				O	Nictitating membrane	Direct	Trendelenburg et al. (1962, a, b)
				O	Vascular smooth muscle	Direct	Persson et al. (1973)
Cocaine	I/O[d]	O/D[e]	D	O	Nictitating membrane	Direct	Trendelenburg et al. (1962a, b)
Chronic denervation	I	I/O	D	O	Nictitating membrane	Mixed	Trendelenburg et al. (1962a, b)

Process					System	Action	References
Release of norepinephrine	O	I/O	–	O	Cardiovascular	Direct	Levitt et al. (1974)
Inhibit reuptake of norepinephrine	O[d]	+/O	+	+	Cardiovascular	Indirect	Iverson (1964), Burgen & Iversen (1965), Swamy et al. (1969), Levitt et al. (1974)
Storage of norepinephrine	O	I/O	(D?)	+	Smooth muscle	Indirect	Swamy et al. (1969)
				O	Cardiovascular	Direct (?)	Shore (1966)
				O	Central nervous system	Direct (?)	Breese et al. (1970)
MAO inhibitors	O/I[f]	I/O	–	I/O	Cardiovascular	Mixed	Gatgounis (1965), O'Mello (1969), Cuthbert et al. (1969), Cuthbert & Vere (1971)
Tachyphylaxis	O	+/O	+	+	Cardiovascular	Indirect (?)	Huidobro & Croxatto (1951)

127

that MAO inhibition potentiates the activity of norepinephrine released by phenylpropanolamine; however, as described above, there is no experimental evidence to demonstrate that phenylpropanolamine does in fact release norepinephrine. It is more likely that since MAO inhibitors prevent the metabolism of norepinephrine, and since phenylpropanolamine inhibits the reuptake of norepinephrine, these two effects are additive when phenylpropanolamine is given in the presence of MAO inhibitors. Studies of the interaction between phenylpropanolamine and MAO inhibitors are discussed in detail in a subsequent section of this chapter (see "Drug Interactions, Potentiation of Phenylpropanolamine by Monoamine Oxidase Inhibitors").

Tachyphylaxis, a decrease in the intensity of drug response when the drug is given repeatedly at brief intervals, is a characteristic of indirect-acting amines. There is one report of tachyphylaxis with IV administration of Propadrine in the cat (Huidobro & Croxatto, 1951). Presumably, one animal was tested at one dose level; however, no details were presented, and it is not possible to evaluate this study. In contrast, no tachyphylaxis developed to the pressor effect of IV phenylpropanolamine in the rat (Moya-Huff et al., 1987). Details of the study of tachyphylaxis to phenylpropanolamine are presented more completely in a previous section of this chapter (see "Effects of Phenylpropanolamine on the Cardiovascular System").

Unfortunately, there are no published reports of studies specifically designed to test for direct effects of phenylpropanolamine on adrenergic receptors in cardiovascular tissue. Since adrenergic receptors in the heart are predominantly β-receptors, and since phenylpropanolamine has predominantly α-adrenergic activity, it is unlikely that phenylpropanolamine has direct effects on receptor activity in the heart. Furthermore, the effects of cocaine or chronic denervation, which can be used to test for direct activity of sympathomimetic drugs, on the cardiovascular activity of phenylpropanolamine have not been reported. Thus, although several lines of evidence indicate that phenylpropanolamine has indirect activity on the cardiovascular system, there is virtually no evidence that would indicate whether phenylpropanolamine also has direct cardiovascular effects.

In contrast, there is evidence that phenylpropanolamine has predominantly direct activity in smooth muscle. Neither reserpine pretreatment (which depletes neuronal stores of norepinephrine) nor administration of cocaine (which inhibits the amine uptake system) altered the ability of phenylpropanolamine to cause contraction of the nictitating membrane in cats (Trendelenburg et al., 1962a,b). *In vitro* experiments using smooth muscle preparations showed that phenylpropanolamine caused contraction of smooth muscle in vas deferens (Minneman et al., 1983), uterus (Ghouri & Haley, 1969), and vascular tissue (Persson et al., 1973; Stevens & Moulds, 1981); in GI smooth muscle, phenylpropanolamine caused inhibition of activity (Ghouri & Haley, 1969). In a test for direct effects of phenylpropanolamine on smooth muscle, it was shown that the effects of phenylpropanolamine on contraction of isolated aortic strips were not altered by pretreatment of the animals with reserpine (Persson et al., 1973), indicating that phenylpropanolamine acts on vascular smooth muscle by direct action. Finally, phenylpropanolamine does bind directly to α-adrenergic receptors in smooth muscle tissue from the rat vas deferens, although with very low affinity (Minneman et al., 1983). Thus the direct effects of phenylpropanolamine on smooth muscle are well established.

Apparently, phenylpropanolamine also has some indirect effects on smooth muscle. Phenylpropanolamine inhibited reuptake of norepinephrine in the vas deferens (Swamy et al., 1969). Whether phenylpropanolamine alters the release or storage of norepinephrine in noradrenergic neurons in smooth muscle has not been reported.

In summary, there is evidence that phenylpropanolamine is a direct-acting amine in smooth muscle and that phenylpropanolamine is an indirect-acting amine in the cardiovascular system. There is incomplete evidence for a direct effect of phenylpropanolamine on the cardiovascular system and some evidence that phenylpropanolamine is a direct-acting amine in vascular smooth muscle. Thus the conventional classification of phenylpropanolamine as a mixed-acting amine with primarily indirect activity in the cardiovascular system and primarily direct activity in smooth muscle may need reconsideration.

MISCELLANEOUS SYMPATHOMIMETIC EFFECTS

Sympathomimetic amines are known to stimulate lipolysis and release of free fatty acids from adipose tissue by a combination of α- and β-adrenergic effects. Phenylpropanolamine was shown to stimulate release of free fatty acids from adipose tissue *in vitro* (Feller & Finger, 1970; Finger & Feller, 1966). Phenylpropanolamine had low potency and low intrinsic activity for release of free fatty acids. The lipolytic activity of a series of sympathomimetic amines was investigated in this study. Because of the experimental design employed, it is not possible to strictly assign the effects of the drugs to α versus β activity, but on the basis of rank order of potency of the drugs, the effects are probably more dependent on β-adrenergic activity.

Sympathomimetic amines may also stimulate release of catecholamines from the adrenal gland. In one study, it was demonstrated that phenylpropanolamine ($8 \times 10^{-5}\ M$) increased the release of catecholamines from isolated, denervated adrenal glands (Rubin & Jaanus, 1966). This effect of phenylpropanolamine was abolished by incubating the glands in either calcium-free medium or a solution of the ganglionic blocker hexamethonium. However, whether this effect of phenylpropanolamine occurs *in vivo* and the role that such an action has on the overall response of the whole animal to phenylpropanolamine are unknown.

Effects of phenylpropanolamine on urinary excretion of water and electrolytes was investigated in one study (Viveros et al., 1970). The 5-hr water diuresis model in rats was used. Phenylpropanolamine (10 mg/kg, PO) had no effect on total urine volume or excretion of potassium but increased excretion of sodium and chloride and raised the Na^+/K^+ ratio. The mechanism of this effect of phenylpropanolamine was not determined. However, in a series of phenylethylamines tested, only amines with α-adrenergic and vasoconstrictor properties increased urinary excretion of electrolytes. More detailed analysis of the mechanism of action of metaraminol on urinary excretion showed that not all the effects of metaraminol could be attributed to α-adrenergic vasoconstriction. The nature of the direct renal and extrarenal effects was not investigated.

Finally, sympathomimetic amines stimulate the secretion of certain glands such as the pancreas and salivary glands. The limited information available suggests that phenylpropanolamine has only minimal effects on insulin secretion and blood glucose in normal animals (Krantz & Hartung, 1931; Resnick et al., 1978; Sandage & Fletcher, 1983). However, phenylpropanolamine may have modest hypoglycemic effects in stressed animals (Fletcher et al., 1982) or in mildly but not severely diabetic animals (Hoebel, 1977; Resnick et al., 1978). The effects of phenylpropanolamine on secretion of the salivary glands has apparently not been investigated.

NASOPHARYNGEAL AND PULMONARY EFFECTS

One of the major clinical uses of phenylpropanolamine is in combination products for cough and cold remedies. Although the rationale for including phenylpropanolamine in these combination products is presumably for its nasal decongestant and antitussive effects, there is limited preclinical information available regarding the efficacy of phenylpropanolamine for these effects. There is, on the other hand, considerable evidence from clinical studies showing that the combination products do provide subjective relief of signs and symptoms of common colds and other mild upper respiratory disorders. The following is a review of the preclinical studies of the efficacy of phenylpropanolamine for nasopharyngeal and pulmonary effects.

The antitussive effects of phenylpropanolamine were tested in dogs and guinea pigs (Winter & Flataker, 1954). Dogs were placed in a closed chamber, and chemically elicited coughing was produced by introducing an irritating vapor (0.5 N H_2SO_4) into the chamber. Coughs were recorded by a microphone attached to the dogs' throats. Phenylpropanolamine (1–8 mg/kg, PO) produced a dose-dependent decrease in coughing. In the guinea pig study, test animals were placed in a restraining chamber and coughing was induced by delivering a 2.8% ammonia vapor through a nebulizer. Phenylpropanolamine produced a dose-dependent decrease in the number of coughs (Table 3.11). In both the dog study and the guinea pig study, the antitussive effects of several drugs were compared. Phenylpropanolamine was nearly as effective as codeine as an antitussive in both species.

The decongestant activity of phenylpropanolamine was investigated in animals (Aviado et al., 1959) and humans (see Chapter 5). Presumably, the decongestant activity is related to local vasoconstriction in the nasal mucosa.

In dogs, decongestant effects were assessed by simultaneously measuring blood pressure, carotid blood flow, and intranasal pressure in anesthetized animals (Aviado et al., 1959). Intranasal pressure was measured by closing off the nasopharynx by means of inflating a balloon in the back of the nasopharyngeal cavity, filling the cavity with saline, and recording the fluid pressure in the cavity via a pressure transducer inserted in the nares. Epinephrine, injected intraarterially (IA) into the carotid, produced an increase in systemic blood pressure that was associated with a biphasic effect on carotid blood flow. There was a brief period of increased carotid flow, followed by a more prolonged decrease in flow. Intraarterial administration of epinephrine produced a decrease in intranasal pressure, indicating a decongestant action. Phenylpropanolamine (100 μg, IA) produced essentially the same response as epinephrine: a decrease in carotid blood flow associated with a decrease in intranasal pressure, indicating a decongestant action. There was one important difference between phenylpropanolamine and epinephrine. For phenylpropanolamine, the decrease in carotid blood flow was greater than the decrease in intranasal pressure, whereas for epinephrine, the sensitivities of the two vascular beds were the reverse.

Another sympathomimetic effect which is potentially beneficial in cough and cold remedies is bronchodilation. However, there is no evidence that phenylpropanolamine produces bronchodilation. Although the effects of phenylpropanolamine on bronchial smooth muscle have not been specifically

TABLE 3.11. Effects of Phenylpropanolamine on Artificially Induced Coughs in Guinea Pigs

Dose of Phenylpropanolamine (mg/kg, SC)	Reduction in Coughs/3 min (No.)
0.5	8.5 ± 2.7[a]
1	18.0 ± 2.8
2	23.7 ± 1.5

Source: Data from Winter and Flataker (1954).
[a]Mean ± SEM. Control—30.6 ± 15.6 coughs/3 min.

tested, it has been demonstrated that norephedrine produced weak broncho-constriction in the isolated trachea-bronchi-lung preparation from the guinea pig (Tainter et al., 1934). In that study, the isomer of norephedrine (identified as Propadrine) was not specified. One of the isomers of norephedrine, d-norpseudoephedrine, was shown to be a weak bronchoconstrictor in the isolated guinea pig whole trachea preparation (Maitai, 1975). In contrast, ephedrine, pseudoephedrine, and epinephrine are effective bronchodilators (Maitai, 1975; Tainter et al., 1934). Furthermore, bronchodilation is a β_2-adrenergic effect. Thus, although the bronchodilator-bronchoconstrictor effects of phenylpropanolamine have not been specifically tested, there is reason to believe that phenylpropanolamine is not a potent bronchodilator.

In summary, there is evidence that phenylpropanolamine is an effective decongestant and antitussive drug, and these effects are the basis for including phenylpropanolamine in combination products for cough and cold remedies. The bronchodilator activity of phenylpropanolamine has not been specifically tested, but phenylpropanolamine is probably not an effective bronchodilator.

ANORECTIC ACTIVITY

MECHANISMS OF REGULATION OF FOOD INTAKE

Regulation of food intake is a complex biological process that involves regulatory mechanisms at biochemical, cellular, organic, organismic, endocrinologic, behavioral, social, and even cultural levels. Obviously, any drug, including phenylpropanolamine, that is used for its anorectic effects could theoretically affect regulation of food intake at any of these levels and may well act at several levels to reduce hunger and decrease food intake. Recent reviews consider the biological mechanisms involved in regulation of food intake (Hoebel, 1977, 1979, 1985). An extensive review of the several theories of regulation of food intake is beyond the scope of this book, and these theories are mentioned only briefly here. Glucostatic theories suggest that hunger and satiety are controlled by changes in blood glucose levels or by related factors such as glucose utilization, insulin, or glucose receptors. Glucose receptors have been identified in the brain, the liver, and the GI tract. According to lipostatic theories, food intake is controlled by either the body fat deposits or related factors such as serum free fatty acids or triglycerides. Central nervous system theories emphasize the role of hunger and satiety centers in the hypothalamus as sites of regulation of food intake. Neurotransmitters, especially norepinephrine and serotonin, are important in regulation of hunger, appetite, and satiety. Miscellaneous factors include hormones (insulin, cholecystokinin), oral and GI factors (taste, gastric contractions, gastric distention), vagal influences, opioid peptides, exercise, and energy balance. Short- and long-term regulation of food intake are generally considered to be controlled by independent mechanisms.

Hunger and appetite are considered to be two distinct physiological phenomena, and the differences between them are important when designing and evaluating experimental studies of regulation of food intake, especially in experimental animals. Hunger is a physiological need of an animal for food, usually occasioned by food deprivation. In contrast, appetite is a psychological motivation for food intake, which is independent of the individual's nutritional state. Hunger and appetite can be distinguished in human subjects by measuring their food intake during a test meal and interviewing them regarding their motivation for food. In experimental animals, motivation for food cannot be determined by interview techniques and more indirect experimental methods must be used. Many of the preclinical studies of anorectic effects of drugs utilize rats as subjects. Under free-running conditions rats are "nibblers," consuming their food in numerous small meals at intervals throughout the day and night, with a predominance for eating during the night, since rats are nocturnal animals. Quantitation of food intake under these conditions is difficult because of the nature of the eating patterns. Meal patterns under free-running conditions probably represent a measure of appetite rather than hunger, but it is possible to train rats to consume their entire daily food intake in a single large "meal" by withholding food for most of the time (usually 18–23 hr/day) and allowing the rats access to food only during the remainder of the day. Measurement of food intake is usually more reliable under such conditions. In addition, since the animals are relatively deprived of food even though their body weights are maintained, food intake during the single meal may be considered a measure of hunger rather than appetite. A further refinement in the attempt to measure motivation for food intake rather than hunger is the use of operant conditioning techniques to measure the animals' willingness to work for a food reward. However, it should be noted that rats on a food-deprivation, restricted-feeding schedule may undergo multiple physiologic adaptations to the relative starvation. The endocrine status of the animals may be especially susceptible to food deprivation. Thus in assessing pharmacodynamic effects of drugs on food intake it is necessary to test the drug effects under several experimental conditions before extrapolating from animal data to predict efficacy in humans.

Finally, it should be noted that regulation of food intake and regulation of body weight are not necessarily causally related. Obviously, body-weight loss or gain is the net result of multiple factors, including food intake, food composition, food utilization, energy utilization, and overall level of activity. Thus in studies of the anorectic efficacy of drugs it becomes important to measure both food intake and body-weight loss (or gain) in order to assess efficacy of the drug treatment.

EFFECTS OF PHENYLPROPANOLAMINE ON BODY WEIGHT

In early experimental studies on the effects of phenylpropanolamine on body weight in rats, Tainter (1944) demonstrated that phenylpropanolamine mixed in the diet and fed to rats for 7 days produced body-weight loss. A wide range of dosage levels was studied, and the maximum body-weight loss was 15% of total body weight in 7 days, although the dose level required to produce such effects was not specified. Furthermore, in pair-feeding experiments, rats given 2.4 mg of phenylpropanolamine per gram of food (approximately 240 mg/kg daily) in the diet for 38 days gained less body weight than did pair-fed controls (Table 3.12). In addition, it was noted that phenylpropanolamine was most effective in reducing food intake during the first week of the study and that tolerance to the anorectic effects developed thereafter. However, the tolerance phenomenon was not investigated quantitatively.

It is interesting to note that whereas one of the primary therapeutic uses of phenylpropanolamine in humans is as an appetite suppressant for use in weight loss programs, in the literature from 1910 to 1986 only two additional studies were published that measured both body-weight loss and food intake in animals and confirmed the results of Tainter (1944). Arch et al. (1982) demonstrated that phenylpropanolamine (9.38 mg/kg daily, PO, for 28 days) decreased weight gain and food intake in normal and genetically obese mice. Only one dosage level was investigated in the study by Arch et al. (1982).

Another study investigated the effects of repeated daily administration of phenylpropanolamine on body weight, food intake, and water intake in rats (Wellman & Sellers, 1986). Rats were given saline or 5, 10, or 20 mg/kg of phenylpropanolamine (IP) twice daily for 12 days. The two lower doses (5 and 10 mg/kg) produced no significant decrease in body-weight gain, food intake, or water intake compared to the control treatment (saline). In contrast, 20 mg/kg of phenylpropanolamine significantly decreased both body-weight

TABLE 3.12. Food Intake and Body Weight Gain in Phenylpropanolamine-Treated and Pair-Fed Control Rats

Group	Food Intake (gm/day)	Weight Gain (gm)
Control[a]	10.1	57.0
Phenylpropanolamine[b]	10.2	25.4

Source: Data from Tainter (1944).
[a]Pair fed to the drug-treated rats.
[b]Phenylpropanolamine (2.4 mg/g of food) in the diet for 38 days.

gain and food intake; phenylpropanolamine did not alter water intake. There was no evidence of tolerance to phenylpropanolamine.

The norephedrine isomer, d-norpseudoephedrine (cathine), produced significant body-weight loss in rats during chronic administration studies (Zelger & Carlini, 1980), but the relevance of these results to the efficacy of phenylpropanolamine is questionable since the various isomers of norephedrine vary considerably in their pharmacological effects (Arch et al., 1982; Fairchild & Alles, 1967; Schonenberger et al., 1976; Swamy et al., 1969).

EFFECTS OF PHENYLPROPANOLAMINE ON FOOD INTAKE

The anorectic efficacy of acutely administered phenylpropanolamine given by various routes in several species has been well documented.

Dose-related decreases in food intake following administration of phenylpropanolamine is best documented in rats. Phenylpropanolamine (1, 5, 10 mg/kg, IP) decreased food intake in rats maintained on a 20-hr fasting, 4-hr feeding schedule (Kornblith & Hoebel, 1976). Food intake during the first hour of the test was decreased, although the overall food intake in 4 hr was not affected; there were no differences between the three doses. At moderate doses, phenylpropanolamine (5, 10, 20 mg/kg, IP) produced a 10–50% decrease in food intake in rats maintained on a 23-hr fasting, 1-hr feeding schedule and maintained at 80% of normal body weight (Wellman & Peters, 1980). Higher doses of phenylpropanolamine (20, 40 mg/kg, IP) decreased food intake in rats maintained on an 18-hr fasting, 6-hr feeding schedule (Epstein, 1959). At these high dose levels, side effects such as piloerection were observed but the general activity level was not altered. Thus doses of phenylpropanolamine ranging from 1 to 40 mg/kg (IP) have been shown to produce anorexia in rats. The estimated ED_{50} (dose that decreased food intake by 50%) was 25 mg/kg (IP) in rats (Katz et al., 1985a). However, the minimum effective dose in rats and the maximum response have not been clearly defined.

Also, repeated administration of 20 mg/kg of phenylpropanolamine (IP) twice daily for 12 days decreased food intake but not water intake in rats (Wellman & Sellers, 1986). Lower doses of phenylpropanolamine (5 or 10 mg/kg, IP) had no significant effect on food intake.

The route of administration influences the anorectic effects of phenylpropanolamine. In rats, phenylpropanolamine decreased food intake at IP doses ranging from 1 to 40 mg/kg (see foregoing), but had no effect on food intake at SC doses as high as 128 mg/kg (Schuster & Johanson, 1985).

In mice, phenylpropanolamine (10 and 40 mg/kg, route not specified) decreased food intake during the first hour after the dose but increased food intake thereafter (Cairns et al., 1984).

In monkeys, phenylpropanolamine was a potent and effective anorectic, with an oral ED_{50} (dose that decreased food intake by 50%) of 4.2 mg/kg (Schuster & Johanson, 1985) or 4.4 mg/kg (Woolverton et al., 1986).

In addition, IV administration of phenylpropanolamine (0.1–30 mg/kg, in a self-administered schedule) produced anorexia in baboons (Griffiths et al., 1978). The daily dose required to reduce food intake by 50% was calculated to be 48 mg/kg.

These studies have measured the effects of phenylpropanolamine on spontaneous food intake; the studies in rats were conducted in rats maintained on artificial fasting-feeding schedules. In addition, studies have shown that phenylpropanolamine also decreased food intake when eating was elicited by electrical stimulation of selected areas of the brain. In rats with electrodes chronically implanted in the lateral hypothalamus, electrically induced feeding was decreased following administration of 5–40 mg/kg phenylpropanolamine (IP) (Hoebel et al., 1975). At the lowest dose (5 mg/kg, IP) phenylpropanolamine selectively decreased food intake with no effect on water intake.

Thus the anorectic effects of phenylpropanolamine have been demonstrated in rats on free-feeding schedules (Epstein, 1959; Kornblith & Hoebel, 1976; Wellman & Peters, 1980) and in an operant conditioning paradigm (Hoebel et al., 1975).

TOLERANCE TO EFFECTS OF PHENYLPROPANOLAMINE ON FOOD INTAKE OR BODY WEIGHT

As discussed previously, tachyphylaxis (rapid tolerance to acutely administered drug) is typical of many actions of sympathomimetic amines. Also, as mentioned earlier, Tainter, (1944) noted tolerance to the anorectic effects of phenylpropanolamine in rats given phenylpropanolamine in the diet. Tolerance developed rapidly during the first week of drug-diet administration. In contrast, no tolerance developed to the anorectic effects of phenylpropanolamine when rats were given 20 mg/kg of phenylpropanolamine (IP) twice daily for 12 days (Wellman & Sellers, 1986). Tolerance to the anorectic effects of d-norpseudoephedrine also developed during the first week of chronic administration in rats (Zelger & Carlini, 1980).

MECHANISM OF ANORECTIC EFFECTS OF PHENYLPROPANOLAMINE: CNS THEORIES

Much of the basic research in regulation of food intake during the past 30 years has focused on neural regulation mechanisms involving primarily hypothalamic loci [see reviews by Hoebel (1977, 1979, 1985)]. This research has been based on identification of satiety mechanisms located in the ventromedial hypothalamus and feeding mechanisms in the lateral hypothalamus.

Electrolytic lesions in the ventromedial hypothalamus in rats produce a syndrome of hyperphagia and obesity, whereas lesions of the lateral hypothalamus produce hypophagia and weight loss. Anatomic and neurochemical studies have demonstrated an ascending adrenergic system that contributes input into the lateral hypothalamus and may inhibit feeding behavior. Pharmacological studies have demonstrated either β-adrenergic inhibition of feeding or a mixed α- and β-adrenergic inhibition of feeding mediated at the level of the lateral hypothalamus.

Since phenylpropanolamine is known to have sympathomimetic effects at peripheral autonomic sites of action, it is logical to investigate whether the anorectic effects of phenylpropanolamine are mediated by adrenergic mechanisms in the hypothalamus. One method for determining the site of action of a drug on the CNS is to ablate the suspected site of action and determine whether this manipulation reduces or abolishes the drug response. To determine whether the anorectic effects of phenylpropanolamine are mediated via activation of satiety mechanisms in the ventromedial hypothalamus, phenylpropanolamine was administered to rats rendered hyperphagic by lesions placed in the ventromedial hypothalamus (Epstein, 1959; Wellman & Peters, 1980). Phenylpropanolamine produced equivalent anorexia in control and in ventromedial hypothalamus-lesioned hyperphagic rats at intermediate doses [5–20 mg/kg, IP (Wellman & Peters, 1980)] and at high doses [20–40 mg/kg, IP (Epstein, 1959)]. These studies suggest that the anorectic effects of phenylpropanolamine are not mediated by an effect on the ventromedial hypothalamus. An additional noradrenergic input into the hypothalamus is via the ventral noradrenergic bundle, which sends norepinephrine-containing axons into the ventromedial hypothalamus. Lesions of the dorsolateral tegmentum disrupt the ventral noradrenergic bundle and produce hyperphagia. However, lesions of the dorsolateral tegmentum had no effect on the anorectic actions of phenylpropanolamine (Wellman & Peters, 1980).

Another technique for investigating sites of drug action in the CNS can be utilized when it has been demonstrated that discrete electrical stimulation of localized brain areas specifically produces a particular behavioral pattern. This technique is to elicit that behavior by electrical stimulation of discrete brain areas and then measure drug effects on the elicited behavior. In rats bearing chronically implanted stimulating electrodes in the lateral hypothalamus, electrical stimulation produces a pattern of eating and drinking in satiated rats. Systemic administration of phenylpropanolamine (5–40 mg/kg, IP) decreased electrically elicited food intake (Hoebel et al., 1975). At high doses and when food and water were both available, phenylpropanolamine decreased food intake and increased water intake. At low doses (5 mg/kg, IP) phenylpropanolamine decreased food intake when food but not water was available, but it had no effect on water intake when only water was available. Thus a differential effect of phenylpropanolamine on food and water intake was demonstrated as a function of the dose and the testing situation.

However, since phenylpropanolamine was administered systemically, no inferences could be made regarding the site of action of phenylpropanolamine in reducing electrically elicited feeding. To investigate the site of action, phenylpropanolamine was administered locally to the brain by an indwelling cannula located at the site of electrical stimulation in the lateral hypothalamus (Hoebel et al., 1975). In this study drug administration and electrical stimulation were accomplished by using a concentric electrode-cannula array. In addition, to control for the possibility that phenylpropanolamine may diffuse from the site of administration to distant sites of action, phenylpropanolamine was administered via a cannula situated in the medial hypothalamus while measuring food intake elicited by stimulation of the lateral hypothalamus electrode. Phenylpropanolamine applied locally to the lateral hypothalamus selectively suppressed food intake but not water intake, whereas local application of phenylpropanolamine to the medial hypothalamus did not affect either food or water intake. These studies suggest that phenylpropanolamine selectively decreases food intake but not water intake, and that this effect is mediated by an effect on the lateral hypothalamic feeding mechanism.

In a further refinement of the lateral-hypothalamus-stimulation-induced feeding paradigm, Kornblith and Hoebel (1976) developed a self-stimulation, stimulation-escape paradigm. In this paradigm, rats bearing electrodes chronically implanted in the lateral hypothalamus were exposed to alternating periods of self-stimulation and stimulation-escape phases. During the self-stimulation phase, the rat had the option to press (or not press) an operant conditioning lever that would deliver electrical stimulation to the lateral hypothalamus and initiate feeding. During the stimulation-escape phase, the electrical stimulation was automatically delivered to the lateral hypothalamus and the rat could press the lever to turn off the stimulus. Thus the self-stimulation responses were a measure of the reward properties of food, whereas the stimulation-escape responses were a measure of the aversion to food. Phenylpropanolamine (5–20 mg/kg, IP) decreased the response during the self-stimulation phase and the lower doses (5–10 mg/kg, IP) increased the response during the stimulation-escape phase (Kornblith & Hoebel, 1976). These studies indicate that phenylpropanolamine decreased the reward properties of food and increased aversion to food.

It has been suggested that the anorectic effects of phenylpropanolamine are mediated by release of norepinephrine or direct noradrenergic effects in the lateral hypothalamus (Hoebel et al., 1975). Phenylpropanolamine does not cause significant release of norepinephrine from noradrenergic neurons except at toxic levels (Levitt et al., 1974). Furthermore, ICV administration of phenylpropanolamine produced no change in brain levels of either norepinephrine or dopamine (Breese et al., 1970). Nonetheless, the results of one study indicate that phenylpropanolamine may produce anorexia via catecholaminergic mechanisms (Cairns et al., 1984). In this study, mice were pretreated with α-methyl-p-tyrosine to deplete endogenous catecholamines; this pretreatment antagonized phenylpropanolamine-induced anorexia. In contrast, another study suggested that l-norephedrine-induced anorexia was not mediated by catecholaminergic mechanisms (Wellman & Ruddle, 1985). In this study, rats were pretreated with various biogenic-amine blocking drugs: phenoxybenzamine, an α-adrenergic blocker; propranolol, a β-adrenergic blocker; haloperidol, a dopamine blocker; or methysergide, a serotonin blocker. None of these pretreatments blocked l-norephedrine-induced anorexia. However, the effects of such pretreatments on phenylpropanolamine-induced anorexia were not specifically tested.

MECHANISM OF ANORECTIC EFFECTS OF PHENYLPROPANOLAMINE: PERIPHERAL MECHANISMS

Given the restricted distribution of phenylpropanolamine to the brain and the low potency of phenylpropanolamine for CNS effects, it is reasonable to consider mechanisms of anorectic effects that may be mediated at peripheral sites. Several peripheral mechanisms of anorexia have been proposed: mechanisms related to alterations in metabolism, effects on gastric transport, and nonspecific mechanisms involving taste aversion.

The early studies by Tainter (1944) demonstrated that phenylpropanolamine (1–5 mg/kg, SC) did not alter the basal metabolic rate in rats. Later, Arch et al. (1982) demonstrated that phenylpropanolamine (0.50 mmol/kg daily, PO, for 28 days) increased thermogenic energy expenditure in normal and genetically obese mice. The increased thermogenesis was associated with decreased food intake, decreased body-weight gain, and decreased total body lipid content.

In general, sympathomimetic drugs increase oxygen consumption and thermogenesis; however, it is unclear whether these effects are related to the use of these drugs for treatment of obesity. The effects of sympathomimetic drugs on food intake, body-weight gain, body composition, and energy expenditure were investigated (Dulloo & Miller, 1984). Seven drugs with different mechanisms of action were selected: ephedrine, methoxyphenamine, yohimbine, tranylcypromine, amitryptyline, iprindole, and theophylline. The drugs were administered in the diet for 7 weeks; the effects were tested in lean and obese mice and in obese rats. Each drug produced more thermogenesis in obese than in lean animals. Of the seven drugs tested, ephedrine and tranylcypromine (an MAO inhibitor) were the most potent in producing thermogenesis. Interestingly, ephedrine decreased body-weight gain and body fat and increased oxygen consumption and heat production, but did not decrease food intake. Apparently, the metabolic effects of ephedrine were unrelated to changes in food consumption.

The thermogenic potential of drugs can be assessed by measuring their effects on heat production in brown adipose tissue of rats (Wellman, 1984). Brown adipose tissue is a specialized form of adipose tissue that is involved in the oxidation of lipids and production of heat. Brown adipose tissue thermogenesis is regulated by the sympathetic nervous system and is stimulated by β-adrenergic agonists. Thermogenesis is estimated in rats by measuring temperature changes in the interscapular brown adipose tissue. Phenylpropanolamine (5 to 40 mg/kg, IP) stimulated brown adipose tissue thermogenesis in anesthetized rats (Wellman, 1984). Phenylpropanolamine also increased rectal temperature but the increase in rectal temperature occurred later than the increase in brown adipose tissue thermogenesis. The relative potency of the phenylpropanolamine isomers was: l-norephedrine > d,l-norephedrine > d-norephedrine (Wellman & Marmon, 1985a). Furthermore, caffeine potentiated the phenylpropanolamine-induced thermogenesis (Wellman & Marmon, 1985c). Reserpine pretreatment to deplete stores of catecholamines abolished the phenylpropanolamine-induced thermogenesis, suggesting that the effect is mediated by release of norepinephrine from sympathetic neurons in the adipose tissue (Wellman & Marmon, 1985b). However, the β-adrenergic blocker propranolol blocked phenylpropanolamine thermogenesis but did not block phenylpropanolamine anorexia, suggesting that stimulation of thermogenesis is not involved in the anorectic activity of phenylpropanolamine (Wellman & Ruddle, 1985).

Sympathomimetic drugs inhibit gastrointestinal smooth muscle. Phenylpropanolamine increased the gastric transport time in rats (Tainter, 1944) and produced a dose-dependent increase in gastric retention of food (Wellman et al., 1986). However, no study has demonstrated conclusively whether inhibition of gastrointestinal smooth muscle contributes to phenylpropanolamine anorexia.

Numerous studies have investigated possible effects of phenylpropanolamine on blood glucose or glucose utilization, although glucostatic mechanisms apparently play only a minor, if any, role in phenylpropanolamine-induced anorexia. More potent sympathomimetic amines have pronounced effects on blood glucose, insulin (Mayer, 1980), and lipolysis (Feller & Finger, 1970). Phenylpropanolamine given to fasted rabbits produced pronounced but variable effects on blood glucose when administered IV (20–30 mg/kg) but was ineffective by the SC (100 mg/kg) or PO (200 mg/kg) routes (Krantz & Hartung, 1931). Variable effects of phenylpropanolamine on blood glucose in normal animals have been reported. In normal rats, phenylpropanolamine (2.5–20 mg/kg, IP) produced a dose-dependent hypoglycemia in one study (Resnick et al., 1978). In another study, norephedrine alone (25 mg/kg, IP; isomer not specified) produced no glycemic effect but reduced epinephrine-induced hyperglycemia (Gourju & Lawson, 1957). In normal mice as well, phenylpropanolamine (200 μmol/kg, IP) produced no glycemic response (Sandage & Fletcher, 1983).

Thus phenylpropanolamine produced no consistent effects on blood glucose in normal animals. Phenylpropanolamine may have significant effects on blood glucose in certain altered physiological states. The hypoglycemic effect of phenylpropanolamine (2.5–20 mg/kg, IP) was greater in diabetic (streptozocin-treated) rats than in control rats (Resnick et al., 1978). In stressed mice, phenylpropanolamine (100–400 μmol/kg, IP) had no effect on blood glucose level in either fasted or fed mice but produced a modest blunting of the blood glucose curve in the glucose tolerance test (Fletcher et al., 1982). Furthermore, phenylpropanolamine increased the glucose-stimulated insulin level and decreased the insulinogenic index (insulin level ÷ plasma glucose level). These latter results indicate that phenylpropanolamine may sensitize the pancreatic beta cells to the effects of glucose loading. In addition, phenylpropanolamine reduced the glucosuria in mildly diabetic monkeys but not in severely diabetic monkeys [unpublished observations cited by Hoebel (1977)].

In summary, phenylpropanolamine stimulates metabolism, inhibits gastrointestinal smooth muscle, and produces small and variable effects on blood glucose and glucose utilization. Such modest effects are not likely to contribute significantly to the anorectic effects of phenylpropanolamine.

Another peripheral mechanism of the anorectic effects of phenylpropanolamine is conditioned taste aversion. Phenylpropanolamine was shown to be an aversive stimulus in the conditioned taste aversion test in rats (Wellman et al., 1981). Phenylpropanolamine (10–40 mg/kg, IP) produced a dose-dependent taste aversion, as well as an inhibition of water intake in an unconditioned suppression test in rats trained to a schedule of 23.5-hr water deprivation, 0.5-hr free access to water. However, the doses used in this study may be toxic doses in water-deprived rats, since the high dose (40 mg/kg) produced catatonia in most rats and death in one rat. In comparison, in normal rats the LD_{50} for IP administration is 160–175 mg/kg. Wellman et al. (1981) suggest that the anorectic effects of phenylpropanolamine may be due to peripheral actions leading to nonspecific malaise or toxicity. According to this mechanism, phenylpropanolamine would decrease both food and water intake. This mechanism is inconsistent with other studies that demonstrated a selective decrease in food intake with no effect on water intake (Hoebel et al., 1975). It should be noted that the increased response during the escape phase of the self-stimulation, stimulation-escape paradigm (Kornblith & Hoebel, 1976) is consistent with a taste aversion mechanism, although the stimulation-escape effect is presumably mediated via central rather than peripheral mechanisms.

COMPARISON OF PHENYLPROPANOLAMINE AND OTHER ANORECTIC DRUGS

The efficacy of phenylpropanolamine as an anorectic drug has been compared with the efficacy of other anorectic drugs, especially with reference to two particular comparisons: comparison to amphetamine and comparison to the isomers of ephedrine and norephedrine.

There is no doubt that amphetamine is a much more potent anorectic than phenylpropanolamine on a weight basis, since the effective doses of amphetamine and phenylpropanolamine are approximately 0.1–2 and 5–40 mg/kg (IP in rats), respectively (Epstein, 1959; Hoebel et al., 1975; Kornblith & Hoebel, 1976; Wellman and Peters, 1980). Amphetamine is approximately 10 times as potent as phenylpropanolamine as an anorectic. However, other important comparisons are the anorectic: CNS stimulation ratio, the anorectic: abuse liability ratio, and the mechanisms of anorectic effects of the two drugs. These comparisons are summarized in Table 3.13. Phenylpropanolamine produces CNS stimulation only at doses higher than the anorectic doses, and only at doses approaching the lethal range. For amphetamine, there is no separation between the anorectic and CNS-stimulating doses, but the lethal dose is much higher. Abuse liability, measured as the ratio between the anorectic dose and the dose that produced self-administration, was negligible for phenylpropanolamine but very high for amphetamine (Griffiths et al., 1978). Finally, while both phenylpropanolamine and amphetamine reduced food intake, the two drugs produced opposite effects in the self-stimulation, stimulus-escape paradigm, in operant conditioning situations, and on water intake. These comparisons suggest that the mechanisms of action of phenylpropanolamine and amphetamine, especially with regard to CNS effects, are considerably different.

Both phenylpropanolamine and amphetamine decreased food intake in mice and the effects were antagonized by pretreatment with α-methyl-p-tyrosine (Cairns et al., 1984). Since α-methyl-p-tyrosine inhibits synthesis of catecholamines, these results might indicate that both phenylpropanolamine and amphetamine produce anorexia by catecholaminergic mechanisms. However, this study compared the effects of 2.5 mg/kg of amphetamine to the effects of 10 mg/kg of phenylpropanolamine. This is a relatively high dose of amphetamine and a relatively low dose of phenylpropanolamine (see Table 3.14). Furthermore, in this study phenylpropanolamine decreased locomotor activity whereas amphetamine increased locomotor activity. Thus, it may be inappropriate to compare the anorectic effects of phenylpropanolamine and amphetamine at the doses used.

TABLE 3.13. Comparison of Phenylpropanolamine and Amphetamine in Rats[a]

	Phenylpropanolamine	Amphetamine	Reference
Anorectic dose	5–40 (IP)	0.1–2 (IP)	Epstein (1959), Kornblith & Hoebel (1976), Wellman & Peters (1980)
CNS stimulation dose	40–80 (SC)	0.3–2.5 (SC)	Schulte et al. (1941)
Lethal dose			
MLD	80 (SC)	10 (SC)	Schulte et al. (1941)
LD_{50}	1490 (PO)	55 (PO)	*Merck Index* (1983)
	160 (IP)	NR	Warren & Werner (1946)
	380–860 (SC)	NR	Warren & Werner (1946)
Effects on food intake			
Free feeding	−	− −	
Self-stimulation	−	(+)	Kornblith & Hoebel (1976)
Stimulus–escape	(+)	(+)	Kornblith & Hoebel (1976)
Operant conditioning for food[b]	−	+	Hoebel et al. (1975)
Effects of water intake	−/o	−	Hoebel et al. (1975), Wellman et al. (1981)

[a]Doses are in mg/kg (route of administration). Symbols: + increased, (+) slightly increased, − decreased, − − greatly decreased, −/o decreased or no effect NR—not reported.
[b]Effects on number of conditioned responses, not on food intake.

TABLE 3.14. Comparison of Effects of Phenylpropanolamine, Amphetamine, and Ephedrine on Locomotor Activity in Rats[a]

| | | Increased Locomotor Activity | | | | | | |
| | | Peak Effect | | Maximum Total Effect | | | | |
Drug	Threshold Dose	Dose	Activity/hr	Dose	Total Activity	Duration (hr)	MLD[b]	MLD/ Threshold Dose
Phenylpropanolamine	40	80	50.4	80	99.7	4	80	2.0
dl-Amphetamine	0.3	2.5	81.2	20	310.4	8	10	33.3
d-Amphetamine	0.125	2.5	86.2	5	234.3	7	10	80
l-Amphetamine	2.5	10	47.8	10	134.2	7	160	64
dl-Ephedrine	16	128	33.0	128	171.3	8	128	8

Source: Data from Schulte et al. (1941).
[a]All doses are in mg/kg (SC). Activity—revolutions.
[b]MLD—minimum lethal dose.

The anorectic potencies of seven appetite suppressants were assessed in rats and monkeys (Schuster & Johanson, 1985). Table 3.15 summarizes the results. In both species, the rank order of potency was d-amphetamine > mazindol > fenfluramine > diethylpropion > phenmetrazine = methylphenidate. However, there appears to be a marked difference in the potency of phenylpropanolamine in monkeys and rats. In rats, phenylpropanolamine produced no effect on food intake at doses as high as 128 mg/kg (SC) but in monkeys, phenylpropanolamine was a potent anorectic with an ED_{50} of 4.2 mg/kg (PO). Phenylpropanolamine was given by different routes in the two species. This may be why the potency estimates are so different, because the potency depends on the route of administration. For example, phenylpropanolamine was more effective in rats when given IP ($ED_{50} = 25$ mg/kg; Katz et al., 1985a) than when given SC.

The anorectic effects of a single PO dose of phenylpropanolamine, three isomers of norephedrine, and four isomers of ephedrine were compared (Arch et al., 1982). One dose level of each isomer was studied, and all the drugs were given at equimolar doses (0.50 mmol/kg). Consequently, the potency and efficacy of the various isomers were not actually determined since potency and efficacy can be determined only from dose-response studies. However, certain comparisons can be made. Phenylpropanolamine ($\pm$-norephedrine) produced greater reduction in food intake than did ($+$)-norephedrine (42 and 29% reduction, respectively). Effects of ($-$)-norephedrine were not investigated. However, since the racemic mixture produced greater effect than the ($+$)-isomer, it can be predicted that ($-$)-norephedrine is a more potent anorectic than ($+$)-norephedrine. However, in the overall comparison of the various ephedrine and norephedrine isomers, there is no consistent difference in

TABLE 3.15. Effects of Drugs on Food Intake

Drug	Effective Dose		
	Rat[a]	Monkey[b]	Human[c]
($+$)-Amphetamine	1.7	0.4	5
Mazindol	3.2	1.0	1
Fenfluramine	5.0	2.2	20
Diethylpropion	10.0	3.0	25
Phenmetrazine	12.9	3.8	25
Methylphenidate	13.5	—[d]	—
Phenylpropanolamine	>128	4.2	25–50

Source: Schuster & Johanson (1985).
[a] ED_{50}, SC.
[b] ED_{50}, PO.
[c] Anorectic dose from *Physician's Desk Reference*.
[d] Not reported.

the effect of the (+)-isomer compared to the corresponding (−)-isomer. There also was no consistent difference in the anorectic effects of ephedrine compared to norephedrine isomers. This lack of stereospecificity of norephedrine and ephedrine isomers with regard to anorectic effects is in sharp contrast to the stereospecificity of the anorectic effects of the isomers of amphetamine. It has been well established that d-amphetamine is much more potent than l-amphetamine in producing anorectic effects.

Another study compared the anorectic potencies of phenylpropanolamine and (+)-norephedrine in rats (Katz et al., 1985a). Adult male rats were deprived of food for 24 hr before administration of the test drug (IP). The ED_{50} (dose required to decrease food intake by 50%) and LD_{50} were determined. The ED_{50}s for phenylpropanolamine and (+)-norephedrine were 25 and 63 mg/kg, respectively. The LD_{50}s were 67 and 343 mg/kg, respectively. These results indicate that (+)-norephedrine was slightly less potent than phenylpropanolamine as an anorectic, but (+)-norephedrine was considerably less toxic.

OTHER CNS EFFECTS

Many sympathomimetic amines exert potent effects on the CNS, producing increased arousal and decreased fatigue, stimulation of respiration, and complex psychogenic effects. Undoubtedly, one of the most potent sympathomimetic amines in terms of stimulation of CNS activity is d-amphetamine. Indeed, the CNS stimulation by amphetamine was the basis for its therapeutic use and is certainly the basis for its abuse as a recreational drug. Thus it is important to consider the effects of phenylpropanolamine on the CNS. However, considering the limited distribution of phenylpropanolamine to the brain (Thiercelin et al., 1976) and the delayed appearance of phenylpropanolamine in brain tissue (Axelrod, 1953; Thiercelin et al., 1976), it is necessary to consider the CNS effects of phenylpropanolamine in relation to the more pronounced peripheral sympathomimetic effects. In most of the early studies, phenylpropanolamine was shown to either have low potency for CNS effects or be inactive in CNS paradigms. Perhaps because of this low potency, there has been a lack of interest in investigating effects of phenylpropanolamine on the CNS, and thus there is relatively limited information available regarding such effects. This is an important area of investigation, especially in light of the common misconception that phenylpropanolamine is an "amphetamine-like sympathomimetic amine."

In *in vivo* dose-response studies for any drug, it is important to measure the drug response at the time of maximum effect. Brain levels of phenylpropanolamine do not reach peak until 1–2 hr after systemic administration, and this would be the optimum time to measure drug response in order to assess

CNS activity. However, many of the studies have measured effects of phenyl-propanolamine at shorter intervals (commonly 30 min after drug administration), which should result in underestimating the potency of the drug.

Also, phenylpropanolamine is a relatively short-acting drug, with a plasma half-life of approximately 3–6 hr in humans (El Egakey & Speiser, 1982; Lonnerholm et al., 1984). Most of the behavioral studies of CNS effects of phenylpropanolamine were conducted using rats as the animal model. The duration of action of most drugs is shorter in rats than in humans, and indeed the plasma half-life of phenylpropanolamine in rats is approximately 1 hr following IV administration (Thiercelin et al., 1976). However, many of the studies have used considerably longer periods of observation—as long as 4 hr in some studies—and again, this would lead to an underestimation of potency.

EFFECTS ON LOCOMOTOR ACTIVITY

Effects of phenylpropanolamine on locomotor activity in rats were investigated in four separate studies. Despite considerable differences in the techniques for measuring locomotor activity and differences in the experimental designs, the conclusions of the studies are consistent. Phenylpropanolamine had very low potency for producing CNS stimulation and increased locomotor activity only in doses approaching lethal levels.

The early studies of the effects of phenylpropanolamine on locomotor activity used the so-called "jiggle cage" method for measuring overall activity. Basically the jiggle cage is a rat cage suspended from a spring. Any movement by the rat(s) in the cage causes the cage to move, and these movements can be recorded by either mechanical or electronic methods. The primary criticism of the jiggle cage method is that it measures all movements including random movements, stereotyped or repetitive movements, and nonpurposeful movements, as well as actual locomotor activity. More recently, sophisticated electronic activity-monitoring devices have been developed that can measure locomotor activity selectively, without interference due to these other kinds of movements. Nonetheless, the results of the two early studies using jiggle cage measurements agree reasonably well with the more recent studies that utilized the more sophisticated methods.

Phenylpropanolamine caused a dose-dependent increase in locomotor activity as measured by the jiggle cage method (Schulte et al., 1941; Warren & Werner, 1945). In an extensive study of the effects of some 75 sympathomimetic amines, Schulte et al. (1941) found that amphetamine and ephedrine were among the most potent and phenylpropanolamine was considerably less potent in increasing locomotor activity (see Table 3.14). More important, the ratio of the effective dose to the minimum lethal dose varied considerably among the various drugs. Phenylpropanolamine increased activity only at doses close to the lethal range, whereas amphetamine increased activity at relatively lower doses. Moreover, the maximum increase in activity was greater for amphetamine than for phenylpropanolamine. These results were confirmed by Warren and Werner (1945), again using the jiggle cage method.

More recently, the effects of phenylpropanolamine on activity were investigated by using activity monitoring devices specifically designed to measure only locomotor activity (Davis & Pinkerton, 1972). These monitoring devices were programmed to eliminate activity counts associated with stereotypic repetitive movements and other random activity not associated with locomotor activity. Phenylpropanolamine (20–51 mg/kg, IP) increased locomotor activity (Davis & Pinkerton, 1972). In separate experiments, relatively high doses of phenylpropanolamine (45–60 mg/kg, IP) produced stereotypic behavior but only in 60–80% of the animals. Phenylpropanolamine also enhanced aggregation lethality in mice, another animal test system for assessing CNS stimulant activity. However, the doses of phenylpropanolamine used in this study were very high and can be considered toxic. A higher dose of phenylpropanolamine (82 mg/kg, IP) was originally included in the study design, but the data were deleted from the results because of the high lethality in this group. Side effects were prominent in the doses used and included piloerection, salivation, exophthalmos, and hyperpnea.

Effects of the various isomers of the ephedrines on locomotor activity in mice were also investigated by using activity monitors that had photoelectric devices programmed to specifically measure locomotor activity (Fairchild & Alles, 1967). Phenylpropanolamine was not investigated in this study. l-Norephedrine was shown to be more potent than d-norephedrine; the LD$_{50}$ levels (and 95% confidence limits) for l- and d-norephedrine were 0.94 (0.720–1.22) and 2.01 (1.75–2.32) mmol/kg (IP), respectively. Norephedrine increased locomotor activity in mice only at doses approaching lethal levels, results consistent with the effects of phenylpropanolamine in rats.

Studies have compared the CNS-stimulant effects of phenylpropanolamine and various isomers of ephedrine. In one study, d-norpseudoephedrine (10 to 50 mg/kg, IP) increased locomotor activity in rats but phenylpropanolamine (10 to 50 mg/kg, IP) did not (Maher et al., 1985); locomotor activity was measured by an open-field method. Furthermore, d-norephedrine (25 to 150 mg/kg, IP) and l-norephedrine (5 to 40 mg/kg, IP) produced no increase in locomotor activity (Eisenberg & Maher, 1987). In another study, slightly higher doses of phenylpropanolamine (20 to 80 mg/kg, IP) increased locomotor activity in rats (Katz et al., 1986); in this study, locomotor activity was measured electronically for 4 hr after administration of the test drugs. d-Norephedrine (20 to 80 mg/kg, IP) also increased locomotor activity.

The mechanism of the CNS stimulation by sympathomimetic drugs is unknown. One study investigated whether sympathomimetic drugs stimulate locomotor activity by a catecholaminergic mechanism (Cairns et al., 1984). In this study, mice were pretreated with dihydroxyphenylalanine (*l*-DOPA) and benserazide to enhance catecholaminergic transmission in the CNS. In untreated mice, phenylpropanolamine (10 and 40 mg/kg, route not specified) produced no increase in locomotor activity. In mice pretreated with *l*-DOPA and benserazide, phenylpropanolamine initially decreased locomotor activity; however, the initial decrease in activity was followed by a pronounced increase in activity. The increased activity was described as qualitatively similar to amphetamine-induced hyperactivity: the mice had gait disturbances, stereotypy, piloerection, and Straub tail. These results suggest that pretreatment with *l*-DOPA and benserazide unmasked an excitatory effect of phenylpropanolamine.

In another study, the locomotor effects of acute and chronic phenylpropanolamine administration were investigated in mice (Stavchansky et al., 1986). Acute administration of phenylpropanolamine (2.5 to 30 mg/kg, IP) produced no significant effect on locomotor activity. In the chronic study, mice were given 5 mg/kg of phenylpropanolamine, 2.5 mg/kg of amphetamine, or saline (IP) daily for 14 days. One day after the last dose, all mice were given 2.5 mg/kg of amphetamine (IP) and amphetamine-induced hyperactivity was measured. In mice chronically treated with phenylpropanolamine the amphetamine-induced hyperactivity was less than in control mice chronically treated with saline. In contrast, in mice chronically treated with amphetamine the amphetamine-induced hyperactivity was enhanced compared to the control response. The authors speculated that chronic administration of amphetamine or phenylpropanolamine produced alterations in dopaminergic neurotransmission in the CNS; however, it is not clear why amphetamine and phenylpropanolamine produced opposite effects on amphetamine-induced hyperactivity.

DRUG DISCRIMINATION STUDIES

Evaluation of psychoactive drugs is a difficult pharmacologic problem. Since psychoactive effects are essentially subjective responses, humans are the subjects of choice for describing these responses. Because of ethical considerations, however, it is often necessary to test psychoactive properties in experimental animals. Drug discrimination studies can be used for this purpose.

The general concept of drug discrimination studies is to train animals to discriminate a known CNS-active drug (the "discriminative cue") from a placebo drug, and then to determine whether a test drug produces a response similar to the discriminative cue. For example, rats can be trained in a two-lever operant conditioning paradigm: After administration of the active drug the rats must press one lever to get a food reward, whereas after vehicle administration they must press the other lever to get the reward. Once the rats have learned to discriminate the active drug from the vehicle, drug testing can begin. On test days, the test drug is substituted for the known CNS-active drug. If the rats preferentially press the "drug lever" after administration of the test drug, then the test drug and the known CNS-active drug are considered to produce similar psychoactive effects, that is, the two drugs have similar discriminative-stimulus properties.

Several studies have evaluated whether phenylpropanolamine produces CNS stimulation. Thus, in the drug-discrimination phase the animals were trained to discriminate a known CNS stimulant (amphetamine or cocaine) from a vehicle. Table 3.16 summarizes the results of these studies. In experimental animals there was either no drug discrimination (i.e., the animals responded on the vehicle lever after administration of phenylpropanolamine) or partial drug discrimination (either the animals responded some of the time on the amphetamine lever, or only some of the animals responded on the amphetamine lever). The response may be species-specific: There was no drug discrimination in mice, partial drug discrimination in rats and monkeys, and complete drug discrimination in pigeons.

In humans the drug discrimination properties of phenylpropanolamine were dose-dependent. At a low dose of phenylpropanolamine (25 mg, PO), there was no drug discrimination against amphetamine; at a higher dose (75 mg), there was discrimination against amphetamine.

When cocaine was the discriminative cue, phenylpropanolamine produced only partial drug discrimination in rats.

One study compared the discriminative-stimulus properties of phenylpropanolamine, ephedrine, or caffeine, alone and in combination, against amphetamine in rats (Holloway et al., 1985). Caffeine, phenylpropanolamine, or ephedrine alone produced partial drug discrimination. However, the triple combination of phenylpropanolamine-ephedrine-caffeine completely substituted for amphetamine as a discriminative-stimulus cue. The authors suggested that the triple combination had either additive or synergistic effects that contributed to the stimulant properties of the combination. This synergism may be the basis for the street drug abuse of such triple combinations.

OPERANT CONDITIONING

One experimental paradigm that has been utilized extensively to evaluate drug effects on complex, higher CNS functioning is to determine the effects of the drug on operant conditioning tasks. Effects of phenylpropanolamine on operant conditioning have been reported. However, there is one major criticism of these studies that limits the interpretation of the results. In many operant conditioning experiments the rats are deprived of food for a period of time before testing, and the operant conditioning consists of the rat learning to press a lever to receive food as the reward. Thus, given the known anorectic effects of phenylpropanolamine, if administration of phenylpropanolamine

TABLE 3.16. Drug Discrimination Studies with Phenylpropanolamine

Species	Discriminative Cue	PPA Dose (mg/kg)	Route	Results	Reference
Mouse	Amphetamine	32	IP	No drug discrimination	Snoddy & Tessel (1985)
Rat	Amphetamine	5–50	IP	Drug discrimination at 10 and 20 mg/kg PPA; antagonized by dopamine blocker pimozide	Stafford & Hoebel (1984)
Rat	Amphetamine	12.8, 22.4	IP	PPA did not completely substitute for amphetamine	Holloway et al. (1985)
Rat	Cocaine	5–20	IP	Partial drug discrimination	Wood & Emmett-Oglesby (1985)
Pigeon	Amphetamine	10	IM	Drug discrimination, but PPA had low potency	Schuster & Johanson (1985)
Monkey	Amphetamine	up to 100	PO	No drug discrimination	Schuster & Johanson (1985)
Monkey	Amphetamine	3–100	IG[a]	Variable results. No drug discrimination in two monkeys; drug discrimination at high doses of PPA in two monkeys	Woolverton et al. (1986)
Human	Amphetamine	25, 75 mg (total dose)	PO	No drug discrimination at 25 mg PPA; Drug discrimination at 75 mg PPA	Chait et al. (1986)

[a]IG — itragastric.

results in a decrease in response during the operant conditioning, it is not possible to determine whether this effect is due to decreased appetite or to an impairment in the operant conditioning behavior per se.

Phenylpropanolamine (3.125–25 mg/kg, IP, administered 10 min prior to the test) produced a dose-dependent decrease in response during a fixed-interval schedule-controlled performance paradigm in rats (MacPhail, 1982). Phenylpropanolamine had no effect on the temporal pattern of response except at the highest dose, which almost totally abolished responding.

Operant conditioning techniques were also used in studies of the anorectic efficacy of phenylpropanolamine (Hoebel et al., 1975). These authors noted an important difference between phenylpropanolamine and amphetamine in terms of effects on operant conditioning for food reward. Phenylpropanolamine reduced food intake during both a free-feeding paradigm and the operant conditioning paradigm. Amphetamine, on the other hand, decreased food intake during free feeding but actually increased responding during the operant conditioning paradigm. The increase in operant conditioning response after amphetamine presumably is due to the increased arousal produced by amphetamine, since the number of lever-pressing responses increased but the rats did not consume the food reward presented in response to lever pressing.

BIOCHEMICAL STUDIES

The sympathomimetic amines that have potent effects on the CNS exert their actions via effects on the synthesis, storage, and release of biogenic amines, especially norepinephrine and dopamine, in brain tissue. For example, amphetamine causes release of norepinephrine and dopamine in the brain, and these effects are related to the effects of amphetamine on arousal and locomotor activity, respectively. However, relatively few studies have investigated the effects of phenylpropanolamine on biogenic amines in the CNS. As mentioned above, the relatively low potency and limited distribution of phenylpropanolamine to the brain are probably responsible for the lack of interest in investigating the effects of phenylpropanolamine on biochemical processes in the CNS.

Effects of phenylpropanolamine on dopamine release in CNS tissue have been studied *in vivo* and *in vitro*. In the *in vivo* study, very small microdialysis probes were implanted in the nucleus accumbens in rats; dopamine and serotonin turnover in this restricted area of the brain was evaluated by analyzing the dialysate (Hernandez & Hoebel, 1986). Unanesthetized rats were given 20 mg/kg of phenylpropanolamine, 2 mg/kg of amphetamine, or saline (route not specified) and the turnover of dopamine and serotonin was evaluated. Both phenylpropanolamine and amphetamine increased the extracellular dopamine concentration; amphetamine decreased the concentration of dopamine metabolites but phenylpropanolamine had the opposite effect. Phenylpropanolamine increased serotonin turnover but amphetamine did not.

In the *in vitro* study, amphetamine, cocaine, and phenylpropanolamine each decreased the uptake of ^{3}H-dopamine in homogenates of the corpus striatum from the rat brain (Baldessarini & Harris, 1974). The IC_{50} (concentration which decreased dopamine uptake by 50%) was 0.20, 0.8, and 6.5 μM for (+)-amphetamine, cocaine, and phenylpropanolamine, respectively; thus, phenylpropanolamine was approximately 1/32.5 as potent as (+)-amphetamine.

However, dopaminergic drugs have produced inconsistent effects on behavioral responses to phenylpropanolamine. In one study, the dopaminergic blocker pimozide antagonized phenylpropanolamine drug discrimination in rats (Stafford & Hoebel, 1984). Since phenylpropanolamine does not produce drug discrimination against amphetamine consistently (see previously), it is unknown whether these results generalize to other behavioral effects of phenylpropanolamine. Other studies failed to demonstrate a dopaminergic mechanism for drug discrimination of psychostimulant phenethylamines related to cathinone and amphetamine (Goudie et al., 1986). Also, one study indicated that phenylpropanolamine may produce anorexia via catecholaminergic mechanisms (Cairns et al., 1984), whereas another study suggested that *l*-norephedrine-induced anorexia was not mediated by catecholaminergic mechanisms (Wellman & Ruddle, 1985). Finally, the results of one study suggested that phenylpropanolamine may stimulate locomotor activity by a catecholaminergic mechanism (Cairns et al., 1984); in this study, a CNS stimulant effect of phenylpropanolamine was demonstrated only when mice were pretreated with dihydroxyphenylalanine (*l*-DOPA) and benserazide to enhance catecholaminergic transmission in the CNS.

In a test of the CNS toxicity of phenethylamines, administration of high phenylpropanolamine doses for 4 days produced no change in brain levels of dopamine, norepinephrine, or serotonin (Woolverton et al., 1986). Rats were given 100 or 200 mg/kg of phenylpropanolamine (SC) twice daily for 4 days. These doses produced body-weight loss during treatment; higher doses (400 or 800 mg/kg) were lethal. (The minimum lethal SC dose of phenylpropanolamine is approximately 350 mg/kg; see Table 4.1.) Fourteen days later, the rats were decapitated, the brains were removed, and the monoamine levels in the frontal cortex, hippocampus, corpus striatum, and hypothalamus were measured. Phenylpropanolamine produced no significant changes in brain monoamine levels. Potent CNS stimulants such as amphetamine produce severe and prolonged depletion of brain monoamines in this bioassay for CNS toxicity.

As discussed earlier (see Mechanism of Action), phenylpropanolamine is a partial α-adrenergic agonist that binds to α-adrenergic receptors in the cerebral cortex, but does not stimulate inositol metabolism in the neuronal membrane (Minneman & Johnson, 1984). These results indicate that even if phenylpropanolamine entered the CNS it would produce no pharmacodynamic effect on the cerebral cortex. In contrast, other sympathomimetic drugs that are full α-adrenergic agonists did stimulate inositol metabolism in the cortex.

Inhibitors of the enzyme MAO can produce changes in CNS function by decreasing metabolism of endogenous monoamines. For example, the therapeutic effectiveness of antidepressant drugs such as tranylcypromine and phenelzine may be related to the inhibition of MAO. Phenylpropanolamine inhibited both brain and liver MAO (Yu, 1986). The inhibition was reversible and competitive; however, phenylpropanolamine was a relatively weak inhibitor with dissociation constants (k_i's) of 150 and 800 μM for type A and type B MAO, respectively. *In vivo,* single low doses of phenylpropanolamine (5 to 20 mg/kg, IP) did not inhibit brain MAO but a relatively high dose (50 mg/kg) did. Administration of 5, 20, or 50 mg/kg phenylpropanolamine (IP) to rats for 7 days produced no cumulative effect on either brain or liver MAO. However, it is unknown whether MAO inhibition contributes to the behavioral effects of phenylpropanolamine.

One experimental method for investigating the effects of phenylpropanolamine on the CNS that circumvents the problem of the limited distribution of the drug to brain tissue is to administer the drug directly into the cerebrospinal fluid by direct intracerebroventricular (ICV) injection. Phenylpropanolamine was administered by the ICV route in one study that showed that 40 μg of phenylpropanolamine (ICV) did not affect the brain levels of either norepinephrine or dopamine (Breese et al., 1970). However, the interpretation of these negative results is limited for several reasons: (1) only one dose level of phenylpropanolamine was administered, and it is possible that this was a subthreshold dose; (2) brain levels of phenylpropanolamine were not measured, and it is possible that the phenylpropanolamine did not diffuse out of the cerebrospinal fluid into the brain tissue; (3) only brain levels of norepinephrine and dopamine were measured (measurement of amine turnover and metabolite concentration would be necessary to evaluate more completely the possible effects of phenylpropanolamine on release of the amines); and (4) neither amphetamine nor mephentermine produced significant effects on brain levels of norepinephrine or dopamine, although other phenylethylamines such as metaraminol, methyloctopamine, and methyltyrosine depleted brain levels of norepinephrine but not dopamine. Since it is known that systemic administration of amphetamine causes release of norepinephrine in the CNS, the lack of effect of amphetamine when administered ICV is puzzling.

Since one of the proposed mechanisms of the anorectic effects of phenyl-propanolamine is release of norepinephrine at the hypothalamic nuclei responsible for suppression of food intake, it would be important to determine by biochemical techniques whether phenylpropanolamine does in fact affect biogenic amine storage and release in the hypothalamus. Such information is not available at this time.

MISCELLANEOUS CNS EFFECTS

While many of the centrally acting sympathomimetic amines produce a central hyperthermia and stimulate the brainstem respiratory centers, there seems to be no clear indication that phenylpropanolamine affects either body temperature or respiratory rate. Wellman et al. (1981) refer to unpublished data indicating that phenylpropanolamine (20 mg/kg, IP) did not induce hyperthermia in rats. Turi et al. (1976), in a bioavailability study in humans given a combination product containing phenylpropanolamine (75 mg) and chlorpheniramine, reported that the combination product did not produce any significant change in either body temperature or respiratory rate. Davis and Pinkerton (1972) reported hyperpnea as a side effect observed following administration of toxic doses of phenylpropanolamine (82 mg/kg, IP) to rats.

Phenylpropanolamine (1–20 mg/kg, SC) increased the threshold for eliciting electrically induced seizures in rabbits (Tainter et al., 1943). Amphetamine also increased the threshold for electrically induced seizures, but ephedrine, tyramine, neosynephrine, and epinephrine were ineffective in altering the seizure threshold.

Phenylpropanolamine caused a dose-dependent decrease in the levels of glycogen in mouse brain *in vivo* (Rogers & Hutchins, 1972). The potency of phenylpropanolamine for decreasing brain glycogen was considerably lower than that of amphetamine. The relevance of this effect of phenylpropanolamine is unknown.

Phenylpropanolamine improved the recovery of function after brain injury in rats and cats (Chen et al., 1986). In rats, motor performance was evaluated by measuring the ability to traverse a narrow elevated beam. The sensorimotor cortex was ablated surgically; this procedure impaired the rat's ability to traverse the beam. A single dose of phenylpropanolamine (0, 10, 15, or 20 mg/kg, IP) was administered 24 hr after cortical ablation. Motor performance was assessed at intervals for up to 15 days. The two highest doses of phenylpropanolamine (15 and 20 mg/kg) improved the rate of recovery from the brain damage. In cats, motor performance was assessed by measuring beam walking and tactile placing reflexes of the forelimbs. The right frontal cortex was ablated surgically and impairment of motor performance was evaluated for 8 days after surgery. Phenylpropanolamine (15 mg/kg) or saline was administered at 4-day intervals from the tenth to the thirtieth day after surgery. Motor performance was rated before each dose and at intervals for up to 2 months after cortical ablation (i.e., 1 month after the last dose of phenylpropanolamine). There was a trend toward improved recovery of function in cats given phenylpropanolamine.

Phenylpropanolamine decreased barbiturate sleep time in mice (Boissier et al., 1965). The ED_{50} (dose that reduced the sleep time by 50%) for this effect was 25 mg/kg (PO); however, higher doses of phenylpropanolamine produced no further shortening of the sleep time.

Intracisternal administration of phenylpropanolamine (1.25 mg/kg) produced excitation, exophthalmos, and rigidity in dogs (Leindorfer, 1950). However, these may represent toxic rather than pharmacological effects at this high dose for intracisternal administration.

METABOLIC EFFECTS

Sympathomimetic amines have significant metabolic effects such as hyperglycemia, stimulation of lipolysis, and increased basal metabolic rate. The effects are the result of a complex set of activities at several sites of action, many of which involve increased intracellular levels of cyclic AMP. Very little is known regarding the metabolic effects of phenylpropanolamine. Early studies indicated that phenylpropanolamine did not alter the basal metabolic rate in rats (Tainter, 1944), and very few studies have been published to confirm or disprove these negative findings. Chronic administration of phenylpropanolamine in the diet (0.50 mmol/kg daily, for 28 days) increased thermogenic energy expenditure in normal and genetically obese mice (Arch et al., 1982). This increase in thermogenesis was associated with a decrease in total body lipid content.

As discussed in a previous section, the thermogenic potential of drugs also can be assessed by measuring brown adipose tissue thermogenesis in rats (Wellman, 1984). Phenylpropanolamine produced a dose-dependent increase in brown adipose tissue thermogenesis (Wellman, 1984). Reserpine pretreatment abolished the phenylpropanolamine-induced thermogenesis, suggesting that the effect was mediated by norepinephrine release from sympathetic neurons (Wellman & Marmon, 1985b). This effect was mediated by a β-adrenergic mechanism because the β-blocker propranolol prevented phenylpropanolamine-induced thermogenesis (Wellman & Ruddle, 1985).

Another study investigated the effects of repeated daily administration of phenylpropanolamine on brown adipose tissue thermogenesis (Wellman & Sellers, 1986). Rats were given saline or 20 mg/kg of phenylpropanolamine (IP) twice daily for 12 days; 2 days after the last chronic dose, the rats were given an acute dose of 20 mg/kg of phenylpropanolamine and the phenylpropanolamine-induced thermogenesis was measured. The baseline brown adipose tissue temperature was slightly elevated in rats chronically treated with phenylpropanolamine, but this effect was statistically insignificant. Also, there was no evidence that tolerance developed to the thermogenic effects of phenylpropanolamine. In a separate study, rats were given 20 mg/kg of d-norephedrine, 20 mg/kg of l-norephedrine, or saline twice daily for 12 days; 2 days after the last chronic dose, the thermogenic effects of an acute dose of norephedrine were measured (each rat was given the same norephedrine isomer during the acute and chronic phases of the study). l-Norephedrine produced approximately twice as much thermogenesis as d-norephedrine. There was no evidence of tolerance to either norephedrine isomer.

Phenylpropanolamine did not produce consistent changes in blood glucose in normal animals (Krantz & Hartung, 1931; Sandage & Fletcher, 1983), although a dose-dependent hypoglycemia in rats given phenylpropanolamine (2.5–20 mg/kg, IP) was reported in one study (Resnick et al., 1978). Phenylpropanolamine may produce a more pronounced hypoglycemic effect in stressed (Resnick et al., 1978) or mildly diabetic animals (Resnick et al., 1978; Hoebel, 1977). While norephedrine (25 mg/kg, IP) had no hyperglycemic effect in adult rats, it did reduce epinephrine-induced hyperglycemia (Gourju & Lawson, 1957).

Phenylpropanolamine (200 μmol/kg, IP) had no effect on blood glucose in normal, lean, or obese mice (Sandage & Fletcher, 1983). In addition, phenylpropanolamine had no statistically significant effect on plasma corticosterone levels in normal mice.

Phenylpropanolamine caused a dose-dependent release of free fatty acids from adipose tissue *in vitro* (Feller & Finger, 1970; Finger & Feller, 1966). Phenylpropanolamine exhibited low potency and low intrinsic activity for stimulation of lipolysis. Phenylpropanolamine also produced dose-dependent depletion of glycogen in the brain *in vivo*, again with very low potency (Rogers & Hutchins, 1972).

STRUCTURE-ACTIVITY RELATIONSHIPS

The early work of Barger and Dale (1910) and of Chen et al. (1929) initiated the systematic investigation of the structure-activity relationships of the phenethylamines. Since that time there has not only been considerable technological advancement in pharmacology, but innumerable derivatives of phenylethylamine have been synthesized as well. Despite these advances, the conclusions of these two early studies continue to be the basis for our understanding of the structural requirements for pharmacological activity at sympathetic sites of action. Because these studies were published long before the introduction of modern-day concepts of α- and β-adrenergic receptors, the results of the studies must be interpreted accordingly.

The study by Barger and Dale (1910) utilized both whole animal and isolated tissue preparations. Blood pressure was recorded in cats with acute spinal cord transections. The isolated tissues were cat uterus and retractor penis muscles of dogs and goats. The following groups of amines were studied: aliphatic amines, aromatic amines without phenolic hydroxyl substitutions (including β-phenylethylamine and phenylpropylamine), amines with one phenolic hydroxyl, and amines with two phenolic hydroxyl groups (i.e., the catecholamines). The conclusions were: (1) the catechol nucleus is not essential for sympathomimetic activity; (2) the primary and secondary amines are the most potent, whereas the quaternary ammonium derivatives have effects at the nicotinic sites as well as at sympathetic sites; (3) the maximum activity within any particular group occurred when a two-carbon chain separated the phenyl group and the amino nitrogen; (4) activity was increased greatly by the 3,4-dihydroxy substitution on the phenyl ring; and (5) the β-hydroxy substitution increased activity of the drug only when the 3,4-dihydroxy substitution was present.

The study by Chen et al. (1929) extended the findings of the study by Barger and Dale (1910). Both *in vivo* and *in vitro* preparations were used, including mydriasis due to topical application in the eye, inhibition of spontaneous contractions in the isolated intestine of the rabbit, oxytocic effects on the guinea pig uterus, pressor effects in cats with acute spinal cord transection, astringent effects on congested nasal mucous membranes in humans (topical application), effects on the frog heart, and lethality in rabbits. The conclusions were:

1. The β-phenylethylamine structure is the common structural requirement for sympathomimetic effects.

2. The α-methyl substitution decreases the activity and prolongs the duration of action of the compounds. α-Methyl substitution may also be required for development of tachyphylaxis. However, increasing the size of the α substitution to α-ethyl further decreased the activity of the amines.

3. Increasing the chain length on either the α-carbon or on the amino-nitrogen in general decreased sympathomimetic activity, but the depressant effect on the heart and lethality in rabbits were increased.

4. The β-hydroxy substitution had complex effects on the pharmacological spectrum. β-Hydroxylation decreased the potency for pressor effects and for cardiac depressor effects but was essential for mydriatic activity. β-Hydroxylation also decreased the lethality of the amines in rabbits.

Chen et al. (1929) also investigated the pharmacological effects of the various optical isomers of ephedrine and pseudoephedrine (Table 3.17). The results showed that the potency of the various isomers differed but that there was no consistent pattern when the two compounds were compared. Thus for ephedrine the l-isomer was more potent than the d-isomer, with a potency ratio of approximately 3 : 1. For pseudoephedrine, the d-isomer was the more potent, and the potency ratio was approximately 7 : 1.

OVERALL STRUCTURE-ACTIVITY RELATIONSHIPS OF PHENETHYLAMINES RELATED TO PHENYLPROPANOLAMINE

Before reviewing the structure-activity studies that relate structure to specific pharmacologic responses, it is important to summarize the general features of the phenylpropanolamine molecule that are responsible for the overall pharmacological profile of phenylpropanolamine and that differentiate phenylpropanolamine from other structurally related compounds.

Phenylpropanolamine contains a two-carbon chain separating the phenyl group and the amino nitrogen, which has been shown repeatedly to be the optimum chain length for sympathomimetic activity.

The β-hydroxyl substitution on phenylpropanolamine decreases the lipid solubility of the drug and greatly decreases the distribution of the drug to the CNS.

The α-methyl substitution renders the compound insensitive to oxidation by monoamine oxidase (MAO). This property is responsible for increasing the duration of action of phenylpropanolamine relative to amines that lack the α-methyl group.

Phenylpropanolamine contains no substitutions on the phenyl ring. Since monohydroxy substitution on the phenyl ring increases potency and dihydroxy substitution confers maximum potency, phenylpropanolamine has rel-

TABLE 3.17. Comparison of Activity of Ephedrine Isomers

Isomer	Mydriasis	Inhibition of Intestine	Contraction of Uterus	Pressor Activity (Relative Ratio)
l-Ephedrine	+ + + + +	+	+	35.15
dl-Ephedrine	+ + + + +	+	+	26.40
d-Ephedrine	+ + +	+	+	11.90
d-Pseudoephedrine	+ + + +	+	+	6.80
dl-Pseudoephedrine	+ + +	+	+	4.00
l-Pseudoephedrine	+	+	+	1.00

Source: Data from Chen et al. (1929).

atively low potency as a sympathomimetic amine. Also, the lack of the 3,4-dihydroxy substitution renders phenylpropanolamine insensitive to metabolism by catechol-O-methyltransferase (COMT). This property increases the oral effectiveness of phenylpropanolamine, since 3,4-dihydroxy-substituted amines are inactivated by MAO in the intestine and in the liver.

Finally, phenylpropanolamine contains no substitution on the amino nitrogen. Since N substitution confers relative selectivity for β rather than for α activity, and the β selectivity is related to the size of the N substitution, phenylpropanolamine has relatively little selectivity for β-adrenergic activity.

In summary, on the basis of these general structure-activity considerations, it could be predicted that phenylpropanolamine would be a sympathomimetic amine with good oral absorption, a relatively long duration of action, low potency—and especially low potency for CNS effects, and relative selectivity for α- rather than β-adrenergic activity. The structure-activity relationships for the various pharmacodynamic responses to phenylpropanolamine are reviewed in the following sections.

STRUCTURE-ACTIVITY RELATIONSHIPS FOR EFFECTS OF PHENYLPROPANOLAMINE ON ADRENERGIC NEURONS

Several studies have demonstrated that the dihydroxy substitution on the phenyl ring and the β-hydroxy substitution are required for optimal effects of sympathomimetic amines on the adrenergic neurons (Bassett et al., 1968; Iversen, 1970; Shore, 1966; Swamy et al., 1969; Trendelenburg et al., 1962a,b).

In the studies of direct and indirect effects of sympathomimetic amines by Trendelenburg et al. (1962a,b), it was demonstrated that the structural requirements for direct action included the dihydroxyphenyl substitution. For monohydroxy-substituted compounds, the m-hydroxy compounds were more potent than the p-hydroxy compounds. The β-hydroxy substitution was relatively less important for determining the direct versus indirect activity.

In a structure-activity study of norepinephrine reuptake in the vas deferens and right atrium of the rat, a series of phenylethylamines, including several of the isomers of norephedrine, was studied (Table 3.18) (Swamy et al., 1969). Activity of the amines in the vas deferens was not correlated to activity in the atrium, presumably because the vas deferens is predominantly α-adrenergic whereas the chronotropic effects in the atrium are β-adrenergic. $(-)$-Norephedrine was more potent than $(+)$-norephedrine in both tissues, although for most isomer pairs, the $(+)$-isomer was the more potent.

The studies by Bassett et al. (1968) also demonstrated that the β-hydroxy and dihydroxyphenyl substituents are required for reuptake of amines by adrenergic terminals in the heart. The dihydroxyphenyl-substituted amines

TABLE 3.18. Potentiation of Norepinephrine in Rat Vas Deferens and Right Atrium

Drug	Vas Deferens			Atrial Rate[a]		
	Rank	Log Unit	Dose Ratio	Rank	Log Unit	Dose Ratio
(−)-Amphetamine	1	0.564	3.67	14	0.637	4.33
(+)-Amphetamine	2	0.488	3.08	12	0.704	5.05
(−)-Norpseudoephedrine	3	0.476	3.00	11	0.747	5.58
(−)-Cocaine	4	0.412	2.59	10	0.778	5.99
(−)-Norephedrine	6	0.399	2.51	4	0.979	9.52
(+)-Norephedrine	21	0.132	1.36	18	0.514	3.26

Source: Data from Swamy et al. (1969).
[a]Reserpine-pretreated rats.

were more potent than the monohydroxyphenyl-substituted amines. Phenyl-propanolamine was not investigated in this study.

The structure-activity relationships for effects of sympathomimetic amines on inhibition of norepinephrine uptake by uptake$_1$ (high-affinity uptake) compared to uptake$_2$ (low-affinity uptake) in the isolated, perfused rat heart were investigated (Burgen & Iversen, 1965; Iversen, 1965). These results were reanalyzed by regression analysis (Ban & Fujita, 1969). The results are summarized in Table 3.19. The results showed that the activity was the sum of (1) a constant attributed to the parent structure, β-phenylethylamine, plus (2) additive contributions of various constituents. Burgen and Iversen (1965)

TABLE 3.19. Effects of Phenylethylamines on Uptake of Norepinephrine

Drug[b]	Inhibition of Norepinephrine Uptake[a]			
	Uptake$_1$		Uptake$_2$	
	Observed[c]	Calculated[d]	Observed	Calculated
(+)-Amphetamine	610	581.9	—	—
Tyramine	245	264.6	75	238.0
(±)-Amphetamine	240	296.9	68	68.0
Phenylethylamine	100	173.4	—	—
(±)-Phenylpropanolamine (SIC)	55	106.2	—	—
(−)-Ephedrine	50	270.2	—	—
(−)-Amphetamine	30	5.8	—	—

[a]Relative to phenylethylamine—100%.
[b]Selected drugs only (total of 59 tested for uptake$_1$, 19 tested for uptake$_2$).
[c]Iverson (1965); Burgen & Iverson (1965).
[d]Ban & Fujita (1969).

concluded that the preponderant constituents affecting the potency of the amines were the α-methyl and the β-hydroxy substitutions. Ban and Fujita (1969) demonstrated that the primary contributions were from the hydrophobic phenyl ring and the positively charged amino group.

STRUCTURE-ACTIVITY RELATIONSHIPS FOR EFFECTS ON SMOOTH MUSCLE ACTIVITY

The structure-activity relationships for smooth muscle activity were investigated in the ileum and the uterus from estrogen-primed rabbits (Ghouri & Haley, 1969). Three structural requirements for α-adrenergic activity in these tissues were identified: (1) the β-hydroxy substitution was required for activity; (2) monohydroxyphenyl substitution increased potency, with the m-hydroxy compounds more potent than the p-hydroxy compounds; and (3) any alkyl substitution on the α-carbon, the β-carbon, or the amino nitrogen decreased the potency. Phenylpropanolamine was shown to have very low potency for α activity in these tissues.

One specialized aspect of the structure-activity relationships for β-hydroxy-substituted phenylethylamines involves the relationship between the potency of the l- and d-isomers. According to the Easson-Stedman hypothesis, the d-isomers are less active than the l-isomers because in the d-isomers the β-hydroxy group stearically hinders binding to the receptor, whereas this does not occur in the l-isomers. To test this hypothesis, Patil et al. (1967a,b) suggested that the d-isomer should be equipotent with the desoxy derivative and tested a series of d- and l-isomers and their desoxy derivatives in the rat vas deferens preparation. There were no differences between the activities of the norephedrine and desoxynorephedrine isomers except that $L(+)$-norpseudoephedrine had very low potency. Patil et al. (1967a,b) suggested that the Easson-Stedman hypothesis was correct for direct-acting amines but not for indirect-acting amines. The results indicated that for phenylethylamines with only one asymmetric carbon, the activities of the isomers differ considerably and that asymmetry around the β-carbon is more important than asymmetry around the α-carbon. However, for drugs with two asymmetric carbons (such as phenylpropanolamine), this does not necessarily hold true. For these compounds, configuration at the β-carbon is important for binding to receptors and increases the potency as direct acting amines. However, the structure-activity relationship for uptake or binding to norepinephrine storage granules (important for indirect-acting amines) may be different from the structure-activity relationships for direct effects. The β-hydroxy substitution may decrease the affinity of the drug for the norepinephrine uptake and/or release mechanism.

MISCELLANEOUS STRUCTURE-ACTIVITY RELATIONSHIP STUDIES

Relatively sparse information is available regarding structure-activity relationships for the CNS stimulation, anorexia, and cardiovascular effects produced by phenylpropanolamine. These are important aspects of the pharmacological activity of phenylpropanolamine, and structure-activity information would be important for a fuller understanding of phenylpropanolamine. The structure-activity relationships for release of free fatty acids from adipose tissue have been well studied, but this is a relatively minor effect of phenylpropanolamine.

The structural requirements for increasing locomotor activity in rats were investigated using the jiggle cage method (Schulte et al., 1941). The basic structure required for CNS stimulant activity was phenyl-1-amino-2-propane. The propyl derivatives had maximum activity, and either increasing or decreasing the length of the side chain decreased the activity. β-Hydroxylation generally decreased activity of the compounds, but this was not always the case for the ephedrines. Monohydroxyphenyl substitution decreased activity, but dihydroxyphenyl substitution increased activity. No conclusion could be drawn regarding the differences between the activity of the optical isomers of various compounds. Finally, it was noted that there was no relationship between the sympathomimetic activity of the drugs and their potency for CNS activity. Phenylpropanolamine was shown to have low potency for increasing locomotor activity in this study.

The CNS stimulating effects of various isomers of ephedrine and related compounds were investigated using locomotor activity in mice as a measure of CNS stimulation (Fairchild & Alles, 1967). The isomers were grouped according to their configuration around the β-carbon (Figure 3.6). In addition, the effects of asymmetry at the α-carbon were investigated. In general, the drugs could be grouped into two categories: drugs that increased locomotor activity at doses considerably less than the LD_{50} and drugs that increased locomotor activity only at doses near the LD_{50}. Both isomers of norephedrine were included in the group in which locomotor activity increased only at doses near the lethal level; furthermore, l-norephedrine was more potent than d-norephedrine. With respect to asymmetry around the β-carbon, the l-isomer was more potent than the d-isomer for both ephedrine and norephedrine.

The structural requirements for CNS depressant and CNS excitant activity of phenylethylamines were investigated in young chickens (Dewhurst & Marley, 1965). Central nervous system depressant and excitant activities were assessed by measurement of sleep activity, cheeping, electrocorticogram activity, and electromyogram activity. According to this classification, phenylpropanolamine had no CNS depressant effect and very low potency for CNS excitant effects. The structure-activity relationships were as follows.

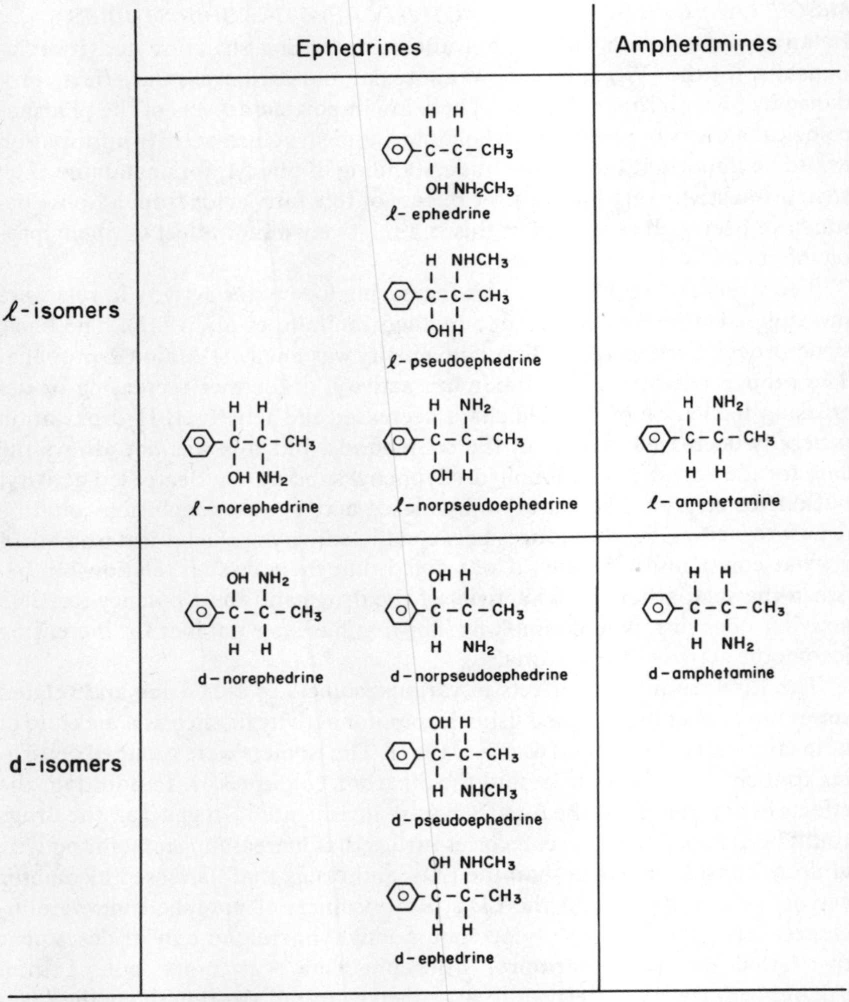

Figure 3.6. Isomers of ephedrines and amphetamines grouped according to configuration around the B-carbon. From Fairchild & Alles (1967).

Substitution at the α-carbon had similar effects on the CNS depressant and excitant activities: methyl substitution decreased the potency and increased the duration of action. On the other hand, the following substitutions had opposite effects on the depressant and excitant activities. N-Methyl substitution increased the potency for depressant effect and decreased the potency for excitant effect. β-Hydroxylation increased the potency for depressant effect and decreased the potency for excitant effect. Finally, 3,4-dihydroxyphenyl substitution increased the potency for CNS depressant effects but abolished CNS excitant activity.

No formal structure-activity study of the anorectic effects of phenylethylamines related to phenylpropanolamine has been published. The anorectic effects of various isomers of ephedrine were compared in normal and genetically obese mice (Arch et al., 1982). Phenylpropanolamine [(±)-norephedrine] produced greater reduction in food intake than did (+)-norephedrine; the effects of (−)-norephedrine were not studied. However, from these results it can be predicted that the (−)-isomer is more potent than the (+)-isomer.

The structural requirements for release of free fatty acids from adipose tissue are as follows (Feller & Finger, 1970; Finger & Feller, 1966). Mobilization of free fatty acids requires β-hydroxylation and ring hydroxylation. In addition, the catechol nucleus is not absolutely required, N-substitution increases the potency, and primary and secondary amines are more potent than tertiary amines. It was not possible to classify the activity of the drugs with respect to α- and β-adrenergic activity, but the response was probably mediated via β-receptor activity. Phenylpropanolamine had very low affinity and low intrinsic activity for release of free fatty acids.

Finally, pattern recognition analysis for classification of sympathomimetic amines indicated that phenylpropanolamine had a mixture of α-adrenergic and CNS stimulant activity (Menon & Cammarata, 1977). This conclusion was based on mathematical analysis of structure-activity relationships of a large number of drugs, including α- and β-adrenergic agonists, cholinergic drugs, and CNS stimulants. The drugs all had the basic structure consisting of X-(C)$_n$-N. The data were preprocessed by principal component analysis to reduce the dimensionality and then subjected to multiple regression analysis for pattern recognition. However, the conclusion that phenylpropanolamine had both α-adrenergic and CNS stimulant activity is questionable, since one of the assumptions of the model was that phenylpropanolamine had precisely this spectrum of activity. Thus the results do not provide additional information regarding the pharmacological activity and structure-activity relationships for phenylpropanolamine.

COMPARISON OF THE ISOMERS OF NOREPHEDRINE

As discussed in Chapter 2 (Chemistry), phenylpropanolamine ($\pm$ norephedrine) has two asymmetric carbon atoms and thus there are four stereoisomers. Many pharmacologic responses are stereospecific (i.e., the response is greater for one stereoisomer than for the other) so it is always important to consider the isomeric form of a drug. Table 3.20 summarizes the studies that compared the pharmacologic activities of these isomers. Effects on locomotor activity, food intake, blood pressure, thermogenesis, and lethality were tested *in vivo;* potentiation of norepinephrine was tested *in vitro* using smooth muscle and cardiac tissues.

Norpseudoephedrine increased locomotor activity at sublethal doses whereas *d*- and *l*-norephedrine increased activity only at near-lethal doses. In the one study that compared phenylpropanolamine and *d*-norpseudoephedrine, phenylpropanolamine was more potent.

Phenylpropanolamine was a more potent anorectic than *d*-norephedrine. No study compared the anorectic potencies of phenylpropanolamine and *l*-norephedrine; however, since the racemic mixture (i.e., phenylpropanolamine) was more potent than the *d*-isomer, *l*-norephedrine is probably more potent than phenylpropanolamine. There are conflicting reports regarding the relative anorectic potencies of phenylpropanolamine and *d*-norpseudoephedrine: In one study phenylpropanolamine was more potent, in another study it was less potent, and in a third study the two were equipotent. *d*-Norpseudoephedrine was more potent than *l*-norpseudoephedrine. Thus, there seems to be no consistent pattern in the potency of the isomer pairs: For norephedrine the *l*-isomer is more potent and for norpseudoephedrine the *d*-isomer is more potent.

For effects on the blood pressure, *l*-norephedrine was more potent than phenylpropanolamine; the other isomers were inactive. For effects on thermogenesis the same order of potency was observed (i.e., the *l*-isomer the most potent, the racemic mixture intermediate, and the *d*-isomer least potent). For potentiation of norepinephrine in smooth muscle or cardiac tissue, *l*-norephedrine was more potent than *d*-norephedrine.

It is difficult to assess quantitatively the stereospecificity of the phenylpropanolamine isomers. For most of the studies summarized in Table 3.20, the ED_{50} values were not reported; in fact, several of the studies compared the isomers only at a single dose and it is impossible to estimate the potencies. For CNS stimulation, *l*-norpseudoephedrine was approximately $1/4$ times as potent as *d*-norpseudoephedrine (Fairchild & Alles, 1967). The LD_{50} for *d*-norephedrine was approximately twice the LD_{50} for *l*-norephedrine (Fairchild and Alles, 1967). The relative potencies for cardiovascular effects cannot be determined directly; however, at the maximum dose tested (10 mg/kg,

IV) phenylpropanolamine increased mean arterial blood pressure 45 mm Hg and *l*-norephedrine increased the pressure 61 mm Hg (Moya-Huff et al., 1987). Thus, there is approximately a two- to four-fold difference in the potencies of the respective stereoisomers.

In general, the pharmacologic responses to the isomers differ only quantitatively. However, it is interesting to note that whereas most phenethylamines inhibited smooth muscle activity, norpseudoephedrine stimulated gastrointestinal smooth muscle (Chen et al., 1929).

In summary, the norpseudoephedrine isomers seem to be more potent than phenylpropanolamine and have less toxicity. For effects on food intake, blood pressure, and thermogenesis, *l*-norephedrine is more potent than phenylpropanolamine and *d*-norephedrine. This is in marked contrast to the stereospecificity of amphetamine since the *d*-isomer of amphetamine is more potent that the *l*-isomer.

DRUG INTERACTIONS

Phenylpropanolamine is available OTC in the United States in appetite-suppressant products and in combination products as cough-cold remedies. Phenylpropanolamine was formerly combined with caffeine in the appetite-suppressant products and is currently combined with antihistamines, anticholinergics, and other agents in the cough-cold remedies. Thus it is important to consider the pharmacological interactions between the components of these products. Furthermore, since these products are available OTC, they can be taken by patients without medical supervision. This accounts for another potential source of drug interactions since the patients may be taking prescription or other OTC drugs at the same time that they take phenylpropanolamine-containing products. The third potential source of drug interactions with phenylpropanolamine is the sale of the so-called amphetamine look-alike drugs, which often contain the triple combination of phenylpropanolamine, caffeine, and ephedrine. Finally, there is a potential for interaction between phenylpropanolamine and certain substances that are consumed in the diet, specifically caffeine and other xanthines in beverages and tyramine in foods. Thus there is considerable potential for drug interactions with phenylpropanolamine.

Investigation of drug interactions involves a considerable amount of research to establish whether a true drug interaction exists and then to determine the nature of the interaction. In order to adequately investigate the interactions between two drugs, the full spectrum of activity of each drug alone must first be investigated; then the activity of one of the drugs must be investigated at a specified dose level (or preferably several dose levels) of the second drug. Only then is it possible to determine whether the two drugs are simply

TABLE 3.20. Comparison of the Isomers of Norephedrine

Isomer(s)[a]	Dose (mg/kg)	Route	Species	Response	Comments	Reference
d-NOR l-NOR d-NORPS l-NORPS d-AMPHET l-AMPHET	Graded doses	IP	Mouse	Locomotor activity Lethality	For drugs that caused CNS stimulation at sublethal doses: d-AMPHET > l-AMPHET > d-NORPS > l-NORPS Drugs that caused CNS stimulation at lethal doses: l-NOR > d-NOR	Fairchild & Alles (1967)
PPA d-NOR l-NOR d-NORPS d-AMPHET	10–50 25–150 5–40 10–50 2	IP	Rat	Locomotor activity	d-NORPS and d-AMPHET increased activity; PPA, d-NOR, l-NOR, no effect	Eisenberg & Maher (1987)
PPA d-NOR	20–80	IP	Rat	Locomotor activity	PPA > d-NOR (except 80 mg/kg)	Katz et al. (1986)
PPA d-NOR d-NORPS l-NORPS	0.50 mmol/kg	PO	Mouse	Food intake Thermogenesis in obese mice	d-NORPS > PPA > d-NOR > l-NORPS d-NORPS > PPA > l-NORPS > d-NOR (l-NOR not reported)	Arch et al. (1982)

Compound	Dose	Route	Species	Effect	Results	Reference
PPA d-NOR	NS	IP	Rat	Food intake	ED_{50}: PPA – 25 mg/kg d-NOR – 63 mg/kg	Katz et al. (1985a)
PPA d-NORPS	10–50	IP	Rat	Lethality Food intake Blood pressure	LD_{50}: PPA – 67 mg/kg d-NOR – 343 mg/kg PPA = d-NORPS PPA – direct effects d-NORPS – indirect effects	Maher et al. (1985)
PPA d-NOR l-NOR d-NORPS l-NORPS	0.3125–10	IV	Rat	Blood pressure (with and without reserpine pretreatment)	l-NOR > PPA, direct effect; d-NOR, d-NORPS, l-NORPS were inactive	Moya-Huff et al. (1987)
d-NOR l-NOR d-NORPS d-AMPHET l-AMPHET	10^{-6} M	in vitro	Rat	Potentiation of norepinephrine responses in vas deferens and atrium	For vas deferens: l-AMPHET > d-AMPHET > d-NORPS > l-NOR > d-NOR For atrial rate: l-NOR > d-NORPS > d-AMPHET > l-AMPHET > d-NOR	Swamy et al. (1969)
PPA d-NORPS l-NORPS d-AMPHET dl-AMPHET	0.0223 mmol/kg	IP	Rat	Brown adipose tissue thermogenesis	l-NOR > PPA > d-NOR; AMPHET > PPA > NORPS	Wellman & Marmon (1985a)

[a] PPA—phenylpropanolamine; NOR—norephedrine; NORPS—norpseudoephedrine; AMPHET—amphetamine; NS—not specified; ED_{50}—dose that decreased food intake 50%; LD_{50}—dose that was lethal in 50% of rats.

additive or subtractive or whether a true synergism (potentiation) or antagonism occurs. The situation is even more complex when one of the drugs is actually a combination product, as is often the case with phenylpropanolamine. In this case, each component of the combination must be tested for possible interactions before the true nature of the drug interaction can be evaluated. Unfortunately, rigorous investigation using appropriate controls is lacking in the majority of the reported cases of drug interactions with phenylpropanolamine. Thus in most cases of such suspected interactions, the interaction should properly be considered a potential drug interaction.

POTENTIATION OF PHENYLPROPANOLAMINE BY MONOAMINE OXIDASE INHIBITORS

Probably the best documented example of drug interactions in humans taking phenylpropanolamine products—and even here the evidence is limited—is the interaction between phenylpropanolamine and monoamine oxidase (MAO) inhibitors. Four case reports have been published reporting that the cardiovascular effects of phenylpropanolamine were potentiated in patients taking MAO inhibitors (Humberstone, 1969; Mason & Buckle, 1968; Smookler & Bermudez, 1982; Terry et al., 1975; Tonks & Lloyd, 1965).

The interaction between phenylpropanolamine and an MAO inhibitor was investigated experimentally in humans (Cuthbert et al., 1969; Cuthbert & Vere, 1971). In one subject, the effects of phenylpropanolamine on blood pressure and heart rate were investigated before and after a 20–30 day course of treatment with the MAO inhibitor tranylcypromine. Phenylpropanolamine was given orally on separate occasions in doses of 50 mg in immediate-release capsules, 50 mg in slow-release form, and 50 mg in a cough linctus preparation. In the control (no MAO inhibition) conditions, phenylpropanolamine in the immediate-release and cough linctus preparations produced a modest elevation of systolic blood pressure and negligible effects on heart rate, whereas phenylpropanolamine in the sustained-release preparation produced no measurable change in the cardiovascular system. Following repeated administration of tranylcypromine, the same doses of phenylpropanolamine produced pronounced increases in both systolic and diastolic blood pressures and a reflex bradycardia. The hypertensive episodes in the case of the immediate-release and cough linctus preparations were so severe that the experiments were terminated by administration of the α-blocking drug phentolamine. Similarly, tranylcypromine potentiated the pressor responses to IV-administered phenylpropanolamine (0.9–20 mg) in three human volunteers (Cuthbert & Vere, 1971). These studies represent the only rigorously documented examples of drug interactions with phenylpropanolamine in human subjects that have been published.

However, the preclinical studies of drug interaction between phenylpropanolamine and MAO inhibitors are not in accord with clinical observations. The structure-activity relationships for interactions between various phenethylamines and MAO inhibition were investigated in dogs (Gatgounis, 1965). Blood pressure and force of contraction of the heart were measured in anesthetized, vagotomized dogs. A series of phenylethylamines were administered IV before and after administration of a dose of 4-phenyl-2-butyl-hydrazine; the dose of this MAO inhibitor was shown to produce near-total inhibition of MAO. The effects of phenylpropanolamine (40 μg/kg, IV) were not potentiated by the MAO inhibitor. The results of the structure-activity analysis indicated that drugs with an α-methyl group are not substrates for MAO, whereas drugs that lack the β-hydroxy group are good substrates for MAO. On the basis of these considerations, phenylpropanolamine would not be expected to be metabolized by MAO.

On the other hand, potentiation of pressor effects of phenylpropanolamine by MAO inhibition was demonstrated in cats with spinal cord transections (D'Mello, 1969). The pressor responses to phenylpropanolamine (100–250 μg, IV) were potentiated by the MAO inhibitor nialamide. However, the pressor responses to phenylpropanolamine were also potentiated by SKF 525A, which is not an MAO inhibitor. The reason for the potentiation of phenylpropanolamine by SKF 525A is not known. Since SKF 525A inhibits hepatic microsomal enzymes, it could potentiate phenylpropanolamine by blocking hepatic metabolism of phenylpropanolamine. Whether this is the mechanism of the interaction is unknown because no study has reported the metabolism of phenylpropanolamine in cats. However, phenylpropanolamine is not metabolized by the liver in monkeys or humans (see Table 3.1); thus it is unlikely that MAO inhibitors potentiate phenylpropanolamine in humans by inhibiting phenylpropanolamine metabolism.

Alternatively, the interaction may be an additive effect on MAO activity *per se*, since recent studies demonstrated that phenylpropanolamine inhibited both brain and liver MAO (Yu, 1986). Phenylpropanolamine inhibited both type A and type B MAO, but was a relatively weak inhibitor. However, no study has tested whether this activity contributes to the hypertensive effects of phenylpropanolamine in the presence of MAO inhibitors.

POTENTIATION OF PHENYLPROPANOLAMINE BY ANTIHYPERTENSIVE DRUGS

Two case reports have been published that indicate that antihypertensive drugs may potentiate the pressor responses to phenylpropanolamine.

CASE 1.   A woman was hospitalized for therapy of hypertension (Misage & McDonald, 1970). Her hypertension was controlled by the adrenergic neuron-blocking drug bethanidine. While in the hospital, she was given three doses of Ornade (phenylpropanolamine, chlorpheniramine, isopropamide) at 12-hr intervals for treatment of a common cold. During the course of the Ornade treatment, her blood pressure again increased back to the prebethanidine levels. Her blood pressure remained elevated for 4 days after cessation of the Ornade, at which time the antihypertensive therapy was changed from bethanidine to methyldopa. The methyldopa was effective in controlling the patient's hypertension. Thus, although the sudden return of hypertension at the onset of Ornade therapy may indicate that the Ornade may be causally related to the hypertension, phenylpropanolamine is a short-acting drug and is not likely to produce a sustained elevation of blood pressure lasting for 4 days after cessation of Ornade therapy. In any case, there are no control data available showing the patient's response to phenylpropanolamine in the absence of bethanidine, so it is not possible to determine whether this is a true potentiation of phenylpropanolamine.

CASE 2.   Interaction between phenylpropanolamine and antihypertensive drugs was observed in a patient taking a combination of methyldopa and the β-blocking drug oxprenolol for control of hypertension (McLaren, 1976). This patient had a history of acute glomerulonephritis at the age of 14 years. At the age of 31 he developed hypertension (blood pressure of 200/120 mm Hg) with uremia. Treatment with methyldopa and oxprenolol was effective in controlling the hypertension, but renal function continued to deteriorate and the uremia became more severe. Triogesic (12.5 mg of phenylpropanolamine, 500 mg of acetaminophen; two tablets, t.i.d.) was prescribed for treatment of a common cold. During the Triogesic treatment, the patient developed headaches, nausea, and paresthesias. His blood pressure was recorded as 220/150 mm Hg, his heart rate was 90 bpm, and the uremia was more severe. One day after cessation of the Triogesic therapy, the blood pressure returned to 140/110 mm Hg, and the paresthesias disappeared. The authors attributed this response to an interaction between phenylpropanolamine and the β-blocker, suggesting that in the presence of the β-blockade the α-adrenergic pressor effect of phenylpropanolamine is unopposed by the β-adrenergic depressor effects. Other interpretations were apparently not considered. Since the pressor effects of phenylpropanolamine in this patient in the absence of antihypertensive therapy is not known, it is not clear whether this is a potentiation of phenylpropanolamine-induced pressor effects.

However, in a controlled clinical study the β-blocker propranolol antagonized the cardiovascular effects of phenylpropanolamine (Pentel et al., 1985). Thus, it is unlikely that the hypertensive episode in Case 2 was due to an interaction between phenylpropanolamine and oxprenolol.

POTENTIATION OF EFFECTS OF TYRAMINE BY PHENYLPROPANOLAMINE

Tyramine is an indirect-acting sympathomimetic amine found in certain foods, including cheeses, pickled herring, and red wine. It is well established that patients taking drugs such as MAO inhibitors may precipitate a hypertensive crisis by eating tyramine-containing foods. In one study in anesthetized dogs, phenylpropanolamine (1 mg/kg, IV) potentiated the pressor response to IV administration of tyramine (Rudzik & Eble, 1967). However, only one dose level of each drug was investigated, and it is not possible to determine whether this was a true potentiation or simply an additive effect since the pressor response to phenylpropanolamine alone was not reported. Also, this was a very high dose of phenylpropanolamine for IV administration.

INTERACTIONS WITH ANTIHISTAMINES

Cough-cold products frequently combine phenylpropanolamine with antihistamines or anticholinergics. Thus, it is important to consider possible drug interactions between phenylpropanolamine and these drugs.

Brompheniramine is a potent antihistamine with little sedative effect, which has been reported to inhibit reuptake of norepinephrine into the nerve terminal. Thus there is potential for interaction between brompheniramine and phenylpropanolamine, since phenylpropanolamine also inhibits reuptake of norepinephrine. Interactions between phenylpropanolamine and brompheniramine were investigated *in vivo* using anesthetized cats, and *in vitro* using isolated aortic strips from rabbits (Persson et al., 1973). Phenylpropanolamine (10–200 μg/kg, IV) produced a dose-dependent increase in carotid blood pressure and heart rate. Antihistaminic doses of brompheniramine had no effect on the responses to phenylpropanolamine, but high doses of brompheniramine decreased the responses to phenylpropanolamine. These results were confirmed by *in vitro* studies. Phenylpropanolamine (0.4–1.6 μg/ml) produced dose-dependent contractions of the aortic strips. Low concentrations of brompheniramine had no effect on the responses to phenylpropanolamine, but higher doses decreased the responses. Thus at antihistaminic doses there was no significant interaction between brompheniramine and phenylpropanolamine, while at high doses there was a nonspecific decrease in the responses to phenylpropanolamine.

INTERACTIONS WITH ANTICHOLINERGIC DRUGS

Anticholinergic drugs such as atropine are often included in cough-cold preparations for their ability to decrease mucus secretions. Interactions between phenylpropanolamine and anticholinergic drugs have been investigated in experimental animals (Davis & Pinkerton, 1972), in healthy volunteers (Mitchell, 1968), and in one case report (Pentel & Mikell, 1982).

Effects of phenylpropanolamine and atropine, alone and in combination, were investigated in rats using four behavioral paradigms (Davis & Pinkerton, 1972). The tests consisted of measurement of locomotor activity and observation of excitatory behaviors such as stereotypy, aggregation lethality (in mice), and acute lethality. The behaviorally effective dose range for phenyl-propanolamine in rats was 20 to 82 mg/kg (IP). Data from the high-dose group were deleted due to the high incidence of lethality from phenylpropa-nolamine alone. Atropine was administered in doses ranging from 0.1 to 1.6 mg/kg (SC), which produced no significant effect on locomotor activity. Atropine had a synergistic effect on the phenylpropanolamine-induced in-crease in locomotor activity; atropine produced a parallel shift of the phenyl-propanolamine dose-response curve to the left. Atropine also synergized with phenylpropanolamine in the aggregation lethality test, but the slope of the dose-response curve was also changed. Atropine had no effect on phenylpro-panolamine-induced stereotypy. Finally, atropine increased the lethality of phenylpropanolamine in some rat strains (Sprague-Dawley and Wistar) but not in others (Long-Evans). Thus the interactions between phenylpropanol-amine and atropine were behavior specific.

In humans, on the other hand, there was no significant interaction be-tween phenylpropanolamine and atropinic drugs on the cardiovascular sys-tem (Mitchell, 1968). Thirty-two normotensive volunteers were investigated in a crossover, randomized, placebo-controlled study. The treatment groups were placebo, phenylpropanolamine (50 mg, sustained-release, b.i.d), and phenylpropanolamine (50 mg, sustained-release) plus belladonna alkaloids, b.i.d. The duration of drug administration was 4 weeks. Blood pressure and heart rate were measured daily, and electrocardiograms were recorded weekly. There were no significant effects of phenylpropanolamine alone on either blood pressure or heart rate. In addition, there were no significant in-teractions between phenylpropanolamine and the belladonna alkaloids with respect to the cardiovascular responses. However, interpretation of the data is limited since no group received belladonna alkaloids alone.

One case was reported of a hypertensive response to phenylpropanolamine that was exacerbated by atropine (Pentel & Mikell, 1982). The patient was a 23-year-old woman with a history of a hypertensive episode in response to a combination decongestant (Contac) containing 50 mg of phenylpropanol-amine, chlorpheniramine, and belladonna alkaloids (Pentel & Mikell, 1982). In a follow-up study, the patient's cardiovascular system was evaluated. This evaluation revealed a previously undiagnosed autonomic dysfunction. Epi-nephrine, administered by IV infusion, produced a pressor response four times the normal response. Phenylpropanolamine doses of 25, 50, and 100 mg (PO) increased the systolic blood pressure by 27, 55, and 71 mm Hg, respectively. These pressor responses to phenylpropanolamine were signifi-cantly greater than pressor responses in normal control patients. In addition, atropine was shown to have an additive effect on the phenylpropanolamine-induced pressor response and produced significant tachycardia. The authors suggest that atropine may contribute to phenylpropanolamine-induced pressor responses by blocking the baroreceptor mediated bradycardia. This interpretation, however, is not supported by the controlled clinical studies of interactions between phenylpropanolamine and atropine.

INTERACTIONS BETWEEN PHENYLPROPANOLAMINE AND CAFFEINE

Phenylpropanolamine has been combined with caffeine and ephedrine in illicit look-alike stimulants. Also, OTC appetite suppressants formerly contained phenylpropanolamine and caffeine; currently, however, no OTC appetite suppressant product contains this combination. Several studies have investigated the potential drug interactions between phenylpropanolamine and caffeine.

Interactions between phenylpropanolamine and caffeine in healthy humans were investigated in a controlled clinical study (Silverman et al., 1980). Supine blood pressures were measured before and at intervals after drug administration for a period of 4 hr. Three groups of subjects were studied. One group received 25 mg of phenylpropanolamine alone (Propadrine). The second group received 25 mg of phenylpropanolamine plus 100 mg of caffeine (Appedrine). The third group received placebo and 25 mg of phenylpropanolamine in a randomized crossover design. The results showed no significant effect of drug treatment on blood pressure or heart rate in any of the treatment groups. Furthermore, there was no significant interaction between phenylpropanolamine and caffeine in regard to blood pressure.

Interactions between CNS effects of phenylpropanolamine and caffeine were investigated (Schlemmer et al., 1984). Effects of phenylpropanolamine (3–300 mg/kg, IP) and caffeine (1–300 mg/kg, IP), alone and in combination, were measured in adult male rats. Caffeine had no effect on phenylpropanolamine-induced increases in locomotor activity or stereotypy, but it potentiated the lethal effects of phenylpropanolamine. Caffeine (10 mg/kg) significantly lowered the LD_{50} of phenylpropanolamine from 72 mg/kg in the controls to 35 mg/kg following caffeine ingestion.

Another study confirmed that caffeine potentiates phenylpropanolamine lethality in rats (Katz et al., 1985b). Lethality was assessed by determining the LD_{50} and the slope of the lethality curve. Furthermore, either the α-adrenergic blocker phentolamine or the β-adrenergic blocker propranolol antagonized the lethality of the phenylpropanolamine-caffeine combination. Propranolol produced no change in the slope of the lethality curve but phentolamine increased the slope, suggesting that the propranolol effect was competitive and the phentolamine effect was noncompetitive.

Synergism between phenylpropanolamine and caffeine was also demonstrated in a drug discrimination test in rats (Holloway et al., 1985). Phenylpropanolamine, caffeine, or ephedrine alone produced only partial drug discrimination against amphetamine. However, the triple combination of phenylpropanolamine-caffeine-ephedrine completely substituted for amphetamine, suggesting additive or synergistic effects on drug discrimination.

Caffeine also potentiated phenylpropanolamine stimulation of brown adipose tissue thermogenesis in rats (Wellman & Marmon, 1985c). Caffeine alone (10 mg/kg, IP) had no effect on thermogenesis.

INTERACTION BETWEEN PHENYLPROPANOLAMINE AND NONSTEROIDAL ANTIINFLAMMATORY DRUGS

In a single case report, a woman taking the Australian appetite suppressant Trimolets (85 mg of D-phenylpropanolamine [SIC]) developed a hypertensive crisis after taking indomethacin (Lee et al., 1979a,b). The drug interaction was later verified by controlled clinical investigation in the same patient. This case report should be evaluated cautiously because the Trimolets formulation was different from the formulation of phenylpropanolamine-containing products sold in the United States. First, Trimolets was an immediate-release formulation containing 85 mg of active ingredient, higher than the recommended dose for immediate-release phenylpropanolamine formulations. Second, some Trimolets formulations contained D-phenylpropanolamine whereas in the United States racemic phenylpropanolamine (i.e., ±-norephedrine) is the approved active ingredient. This is a significant difference because the toxicity of norephedrine isomers varies considerably (see Chapter 4 for a more complete discussion of Trimolets).

CASE. A 27-year-old woman had been taking Trimolets daily for several months with no side effects. A single dose of indomethacin taken after the Trimolets caused a severe bifrontal headache. She was admitted to the hospital with systolic blood pressure of 210 mm Hg; diastolic pressure was unrecordable. One hour later her blood pressure was 150/80 mm Hg and her pulse rate was 72 bpm. The following evening she experienced another brief episode of headache with elevated blood pressure (200/110 mm Hg), which soon subsided to a pressure of 160/90 mm Hg and pulse rate of 56 bpm. On a separate hospital admission for evaluation of recurring headaches, the patient's cardiovascular responses to Trimolets and indomethacin, alone and in combination, were recorded. There was no significant pressor response to Trimolets, indomethacin, or placebo when given individually. When indomethacin was given 40 min after the Trimolets, severe headache, hypertension (blood pressure 200/150 mm Hg), and bradycardia developed. Diazepam (IV) produced sedation but had no effect on the blood pressure. The α-blocker phentolamine (IV) rapidly reduced the blood pressure and headache.

This case history, although well documented, is the only published case of hypertensive crisis produced by combination of phenylpropanolamine with a nonsteroidal antiinflammatory drug (NSAID). There have been no preclinical studies published that have specifically tested this drug interaction.

Given that both phenylpropanolamine and NSAIDs are available OTC and are widely used, it is likely that many individuals take phenylpropanolamine and an NSAID simultaneously. However, review of the literature revealed no other case histories of adverse reactions to this drug combination. Apparently the hypertensive crisis described by Lee et al. (1979a, b) was an idiosyncratic response.

The lack of adverse drug interactions between phenylpropanolamine and another NSAID, aspirin, was confirmed in a 30-day clinical safety study (P.T. Pugliese, unpublished data reviewed in the Federal Register, 1976). In a randomized, placebo-controlled study, 65 adult males and 3 adult females were given 50 mg of phenylpropanolamine with or without 10 gr of aspirin, or placebo four times per day for a total of up to 30 days. There were no significant differences among the treatment groups in vital signs (oral temperature, body weight, pulse rate, blood pressure) or clinical laboratory test results (clinical chemistry, hematology, and urinalysis tests) for any of the observation times. The results of this study confirm the lack of adverse drug interactions between phenylpropanolamine and NSAIDs. (This safety study is described more fully in Chapter 4).

INTERACTIONS BETWEEN PHENYLPROPANOLAMINE AND ADRENERGIC BLOCKING DRUGS

Since phenylpropanolamine is a mixed-acting sympathomimetic amine with at least part of its pharmacodynamic effects mediated via direct effects at α_1-adrenergic receptors, it is reasonable to expect that the effects of phenylpropanolamine would be blocked by α-adrenergic blocking drugs. However, if part of the effects of phenylpropanolamine are due to either norepinephrine release or to inhibition of norepinephrine reuptake, it would be reasonable to expect that some portion of the effects of phenylpropanolamine would be blocked by β-adrenergic blockers, since norepinephrine has both α and β effects. Interactions between phenylpropanolamine and α-blockers were investigated in several studies.

The hypertensive episode produced by phenylpropanolamine in the presence of the MAO inhibitor tranylcypromine was reversed by the α-blocking drug phentolamine (Cuthbert et al., 1969). Phenylpropanolamine caused contraction of smooth muscles in the human urethra both *in vitro* and *in vivo*, and these effects were blocked by the α-blocker phenoxybenzamine (Ek, 1977, 1978). Finally, phenylpropanolamine caused contraction of smooth muscles in the isolated rat vas deferens, and this effect was blocked by the specific α_1-blocker prazosin (Minneman et al., 1983).

The β-adrenergic blocker propranolol antagonized the lethality of phenylpropanolamine; propranolol increased the phenylpropanolamine LD_{50} without changing the slope of the lethality curve (Katz et al., 1985b). Propranolol also antagonized the cardiovascular effects of phenylpropanolamine in humans (Pentel et al., 1985).

INTERACTION WITH OTHER SYMPATHOMIMETIC AMINES

Very few studies have been published that specifically investigated the interactions between phenylpropanolamine and other sympathomimetic amines. Although it would be predicted that phenylpropanolamine and sympathomimetic amines would likely be either additive or synergistic, phenylpropanolamine actually reduced the epinephrine-induced hyperglycemia in rats (Gourju & Lawson, 1957). On the other hand, the isomers of norephedrine potentiated the effects of norepinephrine on the isolated rat vas deferens and right atrium preparations (Swamy et al., 1969), presumably as a result of inhibition of norepinephrine reuptake.

MISCELLANEOUS INTERACTIONS

Cocaine potentiates the effects of many sympathomimetic amines by blockade of the amine uptake mechanism in the noradrenergic neuron terminals. Cocaine did not potentiate the effects of phenylpropanolamine on the nictitating membrane in cats with spinal cord transections (Trendelenburg et al., 1962b). The ED_{50} values (and 95% confidence limits) for phenylpropanolamine-induced contraction of the nictitating membrane before and after acute administration of cocaine were 1160 (547–2470) and 2200 (1700–2840) $\mu g/kg$ (IV), respectively. These are very high doses for IV administration of phenylpropanolamine, since the ED_{50} values for effects on blood pressure and heart rate in control cats were 184 and 145 $\mu g/kg$ (IV), respectively. Interactions between cocaine and phenylpropanolamine on other physiologic responses have not been investigated, so it is not possible to determine whether this lack of potentiation generalizes to other effects of phenylpropanolamine.

In a test of drug effects on psychomotor skills in volunteers, 80 mg of phenylpropanolamine (PO) produced a modest improvement in performance (Nuotto & Seppala, 1984). Phenylpropanolamine also increased the blood pressure (by approximately 8–18 mm Hg) and decreased the heart rate (by approximately 12–17 bpm). Diazepam (10 or 20 mg) antagonized the cardiovascular effects of phenylpropanolamine; diazepam also antagonized the effects of phenylpropanolamine in some psychomotor tests but not in others.

POTENTIAL DRUG INTERACTIONS

Drug interactions between sympathomimetic amines and several other drugs have been documented. Tricyclic antidepressants block reuptake of biogenic amines by the nerve terminals and thus potentiate responses to sympathomimetic amines. β-Adrenergic agonists and ephedrine may have a greater potential for producing cardiac arrhythmias in patients taking digitalis glycosides. Epinephrine, by producing hyperglycemia, may interact with anti-diabetic drugs. Hydrocortisone potentiates the pressor effects of catechol-amines. From these observations, it is reasonable to predict that phenylpro-panolamine would interact with tricyclic antidepressants, digitalis glycosides, antidiabetic drugs, and hydrocortisone [see drug-interaction references such as Hansten (1979) and Lerman and Weibert (1982)]. However, no studies spe-cifically documenting interactions between phenylpropanolamine and any of these drugs have been published.

ABUSE LIABILITY

In view of current concern over the use of phenylpropanolamine in the so-called amphetamine look-alike drugs, it is important to evaluate the abuse liability of phenylpropanolamine. Abuse liability testing is a relatively recent development in the field of pharmacology. Abuse liability testing involves in-vestigation of whether any particular drug has the potential to be abused by human subjects. The term "abuse liability" refers primarily to drug-seeking and drug-taking behavior and is to be considered independently from other aspects of drug abuse such as physical dependence, withdrawal, and tolerance.

Drug abuse is primarily a phenomenon confined to the human condition. Thus abuse liability testing is ideally investigated in humans. One means of testing the abuse liability of drugs in humans is to administer the test drug to volunteers and evaluate their subjective responses to the drug by use of the Addiction Research Center Inventory (ARCI), a subjective-effect question-naire. However, ethical considerations limit the studies that can be conducted in volunteers, especially when dealing with drugs with high abuse liability. Thus animal models of drug abuse have been developed that have contributed significantly to understanding of drug abuse phenomena. Perhaps the most reliable animal model for predicting abuse liability is the drug self-adminis-tration paradigm [see the review by Griffiths et al. (1981)]. In this model, laboratory animals are usually prepared with an indwelling IV catheter for administration of drugs. Then, by means of operant conditioning techniques, the animals are trained to press a lever in order to receive an IV dose of drug. Studies have demonstrated that animals generally will become conditioned to press the lever in order to receive drugs that are frequently abused by humans (e.g., opiates, cocaine, sedative-hypnotics), whereas they will not press the lever in order to receive drugs that are generally not abused by humans. That is, drugs of abuse are generally reinforcers in the self-administration para-digm, whereas other drugs are not. In order to test for the abuse liability of a test drug, the animals are first trained to press the lever to receive doses of known drug reinforcers. Once the drug reinforcement schedule has been established, the IV drug dose is changed from the standard reinforcer to the test drug. A drug is considered to have high abuse liability if the animal continues to press the lever to receive doses of the test drug. On the other hand, if the test drug fails to sustain the operant conditioning, it is considered to have a low abuse liability.

The abuse liability of phenylpropanolamine was determined by means of the self-administration technique in baboons (Griffiths et al., 1978). Phenylpropanolamine (0.1–30 mg/kg, IV) failed to produce reinforcement of drug administration. A maximum of eight doses per day was allowed. Thus the total daily doses of phenylpropanolamine were 0.8–240 mg/kg. In addition, for comparison of abuse liability with therapeutic efficacy, it was demonstrated that phenylpropanolamine in the doses used in the abuse liability testing paradigm did produce anorexia in the baboon. By interpolation of the data, the daily dose of phenylpropanolamine required to reduce food intake by 50% was estimated to be 48 mg/kg.

In order to compare the abuse liability of a series of phenylethylamine anorectic drugs, the reinforcing doses and anorectic doses were compared. The reinforcing dose was defined as the lowest dose of drug that caused reinforcement of operant responding in the self-administration paradigm. The anorectic dose was defined as the dose required to decrease food intake by 50%. Thus the ratio of the reinforcing dose to the anorectic dose is a measure of the relative potency for abuse liability and anorectic efficacy. Drugs with a high reinforcing : anorectic ratio would have high abuse liability and low anorectic efficacy, whereas drugs with a ratio of less than 1.0 would be effective anorectic drugs with low abuse liability. In the series of phenylethylamines tested, phenylpropanolamine and fenfluramine had the lowest reinforcing : anorectic ratios, while diethylpropion and d-amphetamine had the highest ratios. In fact, the reinforcing : anorectic ratio for phenylpropanolamine was zero, since phenylpropanolamine did not reinforce responding at doses as high as 30 mg/kg (IV), q. 3 hr. In comparison, cocaine, which has a high abuse liability, had a reinforcing : anorectic ratio 14.81 higher than that of d-amphetamine.

Monkeys also failed to self-administer phenylpropanolamine (Woolverton et al., 1986). Rhesus monkeys were trained to self-administer cocaine IV; then, phenylpropanolamine (30–300 mg/kg total dose, IV) was substituted for cocaine. These doses of phenylpropanolamine were considered "behaviorally effective" and the monkeys were anorectic after the test. However, the monkeys did not self-administer phenylpropanolamine.

In humans as well, phenylpropanolamine produced no reinforcement of drug ingestion (Chait et al., 1984; Schuster & Johanson, 1985). On four occasions, volunteers were given one of two medications, either an active drug or a placebo. The active-drug and placebo capsules were color coded so that the volunteer could identify the capsule but did not know whether it contained active drug or placebo. The subjects evaluated their subjective responses to the drug. In a subsequent test session, they were asked which capsule they would prefer to take again. The volunteers chose amphetamine, phenmetrazine, and diethylpropion more frequently than placebo. However, they selected phenylpropanolamine (12.5, 25, and 50 mg) no more frequently than placebo.

One additional test to determine whether a drug is likely to be abused is to measure drug self-administration in stressed animals. For example, although rats normally refuse to drink ethanol when given the choice, they will choose to drink ethanol after they have been exposed to environmental stress. However, rats failed to self-administer phenylpropanolamine after exposure to stress (Nash & Maickel, 1986). The rats were given the choice of drinking a saccharin solution with or without 0.05% (w/v) phenylpropanolamine. In the absence of stress, the rats initially drank substantial amounts of the phenylpropanolamine-saccharin solution (equivalent to 22–35 mg/kg/day of phenylpropanolamine). Their intake of phenylpropanolamine declined to a baseline level (approximately 15 mg/kg/day of phenylpropanolamine) after 1 week, then remained fairly constant for up to 4 weeks. Exposure to environmental stress had no significant effect on the consumption of phenylpropanolamine. These results further confirm that phenylpropanolamine has low abuse potential.

Drug-discrimination tests also can be used to assess the abuse liability of drugs. In general, experimental animals will learn to self-administer drugs that are abused frequently by humans, for example, opiates, sedative-hypnotics, CNS stimulants, and cocaine. To determine whether a test drug has abuse potential, experimental animals are trained to discriminate a drug known to be abused by humans, then the test drug is substituted for the known drug. If the test drug maintains drug discrimination it probably has high abuse liability. As discussed in a previous section of this chapter, low doses of phenylpropanolamine do not maintain drug discrimination against amphetamine and high doses produce variable but usually incomplete drug discrimination.

Thus the results from the experimental animal tests suggest that phenylpropanolamine has no abuse liabilty. The abuse liability of phenylpropanolamine has also been investigated in humans (see Chapter 4). Consistent with the results of the animal testing, phenylpropanolamine had low abuse liability in humans.

REFERENCES

Ahlquist, R. P. (1948). A study of the adrenotropic receptors. *Am J Physiol, 153,* 586-600.

Antunes-Rodrigues, J., & McCann, S. M. (1970). Water, sodium chloride, and food intake induced by injections of cholinergic and adrenergic drugs into the third ventricle of the rat brain. *Proc Soc Exp Biol Med, 133,* 1464-1470.

Arch, J. R. S., Ainsworth, A. T., & Cawthorne, M. A. (1982). Thermogenic and anorectic effects of ephedrine and congeners in mice and rats. *Life Sci, 30,* 1817-1826.

Aviado, D. M., Jr., & Schmidt, C. F. (1957). Effects of sympathomimetic drugs on pulmonary circulation: with special reference to a new pulmonary vasodilator. *J Pharmacol Exp Ther, 120,* 512-527.

Aviado, D. M., Jr., Wnuck, A. L., & de Beer, E. J. (1959). A comparative study of nasal decongestion by sympathomimetic drugs. *Arch Otolarynogol, 69,* 598-605.

Axelrod, J. (1953). Studies on sympathomimetic amines. I. The biotransformation and physiological disposition of *l*-ephedrine and *l*-norephedrine. *J Pharmacol Exp Ther, 109,* 62-73.

Axelrod, J. (1955). The enzymatic demethylation of ephedrine. *J Pharmacol Exp Ther, 114,* 430-438.

Baldessarini, R. J. (1971). Release of aromatic amines from brain tissues of the rat in vitro. *J Neurochem, 18,* 2509-2518.

Baldessarini, R. J., & Harris, J. E. (1974). Effects of amphetamines on the metabolism of catecholamines in the rat brain. *J Psychiatr Res, 11,* 41-43.

Ban, T., & Fujita, T. (1969). Mathematical approach to structure-activity study of sympathomimetic amines. Norepinephrine-uptake inhibition. *J Med Chem, 12,* 353-356.

Barger, G., & Dale, H. D. (1910). Chemical structure and sympathomimetic action of amines. *J Physiol* (London), *41,* 19-59.

Barrett, W. E., Hanigan, J. J., & Snyder, D. L. (1981). The bioavailabiltiy of sustained-release tablets which contain phenylpropanolamine and chlorpheniramine. *Curr Ther Res, 30,* 640-654.

Bassett, J. R., Story, M., & Cairncross, K. D. (1968). The influence of orphenadrine upon the actions of a series of sympathomimetic agents. *Eur J Pharmacol, 4,* 198-204.

Beckett, A. H., & Triggs, E. J. (1967). Buccal absorption of basic drugs and its application as an in vivo model of passive drug transfer through lipid membranes. *J Pharm Pharmacol, 19* (suppl), 31s-41s.

Berti, F., & Shore, P. A. (1967). Interaction of reserpine and ouabain on amine concentrating mechanisms in the adrenergic neurone. *Biochem Pharmacol, 16,* 2271-2274.

Bhagat, B., Jackson, C., Wong, H. Y. C., Shein, K., & Bovell, G. (1965). False neurochemical transmitters and response to tyramine in reserpine pretreated preparations. *Life Sci, 4,* 1281-1287.

Boissier, J-R., Simon, P., Fichelle, J., & Hervouet, F. (1965). Action psychoanaleptique de quelques anorexigenes derives de la phenylethylamine. *Therapie, 20,* 297-309.

Breese, G. R., Kopin, I. J., & Weise, V. K. (1970). Effects of amphetamine derivatives on brain dopamine and noradrenaline. *Br J Pharmacol, 38,* 537-545.

Burgen, A. S. V., & Iversen, L. L. (1965). The inhibition of noradrenaline uptake by sympathomimetic amines in the rat isolated heart. *Br J Pharmacol, 25,* 34-49.

Cairns, M. J., Foldys, J. E., & Rees, J. M. H. (1984). The effects of phenylpropanolamine and other sympathomimetics on food consumption and motor activity in mice. *J Pharm Pharmacol, 36,* 704-706.

Caldwell, J., Dring, L. G., Franklin, R. B., Koster, U., Smith, R. L., & Williams, R. T. (1977). Comparative metabolism of the amphetamine drugs of dependence in man and monkeys. *J Med Primatol, 6,* 367-375.

Chait, L. D., Uhlenhuth, E. H., & Johanson, C. E. (1984). Drug preference and mood in humans: mazindol and phenylpropanolamine. In L. S. Harris (Ed.). *Problems of Drug Dependence, 1983,* NIDA Research Monograph 49: DHHS Publication No. (ADM) 84-1316. Washington, DC (pp 327-328).

Chait, L. D., Uhlenhuth, E. H., & Johanson, C. E. (1986). The discriminative stimulus and subjective effects of phenylpropanolamine, mazindol and *d*-amphetamine in humans. *Pharmacol Biochem Behav, 24,* 1665-1672.

Chen, K. K., Wu, C. K., & Henriksen, E. (1929). Relationship between the pharmacological action and the chemical constitution and configuration of the optical isomers of ephedrine and related compounds. *J Pharmacol Exp Ther, 36,* 363-400.

Chen, M. J., Sutton, R. L., & Feeney, D. M. (1986). Recovery of function following brain injury in rat and cat: beneficial effects of phenylpropanolamine [Abstract]. *Proceedings of the Soc Neurosci, 12,* 881.

Cuthbert, M. F., Greenberg, M. P., & Morley, S. W. (1969). Cough and cold remedies: A potential danger to patients on monoamine oxidase inhibitors. *Br Med J, 1,* 404-406.

Cuthbert, M. F., & Vere, D. W. (1971). Potentiation of the cardiovascular effects of some catecholamines by a monoamine oxidase inhibitor. *Br J Pharmacol, 43,* 471p-472p.

Davis, W. M., & Pinkerton, J. T., III (1972). Synergism by atropine of central stimulant properties of phenylpropanolamine. *Toxicol Appl Pharmacol, 22,* 138-145.

Dewhurst, W. G., & Marley, E. (1965). Action of sympathomimetic and allied amines on the central nervous system of the chicken. *Br J Pharmacol, 25,* 705-727.

D'Mello, A. (1969). Interaction between phenylpropanolamine and monoamine oxidase inhibitors. *J Pharm Pharmacol, 21,* 577-580.

Dowse, R., Haigh, J. M., & Kanfer, I. (1983). Determination of phenylpropanolamine in serum and urine by high-performance liquid chromatography. *J Pharm Sci, 72,* 1018-1020.

Dring, L. G., Franklin, R. B., & Williams, R. T. (1975). The fate of amphetamine and norephedrine in the tamarin monkey compared with man. *W Afri J Pharmac Drug Res, 2,* 26-30.

Dulloo, A. G., & Miller, D. S. (1984). Thermogenic drugs for the treatment of obesity: Sympathetic stimulants in animal models. *Br J Nutr, 52,* 179-196.

Eisenberg, M. S., Silverman, H. I., & Maher, T. J. (1987). A comparison of the effects of phenylpropanolamine (PPA), *d*-amphetamine and *d*-norpseudoephedrine on open-field locomotion and food intake in the rat. *Appetite* (in press).

Ek, A. (1977). Innervation and receptor functions of the human urethra. *Scand J Urol Nephrol* (suppl), *45,* 1-50.

Ek, A. (1978). Adrenergic innvervation and adrenergic mechanisms. A study of the human urethra. *Acta Pharmacol Toxicol, 43,* 35-40.

El Egakey, M. A., & Speiser, P. P. (1982). In vitro and in vivo release studies of slow release phenylpropanolamine-polymethylcyanoacrylate entrapment products. *Acta Pharm Technol, 28,* 169-175.

Epstein, A. E. (1959). Suppression of eating and drinking by amphetamine and other drugs in normal and hyperphagic rats. *J Comp Physiol Psychol, 52,* 37-45.

Fairchild, M. D., & Alles, G. A. (1967). The central locomotor stimulatory activity and acute toxicity of the ephedrine and norephedrine isomers in mice. *J Pharmacol Exp Ther, 158,* 135-139.

Federal Register (1976). Establishment of a monograph for OTC cold, cough, allergy, bronchodilator and antiasthmatic drug products. Docket No. 76N-0052. (Reference 10. Pugliese,

P.T., "Sine-Aid II. Human Safety Study," Draft of unpublished data is included in OTC Volume 040298).

Feller, D. R., & Finger, K. F. (1970). Lipolytic activity of structurally related agonists in rat epididymal fat tissue in vitro. *Biochem Pharmacol, 19,* 705-713.

Finger, K. F., & Feller, D. R. (1966). Interaction of various phenethylamines with the adrenergic-adipose tissue receptor system, in vitro. *J Pharm Sci, 55,* 1051-1054.

Fletcher, H. P., Wannarka, G. L., & Sandage, B. W., Jr. (1982). The glycemic effects of sympathomimetics in stressed mice. *Res Commun Chem Pathol Pharmacol, 35,* 377-388.

Fox, A. W., Abel, P. W., & Minneman, K. P. (1985). Activation of α_1-adrenoceptors increases [^{3}H]inositol metabolism in rat vas deferens and caudal artery. *Eur J Pharmacol, 116,* 145-152.

Gatgounis, J. (1965). Structural activity relationships of a series of amines injected before and after monoamine oxidase inhibitor. *Arch Internatl Pharmacodyn Ther, 154,* 412-420.

Ghouri, M. S. K., & Haley, T. J. (1969). In vitro evaluation of a series of sympathomimetic amines and the beta-adrenergic blocking properties of cyclopentamine. *J Pharm Sci, 58,* 882-884.

Goudie, A. J., Atkinson, J., & West, C. R. (1986). Discriminative properties of the psychostimulant *dl*-cathinone in a two lever operant task. *Neuropharmacology, 25,* 85-94.

Gourju, A., & Lawson, A. (1957). The blocking activity of sympathomimetic amines on adrenaline hyperglycaemia. *Biol Chem, 67,* 357-360.

Greiner, T. H., & Garb, S. (1950). The influence of drugs on the irritability and automaticity of heart muscle. *J Pharmacol Exp Ther, 98,* 215-223.

Griffiths, R. R., Brady, J. V., & Bigelow, G. E. (1981). Predicting the dependence liability of stimulant drugs. *Behavioral Pharmacology of Human Drug Dependence.* NIDA Research Monograph No. 37 (pp. 182-196).

Griffiths, R. R., Brady, J. V., & Snell, J. D. (1978). Relationship between anorectic and reinforcing properties of appetite suppressant drugs: Implications for assessment of abuse liability. *Biol Psychiatr, 13,* 283-290.

Hansten, P. D. (1979). *Drug Interactions,* 4th ed. Lea & Febiger, Philadelphia.

Hartung, W. H., & Munch, J. C. (1931). Amino alcohols VI. The preparation and pharmacodynamic activity of four isomeric phenylpropylamines. *J Am Chem Soc, 53,* 1875-1879.

Heimlich, K. R., MacDonnell, D. R., Flanagan, T. L., & O'Brien, P. D. (1961). Evaluation of a sustained release form of phenylpropanolamine hydrochloride by urinary excretion studies. *J Pharm Sci, 50,* 232-237.

Hernandez, L., & Hoebel, B. G. (1986). Microdialysis of the nucleus accumbens: effects of amphetamine and phenylpropanolamine on dopamine and its metabolites in awake rats [Abstract]. *Proceedings of the Soc Neurosci, 12,* 918.

Hoebel, B. G. (1977). Pharmacologic control of feeding. *Ann Rev Pharmacol Toxicol, 17,* 605-621.

Hoebel, B. G. (1979). Hypothalamic self-stimulation and stimulation escape in relation to feeding and mating. *Fed Proc, 38,* 2454-2461.

Hoebel, B. G. (1985). Brain neurotransmitters in food and drug reward. *Amer J Clin Nutr, 42,* 1133-1150.

Hoebel, B. G., Hernandez, L., & Thompson, R. D. (1975). Phenylpropanolamine inhibits feeding, but not drinking, induced by hypothalamic stimulation. *J Comp Physiol Psychol, 89,* 1046-1052.

Holloway, F. A., Michaelis, R. C., & Huerta, P. L. (1985). Caffeine-phenylethylamine combinations mimic the amphetamine discriminative cue. *Life Sci, 36,* 723-730.

Huidobro, F., & Croxatto, R. (1951). Fundamental basis of the specificity of pressor and depressor amines in their vascular effects. *Acta Physiol Latin Am, 1,* 270-290.

Humberstone, P. M. (1969). Hypertension from cold remedies. *Br Med J, 1,* 846.

Innes, I. R., & Kohli, J. D. (1969). Excitatory action of sympathomimetic amines on 5-hydroxytryptamine receptors of gut. *Br J Pharmacol, 35,* 383-393.

Iversen, L. L. (1964). Inhibition of noradrenaline uptake by sympathomimetic amines (Letter). *J Pharm Pharmacol, 16,* 435-437.

Iversen, L. L. (1965). The uptake of catechol amines at high perfusion concentrations in the rat isolated heart: A novel catecholamine uptake process. *Br J Pharmacol, 25,* 18-33.

Iversen, L. L. (1970). Neuronal uptake processes for amines and amino acids. *Adv Biochem Psychopharmacol, 2,* 109-132.

Katz, N. L., Jazwiec, N., King, M., Davis, J. M., & Schlemmer, R. F., Jr. (1985a). Comparative effects of systemically administered racemic phenylpropanolamine (PPA) and its (+)-isomer on rat food intake and lethality. [Abstract]. *Proceedings of the Amer. Soc Pharmacol Exp Ther, 27,* 167.

Katz, N. L., King, M., Jazwiec, N., Williams, E. A., Davis, J. M., & Schlemmer, R. F., Jr. (1985b). Adrenergic blockade antagonizes the lethality in rats by phenylpropanolamine (PPA) alone and in combination with caffeine (C) [Abstract]. *Proceedings of the Federation of Am Soc Exp Biol, 44,* 1637.

Katz, N. L., Hare, M., Davis, J. M., & Schlemmer, R. F., Jr. (1986). Comparison of racemic phenylpropanolamine (PPA) with its (+)-isomer on spontaneous locomotor activity in rats [Abstract]. *Proceedings of the Federation of Am Soc Exp Biol, 45,* 429.

Kopin, I. J. (1972). Aminergic neurons and substitute transmitters in brain. *Res Publ Assoc Res Nerv Mental Dis, 50,* 207-215.

Kornblith, C. L., & Hoebel, B. G. (1976). A dose-response study of anorectic drug effects on food intake, self-stimulation, and stimulation-escape. *Pharmacol Biochem Behav, 5,* 215-218.

Krantz, J. C. Jr., & Hartung, W. (1931). Aminoalcohols VI. A study of the action of phenylpropanolamine upon the blood sugar of rabbits. *J Am Pharm Assoc, 20,* 429-433.

Lands, A. M., Arnold, A., McAuliff, J. P., Luduena, F. P., & Brown, R. G., Jr. (1967). Differentiation of receptor systems activated by sympathomimetic amines. *Nature, 214,* 597-598.

Leaders, F. E., Fortenberry, B., & Kagawa, C. M. (1970). A comparison of mydriatic and ocular hypotensive activities of selected phenylethylamine derivatives administered topically to rabbits. *Arch Internatl Pharmacodyn, 183,* 93-106.

Lee, K. Y., Beilin, L. J., & Vandongen, R. (1979a). Severe hypertension after administration of phenylpropanolamine (Letter). *Med J Aust, 1,* 525-526.

Lee, K. Y., Beilin, L. J., & Vandongen, R. (1979b). Severe hypertension after ingestion of an appetite suppressant (phenylpropanolamine) with indomethacin. *Lancet, 1,* 1110-1111.

Leindorfer, A. (1950). The action of sympathomimetic amines on the central nervous system and the blood sugar: Relation of chemical structure to mechanism of action. *J Pharmacol Exp Ther, 98,* 62-71.

Lerman, F., & Weibert, R. T. (1982). *Drug Interactions Index.* Medical Economics Books, Oradell, NJ.

Levitt, M., Cumiskey, W. R., & Shargel, L. (1974). Studies on the physiologic disposition and activity of phenylpropanolamines in the mouse. *Drug Metab Disposition, 2,* 187-193.

Levy, B., & Ahlquist, R. P. (1957). Inhibition of the adrenergic depressor response. *J Pharmacol Exp Ther, 121,* 414-420.

Liebman, J. (1961). Modification of the chronotropic action of sympathomimetic amines by reserpine in the heart-lung preparation of the dog. *J Pharmacol Exp Ther, 133,* 63-69.

Loman, J., Rinkel, M., & Myerson, A. (1939). Comparative effects of amphetamine sulfate (benzedrine sulfate), paredrine and propadrine on the blood pressure. *Am Heart J, 18,* 89-93.

Lonnerholm, G., Grahnen, A., & Lindstrom, B. (1984). Steady-state kinetics of sustained-release phenylpropanolamine. *Internatl J Clin Pharmacol Ther Toxicol, 22,* 39-41.

Lorhan, P. H., & Mosser, D. (1947). Phenylpropanolamine hydrochloride: Vasopressor drug, for maintaining blood pressure during spinal anesthesia. *Ann Surg, 125,* 171-176.

McIlreath, F. J., De Graw, W., & Kadar, V. (1965). A method for evaluating drug action on the cardiovascular system. *Arch Internatl Pharmacodyn, 157,* 330-338.

McLaren, E. H. (1976). Severe hypertension produced by interaction of phenylpropanolamine with methyldopa and oxprenolol. *Br Med J, 2,* 283-284.

MacPhail, R. C. (1982). Comparison of the effects of phenylpropanolamine and caffeine on schedule-controlled performance [Abstract]. *Proceedings of the Federation of Am Soc Exp Biol, 41,* 1074.

Maher, T., Eisenberg, M., Moya-Huff, F., & Kiritsy, P. (1985). Pharmacological differences between two anorexiants: Phenylpropanolamine (PPA) and d-norpseudoephedrine (d-NOR) [Abstract]. *Proceedings of the Federation of Am Soc Exp Biol, 44,* 1162.

Maitai, C. K. (1975). D-Norpseudoephedrine as an anti-asthmatic: Comparison with l-ephedrine, d-pseudoephedrine. *East Afr Med J, 52,* 330-332.

Marcus, S. (1984). A case for controlled-release drugs in pediatric practice. *Adv Ther, 1,* 159-171.

Mason, W. D., & Amick, E. N. (1981). High-pressure liquid chromatographic analysis of phenylpropanolamine in human plasma following derivatization with O-phthalaldehyde. *J Pharm Sci, 70,* 707-709.

Mason, A. M., & Buckle, R. M. (1968). "Cold" cures and monoamine-oxidase inhibitors. *J Pharm Soc Jpn, 88,* 845-846.

Mayer, S. E. (1980). Neurohumoral transmission and the autonomic nervous system. In A.G. Gilman, L.S. Goodman, & A. Gilman (Eds.). *The Pharmacological Basis of Therapeutics.* Macmillan, New York (pp. 56-90).

Menon, G. K. & Cammarata, A. (1977). Pattern recognition II. Investigation of structure-activity relationships. *J Pharm Sci, 66,* 304-314.

Minneman, K. P., Fox, A. W., & Abel, P. W. (1983). Occupancy of alpha$_1$-adrenergic receptors and contraction of rat vas deferens. *Molec Pharmacol, 23,* 359-368.

Minneman, K. P., & Johnson, R. D. (1984). Characterization of *alpha*-1 adrenergic receptors linked to [^{3}H]inositol metabolism in rat cerebral cortex. *J Pharmacol Exp Ther, 230,* 317-323.

Misage, J. R., & McDonald, R. H., Jr., (1970). Antagonism of hypotensive action of bethanidine by "common cold" remedy. *Br Med J, 4,* 347.

Mitchell, C. A. (1968). Possible cardiovascular effect of phenylpropanolamine and belladonna alkaloids. *Curr Ther Res, 10,* 47-53.

Moya-Huff, F. A., Kiritsy, P. J., & Maher, T. J. (1987). Cardiovascular differences between phenylpropanolamine and its related norephedrine isomers in the rat. *J Pharm Sci, 76,* 114-116.

Moya-Huff, F. A., & Maher, T. J. (1987). Adrenergic receptor subtype activation by (+)-, (−)-, and (±)-norephedrine in the pithed rat. *J Pharm Pharmacol, 39,* 108-112.

Nash, J. F., Jr., & Maickel, R. P. (1986). Effects of exposure to stressful stimuli on the free-choice consumption of various phenethylamines by rats. *Alcohol Drug Res, 6,* 403-415.

Neelakantan, L., & Kostenbauder, H. B. (1976). Electron-capture GLC determination of phenylpropanolamine as a pentafluorophenyloxazolidine derivative. *J Pharm Sci, 65,* 740-742.

Noble, R. E. (1982). Phenylpropanolamine and blood pressure (Letter). *Lancet, 1,* 1419.

Nuotto, E., & Seppala, T. (1984). Phenylpropanolamine counteracts diazepam effects in psychophysiological tests. *Curr Ther Res, 36,* 606-616.

Patil, P. N., LaPidus, J. B., & Tye, A. (1967a). Steric aspects of adrenergic drugs. I. Comparative effects of *DL* isomers and desoxy derivatives. *J Pharmacol Exp Ther, 155,* 1-12.

Patil, P. N., LaPidus, J. B., Campbell, D., & Tye, A. (1967b). Steric aspects of adrenergic drugs II. Effects of *DL* isomers and desoxy derivatives on the reserpine-pretreated vas deferens. *J Pharmacol Exp Ther, 155,* 13-23.

Pentel, P. R, Asinger, R. W., & Benowitz, N. L. (1985). Propranolol antagonism of phenylpropanolamine-induced hypertension. *Clin Pharmacol Ther, 37,* 488-494.

Pentel, P., & Mikell, F. (1982). Reaction to phenylpropalamine/chlorpheniramine/belladonna compound in a woman with unrecognized autonomic dysfunction (Letter). *Lancet, 2,* 274.

Persson, C. G. A., Erjefalt, I., & Keman, M. (1973). Brompheniramine and the cardio-vascular effects of norephedrine and noradrenaline. *Acta Allergol, 28,* 401-415.

Rajan, K. S., Davis, J. M., & Colburn, R. W. (1974). Metal chelates in the storage and transport of neurotransmitters: Interactions of Cu^{2+} with ATP and biogenic amines. *J Neurochem, 22,* 137-147.

Ratnasooriya, W. D., Gilmore, D. P., & Wadsworth, R. M. (1979a). Antifertility effect of sympathomimetic drugs on male rats when applied locally to the vas deferens. *J Reprod Fertil, 56,* 643–651.

Ratnasooriya, W. D., Gilmore, D. P., & Wadsworth, R. M. (1980). Effect of local application of sympathomimetic drugs to the epididymis on fertility in rats. *J Reprod Fertil, 58,* 19-25.

Ratnasooriya, W. D., Gilmore, D. P., & Wadsworth, R. M. (1981). Effect of norephedrine locally applied to the vas deferens on semen quality of rabbits. *Ind J Exp Biol, 19,* 20-25.

Ratnasooriya, W. D., Wadsworth, R. M., & Gilmore, D. P. (1979b). The effect of sympathomimetic drugs on contractility of the vas deferens *in vitro* and *in vivo*. *J Reprod Fertil, 56,* 633-641.

Resnick, S. I., Hernandez, L., Chen, J., & Hoebel, B. G. (1978). Effect of the anorectic drug, phenylpropanolamine, on blood glucose in rats. *Pharmacology, 17,* 157-162.

Rhodes, C. T., Wai, K., & Banker, G. S. (1970). Molecular scale drug entrapment as a precise method of controlled drug release III. In vitro and in vivo studies of drug release. *J Pharm Sci, 59,* 1581-1584.

Rogers, K. J., & Hutchins, D. A. (1972). Studies on the relation of chemical structure to glycogenolytic activity in the brain. *Eur J Pharmacol, 20,* 97-103.

Rubin, R. P., & Jaanus, S. D. (1966). A study of the release of catecholamines from the adrenal medulla by indirectly acting sympathomimetic amines. *Naunyn-Schmiedebergs Arch Pharmakol Exp Path, 254,* 125-127.

Rudzik, A. D., & Eble, J. N. (1967). The potentiation of pressor responses to tyramine by a number of amphetamine-like compounds. *Proc Soc Exp Biol Med, 124,* 655-657.

Sandage, B. W., Jr., & Fletcher, H. P. (1983). Glycemic response to selected sympathomimetics in stressed normal and goldthioglucose mice. *Pharmacology, 27,* 110-116.

Schlemmer, R. F., Heinze, W. J., Asta, C. L., Katz, N. L., & Davis, J. M. (1984). Caffeine potentiates phenylpropanolamine (PPA) lethality but not motor behavior. *Fed Proc, 43,* 572.

Schonenberger, H., Petter, A., Kuhling, V., & Bindl, L. (1976). Synthesis and cardiovascular testing of *N*-(3'-methoxy-benzamidomethyl)-*D*-norephedrine and analogous compounds. *Arch Pharm, 309,* 289-301.

Schulte, J. W., Reif, E. C., Bacher, J. A., Jr., Lawrence, W. S., & Tainter, M. L. (1941). Further study of central stimulation from sympathomimetic amines. *J Pharmacol Exp Ther, 71,* 62-74.

Schuster, C. R., & Johanson, C. E. (1985). Efficacy, dependence potential and neurotoxicity of anorectic drugs. In L. S. Seiden & R. L. Baltser (Eds.), *Behavioral Pharmacology: The Current Status,* 263-279. New York: Alan R. Liss, Inc.

Sherman, P. S., Fisher, S. J., Wieland, D. M., & Sisson, J. C. (1985). Over-the-counter drugs block heart accumulation of MIBG [Abstract]. *J Nucl Med, 26,* 35.

Shore, P. A. (1966). The mechanism of norepinephrine depletion by reserpine, metaraminol and related agents. The role of monoamine oxidase. *Pharmacol Rev, 18,* 561-568.

Silverman, H. I., Kreger, B. E., Lewis, G. P., Karabelas, A., Paone, R., & Foley, M. (1980). Lack of side effects from orally administered phenylpropanolamine and phenylpropanolamine with caffeine: A controlled three-phase study. *Curr Ther Res, 28,* 185-194.

Sinsheimer, J. E., Dring, L. G., & Williams, R. T. (1973). Species differences in the metabolism of norephedrine in man, rabbit and rat. *Biochem J, 136,* 763-771.

Sisson, J. C., Wieland, D. M., Tobes, M., Meyers, L., Mallette, S., Sherman, P., Shen, S-W, Shulkin, B., Shapiro, B., & Beierwaltes, WH. (1985). Kinetics of a norepinephrine analog differ in heart and parotid glands of man [Abstract]. *Clin Res, 33,* 873A.

Smookler, S., & Bermudez, A. J. (1982). Hypertensive crisis resulting from an MAO inhibitor and an over-the-counter appetite suppressant. *Ann Emerg Med, 11,* 482-484.

Snoddy, A. M., Mueller, S. M., & Black, W. L., Jr. (1985). Inhibition of para-hydroxylation does not alter phenylpropanolamine's hypertensive effect in the rat [Abstract]. *Proceedings of the Federation of Am Soc Exp Biol, 44,* 1637.

Snoddy, A. M., & Tessel, R. E. (1985). Prazosin: Effect on psychomotor-stimulant cues and locomotor activity in mice. *Eur J Pharmacol, 116,* 221-228.

Stafford, I., & Hoebel, B. (1984). Cholecystokinin (CCK) and phenylpropanolamine (PPA) share discriminative stimulus properties with amphetamine [Abstract]. *Proceedings of the Soc Neurosci, 10,* 1072.

Stavchansky, S., Riffee, W., & Geary, R. S. (1986). Chronic administration of phenylpropanolamine and caffeine: Effect on locomotor activity. *Res Commun Subst Abuse, 7,* 37-48.

Stevens, M. J., & Moulds, R. F. W. (1981). Heterogeneity of post-junctional alpha-adrenoceptors in human vascular smooth muscle. *Arch Internatl Pharmacodyn, 254,* 43-57.

Stevens, M. J., Rittinghausen, R. E., & Moulds, R. F. W. (1981). Heterogeneity of human vascular pre- and post-synaptic alpha-adrenoceptors. *Clin Sci, 61,* 203s-206s.

Swamy, V. C., Tye, A., Lapidus, J. B., & Patil, P. N. (1969). Steric aspects of adrenergic drugs XIII. Norepinephrine potentiating effects of isomers of sympathomimetic amine in rat vas deferens and atria. *Arch Internatl Pharmacodyn, 182,* 24-31.

Tainter, M. L. (1944). Actions of benzedrine and propadrine in the control of obesity. *J Nutr, 27,* 89-105.

Tainter, M. L., Pedden, J. R., & James, M. (1934). Comparative actions of sympathomimetic compounds: Bronchodilator actions in perfused guinea pig lungs. *J Pharmacol Exp Ther, 51,* 371-386.

Tainter, J. L., Tainter, E. G., Lawrence, W. S., Neuru, E. N., Lackey, R. W., Luduena, F. P., Kirtland, H. B., Jr., & Gonzalez, R. I. (1943). Influence of various drugs on the threshold for electrical convulsions. *J Pharmacol Exp Ther, 79*, 42-54.

Terry, R., Kaye, A. H., & McDonald, M. (1975). Sinutab (Letter). *Med J Aust, 1*, 763.

Thiercelin, J. F., Jacquot, C., Rapin, J. R., & Cohen, Y. (1976). Pharmacokinetics of DL-norephedrine ^{14}C in the rat. *Arch Internatl Pharmacodyn, 220*, 153-163.

Tonks, C. M., & Lloyd, A. T. (1965). Hazards with monoamine-oxidase inhibitors. *Br Med J, 1*, 589.

Trendelenburg, U., Alonso de la Sierra, B. G., & Muskus, A. (1963). Modification by reserpine of the response of the atrial pacemaker to sympathomimetic amines. *J Pharmacol Exp Ther, 141*, 301-309.

Trendelenburg, U., Muskus, A., Fleming, W. W., & Alonso de la Sierra, B. G. (1962a). Modification by reserpine of the action of sympathomimetic amines in spinal cats: A classification of sympathomimetic amines. *J Pharmacol Exp Ther, 138*, 170-180.

Trendelenburg, U., Muskus, A., Fleming, W. W., & Alonso de la Sierra, B. G. (1962b). Effect of cocaine, denervation and decentralization on the response of the nictitating membrane to various sympathomimetic amines. *J Pharmacol Exp Ther, 138*, 181-193.

Turi, P., Dauvois, M., & Michaelis, A. F. (1976). Continuous dissolution rate determination as a function of the pH of the medium. *J Pharm Sci, 65*, 806-810.

Vidrio, H., & Pardo, E. G. (1973). Antihypertensive effects of sympathomimetic amines. *J Pharmacol Exp Ther, 187*, 308-314.

Viveros, A., Vidrio, H., & Vargas, R. (1970). Diuretic effects of various sympathomimetic amines. *Bol Estud Med Biol Mex, 26*, 239-245.

Warren, M. R., & Werner, H. W. (1945). The central stimulant action of some vasopressor amines. *J Pharmacol Exp Ther, 85*, 119-121.

Warren, M. R., & Werner, H. W. (1946). Acute toxicity of vasopressor amines. II. Comparative data. *J Pharmacol Exp Ther, 86*, 284-286.

Wellman, P. J. (1984). Influence of dl-phenylpropanolamine on brown adipose tissue thermogenesis in the adult rat [Abstract]. *Physiol Psychol, 12*, 307-310.

Wellman, P. J., Arasteh, K., Ruddle, J. L., & Strickland, M. D. (1986). Effects of phenylpropanolamine on gastric retention in the adult rat. *Brain Res Bul, 17*, 127-128.

Wellman, P. J., Malpas, P. B., & Wikler, K. C. (1981). Conditioned taste aversion and unconditioned suppression of water intake induced by phenylpropanolamine in rats. *Physiol Psychol, 9*, 203-207.

Wellman, P. J., & Marmon, M. M. (1985a). Comparison of brown adipose tissue thermogenesis induced by congeners and isomers of phenylpropanolamine. *Life Sci, 37*, 1023-1028.

Wellman, P. J., & Marmon, M. M. (1985b). Effects of reserpine and adrenal demedullation on brown adipose tissue thermogenesis induced by dl-phenylpropanolamine. *Res Comm Chem Pathol Pharmacol, 47*, 211-220.

Wellman, P. J., & Marmon, M. M. (1985c). Synergism between caffeine and dl-phenylpropanolamine on brown adipose tissue thermogenesis in the adult rat. *Pharmacol Biochem Behav, 22*, 781-785.

Wellman, P. J., & Peters, R. H. (1980). Effects of amphetamine and phenylpropanolamine on food intake in rats with ventromedial hypothalamic or dorsolateral tegmental damage. *Physiol Behav, 25*, 819-827.

Wellman, P. J., & Ruddle, J. R. (1985). Effects of pharmacological blockade on phenylpropanolamine anorexia [Abstract]. Paper presented at a satellite meeting of the 15th annual meeting of the Soc Neurosci, San Antonio, Tx.

Wellman, P. J., & Sellers, T. L. (1986). Weight loss induced by chronic phenylpropanolamine: Anorexia and brown adipose tissue thermogenesis. *Pharmacol Biochem Behav, 24,* 605-611.

Westlake, W. J. (1975). Demonstration of claimed "controlled-release" properties of a drug formulation. *J Pharm Sci, 64,* 1075-1077.

Wilkinson, G. R., & Beckett, A. H. (1968). Absorption, metabolism and excretion of the ephedrines in man. I. The influence of urinary pH and urine volume output. *J Pharmacol Exp Ther, 162,* 139-147.

Winter, C. A., & Flataker, L. (1954). Antitussive compounds: Testing methods and results. *J Pharmacol Exp Ther, 112,* 99-108.

Wood, D. M., & Emmett-Oglesby, M. W. (1985). Discriminative stimulus properties of anorectic drugs compared to the discriminative stimulus properties of cocaine [Abstract]. *Proceedings of the Soc Neurosci, 11,* 630.

Woolverton, W. L., Johanson, C. E., de la Garza, R., Ellis, S., Seiden, L. S., & Schuster, C. R. (1986). Behavioral and neurochemical evaluation of phenylpropanolamine. *J Pharmacol Exp Ther, 237,* 926-930.

Yu, P. H. (1986). Inhibition of monoamine oxidase activity by phenylpropanolamine, an anorectic agent. *Res Comm Chem Pathol Pharmacol, 51,* 163-171.

Zelger, J. L., & Carlini, E. A. (1980). Anorexigenic effects of two amines obtained from *Catha edulis* Forsk. (Khat) in rats. *Pharmacol Biochem Behav, 12,* 701-705.

4

SAFETY

Drug safety is a major pharmaceutical issue in contemporary society. Before a new drug can be approved for marketing, it must be subjected to a lengthy series of preclinical drug screening tests as well as clinical trials to evaluate its potential to produce toxic effects in humans. This has not always been the case. Phenylpropanolamine was used clinically for many years before the institution of FDA regulations requiring such preclinical and clinical toxicity testing. As a result, until about 1970 there was a considerable body of experience on the clinical use of phenylpropanolamine and phenylpropanolamine-containing products with relatively sparse systematic and well-controlled data on toxicity and safety testing. Beginning in the early 1970s, several factors led to a reevaluation of the safety of phenylpropanolamine-containing products. One factor was the increasing recognition of the importance of FDA responsibility in regulating both the safety and efficacy of commercial drug products. Another factor was the sudden increase in consumption of phenylpropanolamine products (see Chapter 1). Phenylpropanolamine had been used for years as a nasal decongestant and was commonly combined with other drugs such as antihistamines and anticholinergics in cough-cold preparations. In the early 1970s, the manufacture and sale of amphetamine was severely restricted. Subsequently, phenylpropanolamine was marketed extensively as an appetite suppressant and soon became one of the most popular OTC diet aids. At that time, OTC appetite suppressants contained a combination of phenylpropanolamine and caffeine. Street drug abuse of look-alike drugs (pick-me-ups, pseudospeed) then became a problem; often these products contained the triple combination of phenylpropanolamine, ephedrine, and caffeine. To cooperate with the FDA in its efforts to control these look-alike drugs, manufacturers and marketers of OTC phenylpropanolamine-caffeine combination products voluntarily agreed to cease manufacturing such combinations (Federal Register, 1983). Consequently, phenylpropanolamine-containing appetite suppressants currently sold in the United States are caffeine-free formulations.

As a consequence of these various factors, the consumption of phenylpropanolamine escalated rapidly. Perhaps not surprisingly, the number of adverse drug reaction reports citing phenylpropanolamine as a possible source of toxicity has increased in recent years. Of the approximately 60 adverse reaction reports in the published literature, only five were published before 1970, in the 1960s. Thus, phenylpropanolamine had been used clinically for over 40 years and was considered a safe drug. More recently, adverse drug reaction reports suggested that phenylpropanolamine may have been associated with cardiovascular effects (hypertension and stroke) and central nervous system effects (psychotic reactions and seizures). These may be misleading conclusions because reports of adverse reactions to Trimolets (a high-dose, immediate-release formulation marketed in Australia) drew considerable attention to the safety of "phenylpropanolamine." Since it is not entirely clear whether Trimolets actually contained phenylpropanolamine or an isomer of ephedrine, these adverse drug reactions cannot unequivocally be attributed to phenylpropanolamine (Morgan, 1985b). This issue is described fully in a later section of this chapter (See Appetite Suppressants: Trimolets). Nonetheless, the Trimolets reports drew attention to the possibility of an association between phenylpropanolamine and hypertension (these reports are cited in most of the case reports discussed in this chapter). As Morgan (1985a) points out "... phenylpropanolamine ingestion and high blood pressure are extremely common events. When they appear together, how often is the linkage merely coincidental?"

In contrast, although these few adverse drug reaction reports suggest that phenylpropanolamine may cause adverse reactions, controlled clinical trials have repeatedly demonstrated that phenylpropanolamine, taken at recommended doses in approved formulations (which in fact contain phenylpropanolamine and not another isomer), is a safe drug. In safety studies specifically designed to test cardiovascular and CNS effects, a total of more than 1000 patients were given phenylpropanolamine at recommended doses; phenylpropanolamine produced no significant adverse effects (these studies are reviewed later in this chapter). In addition, more than 50 controlled clinical trials of the efficacy of phenylpropanolamine-containing products for use as nasal decongestants, appetite suppressants, or in treatment of urinary incontinence confirm the low incidence of side effects when phenylpropanolamine-containing products are taken in recommended doses (these studies are reviewed in Chapter 5). Furthermore, studies have shown that, even when taken at doses as high as 3 to 10 times the recommended dose, phenylpropanolamine produced no significant side effects (these studies are reviewed in this chapter). Finally, evaluation of overdose cases reported to a poison control center confirms the safety of phenylpropanolamine (Ekins and Spoerke, 1983).

ANIMAL TOXICOLOGY STUDIES

ACUTE TOXICITY

The acute toxicity (LD_{50} and minimum lethal dose, MLD) of phenylpropanolamine hydrochloride is summarized in Table 4.1. These data indicate that the oral LD_{50} and MLD of phenylpropanolamine hydrochloride in mice, rats, and dogs are very high; that is, the toxicity is very low. Thus by the oral route of administration, this drug would be expected to have a very wide margin of safety in humans.

Although phenylpropanolamine is invariably administered orally or intranasally, Table 4.1 provides comparative toxicity data in laboratory animals by other routes of administration. Phenylpropanolamine has a wide margin of safety by all routes administered. As would be expected, the relative toxicity depends on the route of administration as well as species.

For comparison, the acute toxicity of phenylpropanolamine base [(−)-norephedrine] is shown in Table 4.1. According to the one reported study in which the drug was administered by the intraperitoneal route to rats, the LD_{50} was about 1/2.5 that of the salt (hydrochloride). This may be due to use of older rats in this study. When administered IP to mice, the LD_{50} of the phenylpropanolamine base was lower than the LD_{50} of the salt. When administered IP to rabbits or IV to rabbits or mice, the toxicities of the salt and the base were essentially the same. The toxicity of the phenylpropanolamine base by the oral route for laboratory animals has not been reported.

The minimum lethal dose of phenylpropanolamine when administered intranasally to children was estimated to be about 200 mg/kg, with the adult MLD at least 10 times higher (Dreisbach, 1983). The probable lethal dose of phenylpropanolamine administered to humans by the oral route was estimated to be 5–50 mg/kg, similar to that for ephedrine (Gosselin et al., 1984).

The effects of extremely high doses of phenylpropanolamine HCl were in-

TABLE 4.1. Acute Toxicity of Phenylpropanolamine HCl in Animals

Species	Route	LD_{50} (mg/kg)	Reference
Mouse	PO	450	Sunshine (1969)
Mouse	PO	1060	Groves et al. (1970)
Rat	PO	1490	RTECS[a]
Rat	PO	1538	Groves et al. (1970)
Mouse (isolated)	IP	412	Davis & Pinkerton (1972)
Mouse (aggregated)	IP	266	Davis & Pinkerton (1972)
Mouse (aggregated)	IP	320	Davis & Pinkerton (1972)
Mouse	IP	428	RTECS
Rat	IP	MLD 175	Hartung & Munch (1929)
Rat (300–500 g)	IP	160	Warren & Werner (1946b)
Rat	IP	MLD 175	RTECS
Dog	IP	MLD > 500	Hartung & Munch (1929)
Mouse	SC	600	Warren & Werner (1946b)
Mouse	SC	MLD 700	RTECS
Rat (300–500 g)	SC	380	Warren & Werner (1946b)
Rat (190–250 g)	SC	860	Warren & Werner (1946b)
Rat	SC	MLD 350	RTECS
Guinea pig	SC	MLD 600	Hartung & Munch (1929)
Guinea pig	SC	MLD 350	RTECS
Rabbit	SC	255	Warren & Werner (1946b)
Rabbit	IM	320	Warren & Werner (1946b)
Mouse	IV	114	Sunshine (1969)
Mouse	IV	180	RTECS
Rat	IV	55	Hartung (1946)
Rabbit	IV	MLD 75	Hartung & Munch (1929)
Rabbit	IV	MLD 75–90	Hartung (1946)
Rabbit	IV	50	Warren & Werner (1946b)
Rabbit	IV	75	Sunshine (1969)
Rabbit	IV	MLD 75	RTECS

Acute toxicity of phenylpropanolamine base
[(−)-norephedrine] in animals

Mice	IP	266	RTECS
Mice	IP	200	RTECS
Rats	IP	60	RTECS
Mice	IV	114	RTECS
Rabbits	IV	75	RTECS

[a]MLD—minimum lethal dose. RTECS—Registry of Toxic Effects of Chemical Substances.

TABLE 4.2. Dose–Response Relationships for Phenylpropanolamine HCl in Mice, Rats, and Dogs

Species	Route	Dose (mg/kg)	Dose Ratio[a]	Overt Effects	Comments
Mice	PO	44.5	125	Piloerection, lacrimation, spontaneous motor activity	Onset 10 min; duration 35–50 min; no deaths
		89	249	Same	Onset 10 min; duration 45–75 min; no deaths
		178	499	Same	Onset 10 min; duration 50–110 min; no deaths
		356	998	Same	Onset 10 min; duration 50–110 min; no deaths
Rat	PO	42.7	120	Piloerection, tachypnea	Onset 15 min; duration 105 min; no deaths
		85.5	239	Piloerection, tachypnea, salivation (1/3)	Onset 15 min; duration 225 min; no deaths
		171.0	480	Piloerection, tachypnea, salivation	Onset 15 min; duration 225 min; deaths NS[c]
		342.0	958	Piloerection, tachypnea, increase or decrease, spontaneous motor activity, salivation	Onset 15 min; duration >5 hr; 1/3 dead
Dog	PO	28.5	80	Salivation, tachypnea, peripheral vasodilation	Onset 30 min; duration
		28.5	80	Salivation, peripheral valodilation, mydriasis, anorectic	Onset 90 min; duration >300 min
		57.0	160	Salivation, peripheral vasodilation	Onset 30 min; duration 225 min
		57.0	160	Emesis, peripheral vasodilation, salivation	Onset 15 min; duration 225 min
Dog	PO	100[b]	280	Emesis	—
		500[b]	1400	Emesis (1/2)	—
		1000[b]	2800	Emesis	1/2 dead

Source: SKF preclinical data.

[a]Dose in animals: recommended human dose of 25 mg/70 kg body weight.

[b]Five of the six dogs had emesis; therefore, the actual retained dose was less.

[c]NS—not specified.

vestigated in mice, rats, and dogs (Table 4.2). In all three species, no deaths occurred at dose levels up to about 900 times the recommended oral human dose of 25 mg/70 kg.

Two studies investigated whether phenylpropanolamine produces myocardial necrosis (Rosenblum et al., 1965; Pentel et al., 1984). In one study, 15 sympathomimetic drugs were tested (Rosenblum et al., 1965); each drug was given IP to rats 3 times at 24-hr intervals. The hearts were collected for histological analysis 12 hr after the last dose. Ten of the 15 drugs produced cardiac necrosis in more than 50% of the animals. Phenylpropanolamine produced no cardiac necrosis when given at doses of 2.21 and 22.1 mg/kg, but 221.0 mg/kg of phenylpropanolamine produced necrosis in 6 of 6 rats. The latter is a near-lethal dose (see Table 4.1). Comparison of the various sympathomimetic drugs suggested that no single common mechanism was responsible for the cardiac lesions; the necrosis was unrelated to elevation of blood pressure, tachycardia, increased force of contraction, or changes in metabolism. Furthermore, the sympathomimetic-induced cardiac necrosis seemed to be species-specific: Isoproterenol produced cardiac necrosis in rats, hamsters, and cats, but no necrosis in dogs or domestic pigs.

In the second study, rats were given single phenylpropanolamine doses IP (Pentel et al., 1984). Phenylpropanolamine (4 mg/kg) increased systolic blood pressure by 51 ± 15 mm Hg; the response lasted approximately 0.5–1.0 hr. A higher phenylpropanolamine dose (8 mg/kg) increased serum creatinine kinase; the maximum increase was observed 1.5 hr after the dose and the values returned to the control level 6 hr after the dose. Rats were killed 24 hr after the dose and their hearts were examined by light microscopy. Dose-related diffuse myocardial necrosis was observed; the doses of phenylpropanolamine were not specified.

The margin of safety for four phenylethylamines was assessed in rats (Weiss & Vick, 1985). Phenylpropanolamine, ephedrine, d-amphetamine, and p-chloroamphetamine were given PO and the heart rate was measured every 30 min for 3 hr in unrestrained male rats. The cardiovascular risk was assessed by calculating the ratio of the minimum lethal dose to the change in heart rate. Phenylpropanolamine had the highest margin of safety of the four drugs; the rank order of safety was phenylpropanolamine > d-amphetamine > ephedrine > p-chloroamphetamine.

To assess the potential CNS neurotoxicity, rats were given very high doses of phenylpropanolamine (100 or 200 mg/kg) SC twice daily for 4 days (Woolverton et al., 1986). Two weeks later the rats were killed, decapitated, and the brains were removed; the concentrations of dopamine, norepinephrine, and serotonin in frontal cortex, hippocampus, striatum, and hypothalamus were measured. Phenylpropanolamine produced no significant change in monoamine levels in the brain except that dopamine was slightly decreased (17–29%) in the frontal cortex only at the higher dose. These results indicate that phenylpropanolamine produces no severe CNS neurotoxicity. Other drugs, such as amphetamine, which produce severe neurotoxicity cause severe, prolonged depletion of brain monoamines in this *in vivo* bioassay procedure.

COMPARATIVE TOXICITY

The effect of environmental temperature on the toxicity of various pressor amines was investigated (Warren & Werner, 1946a). Mice weighing 10–19 g and housed at 26°C were used; when subjected to 32°C they were conditioned to that temperature for 2 hr before drug administration. The hydrochlorides of the amines were used.

When the environmental temperature was increased to 32°C, the acute subcutaneous toxicity of ephedrine was markedly increased (7.2-fold), that of amphetamine moderately increased (4.1-fold), and phenylpropanolamine slightly increased (2.8-fold), whereas the toxicity of tuaminoheptane, phenylpropylmethylamine, and naphazoline (1.5-, 1.4-, and 1.1-fold, respectively) were not significantly increased (see Table 4.3). Comparison of the effects of ephedrine or phenylpropylmethylamine by IV and SC routes indicates that the effects of environmental temperature were not due to alterations in rates of absorption. The mouse is a species with a stable body temperature at environmental temperatures of up to 33°C.

Additional studies on younger (180–240 g) and older (300–500 g) rats injected SC with these amines indicate that the toxicity of the amines is markedly increased in the older, heavy rats (Warren & Werner, 1946a). These older animals have comparatively low thermal stability, and the temperature increases due to the amines are sufficient to upset their temperature regulation to a serious degree.

TABLE 4.3. Effect of Environmental Temperature on Toxicity in Mice[a]

Drug (Hydrochloride)	LD_{50} at 26°C (mg/kg)	LD_{50} at 32°C (mg/kg)
Ephedrine	600 ± 54.8	83 ± 8.9
Phenylpropanolamine	600 ± 49.0	214 ± 26.3
Amphetamine	42 ± 4.2	15 ± 1.6
Tuaminoheptane	115 ± 11.6	76 ± 6.5
Phenylpropylmethylamine	540 ± 48.0	400 ± 37.0
Naphazoline	170 ± 13.8	150 ± 11.0

Source: Data from Warren and Werner (1946a).
[a]All drugs given SC.

These results indicate that fluctuations in environmental temperature and age and weight of laboratory animals alter the toxicity of certain vasopressor amines.

Further studies on the comparative acute toxicity of seven vasopressor amines indicate there are marked differences in toxicity according to species, route of administration, and age of the animal tested (Warren & Werner, 1946b). The following subjects were used in this study: 610 New Zealand white rabbits weighing 2–3 kg; 220 Swiss white mice weighing 16–20 g; and 839 Wistar white rats in two groups—young mature animals weighing 190–250 g and older heavier animals weighing 300–500 g. These animals were housed in rooms at a temperature of $26 \pm 1°C$. Deaths were recorded for the 14-day observation period, and LD_{50} levels were calculated according to the method of Miller and Tainter.

By all routes of administration tested, phenylpropylmethylamine, ephedrine, and phenylpropanolamine were considerably less toxic—with higher LD_{50} levels—than the four other vasopressor amines, and by the IM and SC routes phenylpropanolamine was the least toxic of all amines tested (Table 4.4).

There were some significant differences in toxicity between the light (190–

TABLE 4.4. Comparative Toxicity

Drug	Species: Route:	Heavy rats, IP	Rabbit, IV	Rabbit, IM
		LD_{50} (mg/kg)		
Phenylpropylmethylamine		154 ± 9.2	72 ± 1.7	220 ± 15.0
Ephedrine		165 ± 15.2	60 ± 2.2	175 ± 9.2
Phenylpropanolamine		160 ± 6.7	50 ± 3.1	320 ± 29.2
Tuaminoheptane		34 ± 2.2	22 ± 1.4	85 ± 5.7
Amphetamine		36 ± 3.0	10 ± 1.6	10 ± 0.8
Naphazoline		50 ± 3.6	0.5 ± 0.09	0.95 ± 0.23
Phenylephrine		17 ± 1.1	0.5 ± 0.15	7.2 ± 0.35

Drug	Species: Route:	Mice, SC	Light Rat, SC	Heavy Rat, SC	Rabbit, SC
Phenylpropylmethylamine		540 ± 48.0	850 ± 36.7	860 ± 34.3	205 ± 15.9
Ephedrine		600 ± 54.8	650 ± 109.4	380 ± 40.0	165 ± 12.3
Phenylpropanolamine		600 ± 49.0	860 ± 51.6	380 ± 27.1	265 ± 10.3
Tuaminoheptane		115 ± 11.6	135 ± 0.1	160 ± 13.0	130 ± 14.4
Amphetamine		42 ± 4.2	165 ± 16.5	39 ± 2.3	11 ± 1.2
Naphazoline		170 ± 13.8	385 ± 39.6	325 ± 22.5	0.85 ± 0.13
Phenylephrine		22 ± 4.3	27 ± 2.9	33 ± 2.0	22 ± 2.2

Source: Data from Warren and Werner (1946b).

250 g) and heavy (300–500 g) rats administered the amines by the SC route. Phenylpropanolamine was 2.2 times more toxic in the older, heavier rats than in the younger rats. Amphetamine was much more toxic, ephedrine considerably more toxic, and naphazoline slightly more toxic in the heavier rats. The three other amines tested were slightly less toxic in the heavier animals.

The most toxic of the amines were tuaminoheptane, amphetamine, naphazoline, and phenylephrine, with the two latter compounds having low LD_{50} levels by the IV route in rabbits. Naphazoline was particularly toxic for the rabbit by all routes administered but was the least toxic of the four in this group following SC administration to rats and mice. Phenylpropanolamine was less toxic than naphazoline when administered SC to heavier rats; by all other routes in rats, rabbits, or mice, phenylpropanolamine was markedly less toxic than naphazoline.

The acute toxicity and central locomotor stimulatory activity in mice of the isomers (both enantiomorphs and diastereoisomers) of ephedrine and norephedrine were compared with the optical isomers of amphetamine (Fairchild & Alles, 1967). Central locomotor stimulation was definitely produced by 5 of the 10 compounds (*d*- and *l*-amphetamine, *d*- and *l*-norpseudoephedrine, and *l*-ephedrine), with *d*-amphetamine the most potent compound. Both *d*- and *l*-norephedrine, *d*- and *l*-pseudoephedrine, and *d*-ephedrine, produced measurable locomotor stimulation only at levels approaching lethal doses.

To determine the acute toxicity of the isomers, a total of 32 or 40 adult male Swiss albino mice, in four or five dosage groups of eight animals each, were injected IP with the test compounds. Mice were housed four to a cage having a floor area of 463 cm^2 at an ambient temperature of 25°C. A dose-lethality curve was plotted, and the LD_{50} and 95% confidence limits, calculated by the method of Litchfield and Wilcoxon, were based on the number of animals dying within 24 hr.

d-Amphetamine, with an LD_{50} of 0.065 mmol/kg, had the greatest toxicity in mice (Table 4.5). With *d*-amphetamine used as the reference standard with its LD_{50} value equated to unity, all other compounds in the series were compared, with their toxicity dose ratios expressed to the nearest whole number. Thus *l*-amphetamine, the second ranked compound, had a toxicity ratio of 9. The most toxic ephedrine isomers were *d*-norpseudoephedrine, *l*-norephedrine, and *d*-pseudoephedrine, with dose ratios of 13, 14, and 15, respectively. Clearly, the least toxic compounds in the series were *d*-norephedrine and *l*-norpseudoephedrine, with dose ratios of 31 and 32, respectively. Phenylpropanolamine per se was not investigated in this study; phenylpropanolamine is the racemic mixture of *d*- and *l*-norephedrine.

The lethality of phenylpropanolamine [i.e., (±)-norephedrine] and (+)-norephedrine were compared in rats (Katz et al., 1985a). The IP LD_{50}s for

TABLE 4.5. Acute Toxicity in Mice

Drug	LD_{50} (mmol/kg)	Confidence Limits (90%)	Toxicity Ratio
d-Amphetamine SO₄	0.065	(0.049–0.086)	1.0
l-Amphetamine SO₄	0.630	(0.350–1.16)	9
d-Ephedrine HCl	1.23	(1.15–1.32)	19
l-Ephedrine HCl	1.21	(1.04–1.36)	18
d-Norephedrine HCl	2.01	(1.75–2.32)	31
l-Norephedrine HCl	0.94	(0.72–1.22)	14
d-Pseudoephedrine HCl	1.00	(0.84–1.19)	15
l-Pseudoephedrine HCl	1.41	(1.30–1.52)	22
d-Norpseudoephedrine HCl	0.865	(0.605–1.24)	13
l-Norpseudoephedrine HCl	2.06	(1.96–2.16)	32

Source: Data from Fairchild and Alles (1967).

phenylpropanolamine and (+)-norephedrine were 67 and 343 mg/kg, respectively, demonstrating that the (+)-isomer is less toxic than the racemic mixture.

DRUG COMBINATIONS

Many commercial OTC products combine phenylpropanolamine with other drugs. Cough-cold preparations frequently combine phenylpropanolamine with antihistamines and/or anticholinergics to produce a wider spectrum of symptomatic relief. Formerly, diet preparations contained phenylpropanolamine and caffeine, although this combination is now prohibited. The so-called amphetamine look-alikes or pseudospeed may contain phenylpropanolamine, ephedrine, and caffeine. Thus it is important to consider the toxicity of such drug combinations.

Since antimuscarinic agents, such as atropine and scopolamine, augment the behavioral stimulatory effects of amphetamine, the toxicity of phenylpropanolamine and atropine alone and in combination was investigated to determine whether the two drugs produced additive or synergistic effects (Davis & Pinkerton, 1972). Sprague-Dawley, Long-Evans, and Wistar rats and Swiss-Webster albino mice were used in this study. All animals were housed at a room temperature of 24°C. Mice were studied in both isolation and aggregation. In isolation, the mice were housed singly in a cage with a floor dimension of 9 × 12 cm and a height of 8 cm. In aggregation, five mice were placed in a cage of the same size. When an aggregated mouse died it was replaced with an untreated mouse to maintain the same degree of aggregation. Phenylpropanolamine hydrochloride was administered IP; atropine (0.4 mg/kg to rats and 10 mg/kg to mice) was administered SC 5–10 min before the phenylpro-panolamine. Mouse LD_{50} levels were estimated by the method of Litchfield and Wilcoxon. Lethality of rats was determined incidental to behavioral and activity studies.

In rats, lethality following a dose of 60 mg/kg of phenylpropanolamine was low; deaths occurred after about 3 hr of hyperactivity (Table 4.6). When 0.4 mg/kg of atropine was given before phenylpropanolamine, the toxicity was increased sixfold in Sprague-Dawley rats. In Wistar rats, there were no deaths with or without atropine at a dose of 45 mg/kg of phenylpropanol-amine, but at a dose of 60 mg/kg there was synergism in lethality by atropine and phenylpropanolamine. In Long-Evans rats there was no synergism be-tween phenylpropanolamine and atropine. At a dose of 75 mg/kg of phenyl-propanolamine, lethality in Wistar rats was further enhanced by atropine.

The acute toxicity of phenylpropanolamine was higher in aggregated mice than in isolated mice, but this effect was not as pronounced as that for *d*-amphetamine (Table 4.7). Pretreatment of aggregated mice with atropine significantly enhanced the lethality of phenylpropanolamine and also in-creased the slope of the dose-response curve.

Thus atropine increased the lethality of phenylpropanolamine in rats. Phenylpropanolamine also caused greater lethality among aggregated mice than among isolated mice, and this effect was considerably enhanced by pre-treatment with the anticholinergic drug atropine.

The toxicity of phenylpropanolamine combined with chlorpheniramine and isopropamide, components of the cough-cold preparation Contac or Or-nade, was investigated (Groves et al., 1970). Chlorpheniramine is an antihis-tamine, and isopropamide is an anticholinergic. The dose lethality curves were

TABLE 4.6. Acute Toxicity of Phenylpropanolamine and Atropine in Rats

Rat Strain	Dose (mg/kg)		Incidence of Death
	Phenylpropanolamine	Atropine	
Sprague–Dawley	60	—	2/25
	60	0.4	12/25[a]
Long–Evans	60	—	2/20
	60	0.4	4/20
Wistar	45	—	0/25
	45	0.4	0/25
Wistar	60	—	0/25
	60	0.4	6/25[a]
Wistar	75	—	4/45
	75	0.4	18/45[a]

Source: Data from Davis and Pinkerton (1972).
[a]Significantly increased compared to phenylpropanolamine alone.

TABLE 4.7. Acute Lethality in Isolated and Aggregated Mice

Treatment	Housing Condition	LD_{50} (mg/kg)	95% Confidence Limits	Slope Function
Phenylpropanolamine	Isolated	412	382–445	1.22
	Aggregated	320	296–356	1.25
d-Amphetamine	Isolated	27.5	25.1–30.1	1.29
	Aggregated	9.1	8.4–10.0	1.25
Phenylpropanolamine	Isolated	415	370–465	1.31
	Aggregated	266	236–299	1.33
Phenylpropanolamine + atropine	Isolated	297	129–683	7.88[a]
	Aggregated	17.5	8.1–35.7	6.15[a]

Source: Data from Davis and Pinkerton (1972).
[a]Slope function differed significantly from phenylpropanolamine alone ($p < .05$).

determined for each component alone and the triple combination, given to mice and rats. All drugs were given orally. In mice, the LD_{50} (with 95% fiducial limits) for oral phenylpropanolamine alone was 1060 (910–1236) mg/kg. Overt signs of toxicity at these lethal doses were decreased spontaneous activity, salivation, dyspnea, and clonic convulsions. Comparison of the observed and predicted potencies of the three individual drugs and the triple combination indicated that the combination neither potentiated nor antagonized the toxicity of any of the individual components. The results in rats were different. In rats, the LD_{50} (with 95% fiducial limits) for oral phenylpropanolamine was 1538 (1177–166,231) mg/kg. Overt signs of toxicity were piloerection, salivation, and mydriasis. In this species, the triple combination potentiated the toxicity of the individual active drugs. However, the authors noted that the lethal doses used were extremely high compared to the proposed therapeutic doses and that it was not possible to predict whether any interaction would occur at therapeutic dose levels.

The effects of phenylpropanolamine and caffeine alone, and in combination, on the lethality and motor behavior in rats were reported (Schlemmer et al., 1984). The drugs were administered IP to male Sprague-Dawley rats weighing 225–450 g, with 8–25 rats at each dose level. The LD_{50} for phenylpropanolamine (base) was 72 mg/kg and for caffeine, 233 mg/kg. At all doses tested, caffeine potentiated the lethality of phenylpropanolamine. For example, 10 mg/kg of caffeine reduced the phenylpropanolamine LD_{50} to 35 mg/kg. The same 10-mg/kg dose of caffeine did not significantly potentiate locomotor activity and stereotypy induced by phenylpropanolamine. The authors postulate that cases of toxicity from drugs containing phenylpropanolamine and caffeine may result from caffeine potentiation of phenylpropanolamine toxicity without enhancement of behavioral changes.

A second study confirmed that caffeine potentiates phenylpropanolamine lethality (Katz et al., 1985b). Furthermore, pretreatment with the α-blocker phentolamine antagonized the lethality of the phenylpropanolamine-caffeine combination and increased the slope of the lethality curve. The β-blocker propranolol likewise antagonized the lethality of the combination but produced no change in the slope of the curve. In this study the overt effects observed at lethal phenylpropanolamine doses were convulsions and hemorrhaging from the eyes, nose, and mouth.

The effect of phenylpropanolamine in combination with caffeine was investigated in normotensive, spontaneously hypertensive, and stroke-prone spontaneously hypertensive rats (Mueller et al., 1984). Repeated IP injections of phenylpropanolamine (6 mg/kg) plus caffeine (24 mg/kg) in normotensive and spontaneously hypertensive rats resulted in increased activity within 2 hr. After injection of stroke-prone spontaneously hypertensive rats, two were actively fighting the first day, one died the first night (after two injections) of extensive tubular necrosis, and one died (after three injections) of cerebral hemorrhage. Of the four remaining in this group, one was hyperactive and had dried blood around his nose, and one bled from the rectum.

After IP injection of phenylpropanolamine plus caffeine, maximal blood pressure increases were: normotensive rats ($n = 6$), 43 ± 7 mm Hg; spontaneously hypertensive rats ($n = 7$), 22 ± 2 mm Hg; and stroke-prone spontaneously hypertensive rats ($n = 2$), 73 ± 1 mm Hg. Blood pressures of the control animals for the three groups ($n = 5$ or 6) were 135 ± 7 mm Hg, 163 ± 11 mm Hg, and 193 ± 9 mm Hg, respectively.

Of the 11 spontaneously hypertensive rats given phenylpropanolamine and caffeine, two showed histological evidence of subarachnoid hemorrhage, one of which, a 12–14-month-old male, had leptomeningeal extravasation. There was no direct correlation between the acute increase in blood pressure and cerebral hemorrhage.

The interpretation of the results from this study (Mueller et al., 1984) is limited by several problems. First, the isomer of phenylpropanolamine was not specified. Since the toxicity of the isomers of norephedrine varies widely (Table 4.5), this could be an important factor. Second, the rats in some of the treatment groups were old; of the six spontaneously hypertensive rats, four were 12–14 months old. The toxicity of phenylpropanolamine is higher in older rats than in younger rats (Table 4.4 and Morgan, 1985b). The finding of extensive tubular necrosis of the kidneys in spontaneously hypertensive rats is difficult to attribute to drug administration; such toxicity would not be expected to develop and cause death within 18 hr.

HUMAN SAFETY STUDIES

There are 17 reports, including 21 separate studies, of clinical safety trials. These studies were specifically designed to test the safety of phenylpropanolamine with special reference to cardiovascular or CNS effects. In addition, nearly 50 controlled clinical trials of the efficacy of phenylpropanolamine for various indications have been conducted. Observation of side effects during these efficacy studies constitute additional evidence for the safety of phenylpropanolamine; these studies are reviewed in Chapter 5. Finally, numerous preclinical studies attest to the low potency of phenylpropanolamine for cardiovascular and CNS stimulation (reviewed in Chapter 3). In this section, those studies specifically designed to test the safety of phenylpropanolamine or phenylpropanolamine-containing products are reviewed.

SAFETY OF PHENYLPROPANOLAMINE ALONE

CARDIOVASCULAR STUDIES

More than 50 studies have been conducted to assess the cardiovascular responses to phenylpropanolamine in humans; Table 4.8 summarizes these studies.

Effects of acute administration of 50, 75, 150, and 250 mg of phenylpropanolamine (immediate-release formulation) and placebo on blood pressure and heart rate were measured in healthy male volunteers (Ryan et al., 1987). The increase in supine and standing blood pressure was related to the phenylpropanolamine dose: 50 and 250 mg of phenylpropanolamine produced maximum increases in blood pressure of 28/13 and 87/30 mm Hg, respectively; there was no statistical analysis of the results. The response to the two highest doses of phenylpropanolamine was biphasic, with an initial increase followed by a later postural decrease in blood pressure. Phenylpropanolamine produced no change in heart rate, conduction, or rhythm.

The effects on blood pressure of a single dose of phenylpropanolamine (37.5 mg in immediate-release form) were compared with placebo in a randomized, double-blind, crossover study with a washout period of at least one week between treatments (Pentel et al., 1985a). Four males and six females (18–35 years old), who were healthy, normotensive, and not obese, participated. Before dosing subjects remained supine for 30 min, after which blood pressure was measured in supine, sitting, and standing positions. Subjects remained supine during the study except when sitting and standing pressures were measured. Blood pressure was measured every 15 min after dosing for 4 hr. The mean increase in supine systolic blood pressure was greater after phenylpropanolamine (18.5 ± 10.7 mm Hg) than after placebo (5.1 ± 5.4 mm Hg). Increases in systolic blood pressure were noted in all 10 subjects and ranged from 8 to 43 mm Hg. Maximum blood pressure was noted in most subjects 1–2 hr after dosing, and all had returned to within 10 mm Hg of their baseline systolic pressure by 4 hr. The increases in blood pressure associated with phenylpropanolamine were postural, and no changes were noted in sitting or standing pressures.

The effects of phenylpropanolamine (75 mg/day in sustained-release form) on ambulatory blood pressure during rest and during unrestricted daily activity were investigated by Goodman et al. (1986) in 18 healthy male volunteers (22–34 years old). The study was a randomized, double-blind, placebo-controlled, crossover design with a minimum 2-week washout period between the two 7-day test periods. Twenty-four-hour ambulatory blood pressure monitoring was performed on days 1 and 6 (blood pressure was measured every 15 min from 6 A.M. to midnight and at 30-min intervals from midnight

TABLE 4.8. Clinical Studies With Phenylpropanolamine (PPA): Cardiovascular Findings[a]

Reference	Experimental Design	PPA Dose	Formulation/ Trade Name	Dosing Regimen	n[b]	Health Status	Frequency of Observation	Findings
			Single-Dose Studies: Immediate release formulations					
McLaurin et al. (1961)	DB PC Crossover	25 mg	25 mg PPA Propadrine Placebo	1 doses at 5–6 hr interval	88	Nasal obstruction	1 hr after first dose, and the next day	PPA did not produce a significant change in BP or HR compared to placebo treatment.
Silverman et al. (1980)	SB	25 mg	25 mg PPA Propadrine	1 dose	15	Healthy	Hourly for 3 hr	In all 3 studies, there was no significant difference in mean supine BP for subjects taking PPA compared to pretreatment values or to placebo treatment (as appropriate). There were no significant differences in HR after PPA, except that the HR decreased at 2 and 3 hr after 25 mg PPA in the SB study only.
	Open study	25 mg	25 mg PPA, 100 mg caff Appedrine	1 dose	10	Healthy	30-min intervals for 4 hr	
	DB PC Crossover	25 mg	25 mg PPA Propadrine Placebo	1 dose	12	Healthy	30-min intervals for 4 hr	
Biaggioni et al. (1986)	Open study No placebo	25 mg	NS IR	1 dose	9	Orthostatic hypotension	5-min intervals	PPA produced a significant increase in BP (+32/+15 mm Hg; mean pressure, +21 mm Hg) but no change in HR.

Reference	Design	Dose	Formulation	Regimen	N	Population	Sampling	Results
Pentel et al. (1985a)	DB PC Crossover	37.5 mg	IR Placebo	1 dose	10	Normotensive	15-min intervals for 4 hr	The maximum increase in supine systolic BP was greater for PPA (+18.5 mm Hg) than for placebo (+5.1 mm Hg); the maximum increase occurred 1–2 hr after administration of PPA. PPA produced no significant change in diastolic BP or HR. PPA produced no significant changes in sitting or standing BP.
Cuthbert et al. (1969)	Open study	50 mg 100 mg	Generic (IR) Generic (IR)	1 dose	3	Healthy	20-min intervals	50 mg of PPA produced a modest increase in systolic BP (range +18 to +26 mm Hg) and no change in diastolic BP or HR. 100 mg PPA increased BP (+27/+15 mm Hg) and decreased HR (−18 bpm).[c] SR preparations produced no change in BP or HR (no data presented).
Pentel et al. (1985b)[d]	DB Crossover	37.5 mg 75 mg	NS (IR) NS (IR)	1 dose	6	Normotensive	Every 30 min for up to 5 hr	PPA increased supine BP; the increase was greater after 75 mg of PPA (+31/+20 mm Hg) than after 37.5 mg of PPA (+10/+8 mm Hg). PPA decreased the HR (−10.8 and

TABLE 4.8. Continued.

Reference	Experimental Design	PPA Dose	Formulation/ Trade Name	Dosing Regimen	n^b	Health Status	Frequency of Observation	Findings
								−9.4 bpm for 75 and 37.5 mg, respectively). 75 mg of PPA increased left ventricular fractional shortening, stroke volume, ejection fraction, cardiac output, and systemic vascular resistance.
Wenger & Lapsa (1970)	DB PC	NS^e	PPA, pheniramine, pyrilamine Triaminic	1 dose	46	Rhinitis	0.5, 2, 4, 6, 8 hr	"There was no significant change in blood pressures." No data are presented.
	Open study	Placebo NS^e	Triaminic		34 45			
Single-Dose Studies: Trimolets								
Horowitz et al. (1979)	DB PC Crossover	85 mg Placebo	Trimolets Placebo	1 dose	6 6	Normotensive	Hourly for 6 hr	Trimolets produced a significant increase in systolic and diastolic BP (maximum 151/100 mm Hg) and decrease in HR (−15.8 bpm) com-

Study	Design	Dose	Treatment		N	Subjects	Schedule	Comments
Horowitz et al. (1980)	DB PC Crossover	85 mg	Trimolets	1 dose	37	Healthy	Every 30 min for 3 hr	...pared to pretreatment values. Trimolets produced a significant increase in diastolic BP (+24 mm Hg) compared to placebo treatment. Trimolets decreased the HR. Peak effect occurred after 1.5–3.0 hr.
			Placebo		35			

Single-Dose Studies: Sustained release formulations

Study	Design	Dose	Treatment		N	Subjects	Schedule	Comments
Horowitz et al. (1980)	DB PC Parallel groups	50 mg	50 mg PPA, 0.25 mg BA Contac 500	1 dose	34	Healthy	Every 30 min for 3 hr	Contac 500 produced a modest, significant increase in diastolic BP (+5 mm Hg) compared to placebo treatment.
			Placebo		35			
Liebson et al. (1982b)	DB PC Crossover	75 mg	(SR) NS Placebo	1 dose	59	Normotensive	0.5–2 hr intervals for 12 hr	75 mg of PPA (SR) produced statistically but not clinically significant increases in BP (mean differences ranged from 0.83 to 3.37 mm Hg), but no significant change in HR.
Mitchell (1968)	DB PC Crossover	100 mg	50 mg PPA, 0.25 mg BA (SR) NS Placebo	2 capsules	6	Normotensive	Every 15 min for 90 min, then every 30 min for 90 min	Drug treatment did not produce any significant change in BP or HR compared to placebo treatment.

TABLE 4.8. Continued.

One-day studies: Comparison of immediate release and sustained release formulations

Reference	Experimental Design	PPA Dose	Formulation/ Trade Name	Dosing Regimen	n^b	Health Status	Frequency of Observation	Findings
Liebson et al. (1982a)[f]	DB PC Parallel groups	25 mg 75 mg	IR SR Placebo	t.i.d. o.d.	50 50 50	Normotensive	0.5–2 hr intervals for 12 hr	Neither 25 mg of PPA (t.i.d.) nor 75 mg of PPA (SR) produced any significant changes in standing, sitting, or supine BP or HR.
Noble (1983)[f]	DB PC Parallel groups	25 mg 75 mg	IR SR Placebo	t.i.d. o.d.	72 72 72	Weight stratified	0.5–2 hr intervals for 12 hr	Neither 25 mg of PPA (t.i.d.) nor 75 mg of PPA (SR) produced significant changes in standing, sitting, or supine BP or HR.
Morgan (1985)[g]	DB PC Parallel groups	25 mg 75 mg	IR SR Placebo	t.i.d. o.d.	81 74 69	Weight stratified	0.5–2 hr intervals for 12 hr	Neither 25 mg of PPA (t.i.d.) nor 75 mg of PPA (SR) produced significant changes in standing, sitting, or supine BP or HR.
Blackburn (1984)[h]	DB PC Parallel groups	25 mg 75 mg	IR SR Placebo	t.i.d. p.d.	72 72 72	Weight stratified	0.5–2 hr intervals for 12 hr	Neither 25 mg of PPA (t.i.d.) nor 75 mg of PPA (SR) produced significant changes in standing, sitting, or supine BP or HR.
Robertson (1983)[i]	DB PC Parallel groups	25 mg 75 mg	IR SR Placebo	t.i.d. o.d.	73 78 73	Weight stratified	0.5–2 hr intervals for 12 hr	25 mg of PPA (t.i.d.) produced no significant change in BP or HR compared to placebo. 75 mg of PPA (SR) produced

Repeated-dose studies: Immediate release formulations

		25 mg	NS (IR)	t.i.d. for 4 days	14	Normotensive	0, 0.5, 1, 2 hr on days 1, 2, 3, and hourly for 12 hr on day 4	small but statistically significant increases in supine BP (+4.5/+3.7 mm Hg), but no significant change in HR.
Saltzman et al. (1983)	PC Crossover							
Griboff et al. (1975)	DB PC Parallel groups	25 mg	50 mg PPA, 100 mg caff Anorexin Placebo	t.i.d. for 4 weeks	33/37 33/40	Obese	Every 2 weeks	The mean diastolic BP before treatment was 69 mm Hg; on day 4 the mean peak diastolic BP was 82 mm Hg. Changes in BP were unrelated to plasma PPA concentration. Anorexin produced no significant change in BP ($-4/-1$ mm Hg) or HR (-1.6 bpm) compared to pretreatment values.
Altschuler et al. (1982)	DB PC Parallel groups	25 mg	25 mg PPA, 100 mg caff (IR) Appedrine	t.i.d. for 8 weeks	25/31	Obese	Every 2 weeks	Appedrine produced no change in BP (0/+2 mm Hg) or HR (+0.7 bpm) compared to pretreatment values.
Bradley & Raines (1987)	SB PC Crossover (pilot study)	25 mg 75 mg	25 mg PPA, 100 mg caff (IR) NS 75 mg PPA (SR) NS Placebo	t.i.d. for 2 weeks o.d. for 2 weeks	10/12	Obese; controlled, stable hypertension	0.5, 1, 2, 4 hr after first dose; then weekly	No significant differences in BP or HR after 2 weeks of treatment compared to pretreatment values. Statistically but not clinically significant increases in BP or HR at 0.5–4 hr after the initial dose.

TABLE 4.8. Continued.

Reference	Experimental Design	PPA Dose	Formulation/ Trade Name	Dosing Regimen	n^b	Health Status	Frequency of Observation	Findings
Bradley & Raines (1987)	DB PC	25 mg	NS (IR) Placebo	t.i.d. for 6 weeks	28/36 32/36	Obese; controlled, stable hypertension	0.5, 1, 2, 4 hr after first dose; then weekly	No significant differences in BP or HR at week 2, 4, or 6 compared to pretreatment values. Statistically but not clinically significant increase in supine systolic BP (+3 mm Hg), decrease in standing diastolic BP (−3 mm Hg) and supine HR (−5.9 bpm) after the initial dose.
Barrett et al. (1981)	DB Crossover	25 mg	25 mg PPA, 4 mg CPM (IR) generic	Every 4 hr for 4 days	18	Healthy	Daily	Drug treatment produced no change in BP (−6/−3 mm Hg) or HR (+2.2 bpm) compared to pretreatment values.
Unger et al. (1967)	Open study	25 mg	25 mg PPA, 100 mg GG, 300 mg TSG, Asbron	t.i.d. for 1–3 weeks	21	Asthmatic, hypertensive	Pretreatment and 1 hr after final dose	25 mg of PPA (t.i.d.) produced no significant change in BP (0/−1 mm Hg) compared to baseline values.
Black (1937)	Open study	24–48 mg	24 or 48 mg of PPA Propadrine	Every 3 hours	131[i]	Asthma, hay fever, urticaria, angioneuredema	NS	In 41 normotensive patients, a single 48 mg dose produced a maximum increase of +15 mm Hg systolic and no change in diastolic pressure. In 5 patients who took 8

Repeated dose studies: Sustained release formulations

Study	Design	Dose	Treatment	N	Patient	Duration	Comments
Cutting (1943)	Open study	25–50 mg	25 mg of PPA t.i.d., increasing to as much as 50 mg of PPA every hour (IR) Propadrine	13	Obese	NS	doses of 48 mg each in 2 days (total of 384 mg), the maximum increase was +10 mm Hg systolic. In 1 hypertensive patient, a single 24 mg dose produced a decrease of −10 mm Hg systolic and no change in diastolic pressure. Only 1/13 patients had tachycardia; "there was no significant change in blood pressure at any time" (no data presented).
Altschuler et al. (1982)	DB PC Parallel groups	37.5 mg	37.5 mg of PPA 140 mg caff (SR), Prolamine Placebo	28/36 28/36	Obese	2 weeks	Prolamine produced no change in BP (−1/0 mm Hg) or HR (−0.5 bpm) compared to pretreatment values.
Sebok (1985)	DB PC Parallel groups	35 mg	35 mg of PPA 140 mg caff (SR), Prolamine Placebo	26/35 23/35	Obese	NS	Prolamine produced no clinically significant change in BP or HR.
Renvall & Lindquist (1979)	DB PC	50 mg	50 mg of PPA (SR), Monydrin Placebo	25 26	Chronic nonallergic rhinitis	Pretreatment and day 4	Monydrin twice daily for 4 days produced no change in BP (0/0 mm Hg) compared to pretreatment values.

TABLE 4.8. Continued.

Reference	Experimental Design	PPA Dose	Formulation/ Trade Name	Dosing Regimen	n^b	Health Status	Frequency of Observation	Findings
Noble (1982)	DB PC	50 mg	NS	t.i.d. for 12 weeks	n.s.	Obese	NS	50 mg of PPA (t.i.d.) produced no significant increase in BP.
Altschuler et al. (1982)	DB	50 mg	50 mg of PPA, 200 mg caff (SR), Dexatrim	o.d. for 6 weeks	27/34	Obese	Every 2 weeks	Dexatrim produced no change in BP (0/+2 mm Hg) or HR (−1 bpm) compared to pretreatment values.
Broms & Malm (1982)	DB PC Crossover	50 mg	50 mg of PPA, 12 mg BPM (SR), Lunerin	b.i.d. for 10 days	19	Nonallergic rhinitis	NS	Lunerin produced no change in BP or HR compared to pretreatment values.
Mitchell (1968)	DB PC Crossover	50 mg	NS (SR) 50 mg of PPA, 0.25 mg BA (SR), NS	b.i.d. for 5 days	32	Normotensive	Daily	The mean aterial pressure was not significantly different from the control value (87 mm Hg) in patients given placebo, PPA, or PPA and belladonna (88, 88, or 87 mm Hg, respectively). HR was significantly decreased compared to control HR only in patients given PPA and belladonna.
Saltzman et al. (1983)	PC Crossover	75 mg	(SR) NS	o.d. for 4 days	14	Normotensive	0, 0.5, 1, 2, hr on days 1, 2, 3, and hourly for 12 hr on day 4	Pretreatment values for BP were not reported, and no placebo was used. The maximum BP recorded on day 4 was 117/68 mm Hg; the mean peak diastolic BP was 60 mm Hg.

214

Reference	Design	Dose	Treatment	Dosage schedule	N	Population	Measurement frequency	Results
Goodman et al. (1986)	DC PC Crossover	75 mg	(SR) Control	o.d. for 7 days	18	Normotensive	4 times per week; and 24-hr monitoring of ambulatory BP on days 1 and 6	PPA produced no significant change in BP or HR compared to placebo-treatment values.
Weintraub et al. (1986)	DB PC Parallel groups	75 mg	75 mg of PPA, Acutrim (OROS) Placebo	o.d. for 12 weeks	40/53 38/53	Obese	Biweekly	Acutrim produced a slight decrease in BP both in patients given PPA (−4/−1 mm Hg) and placebo (−3/−1 mm Hg) compared to baseline values; the HR slightly increased in both groups.
Krosnick et al. (1982)	DB PC Crossover	75 mg	(SR) NS Placebo	b.i.d. for 2 weeks	6	Obese; maturity-onset diabetes; hyperglycemic	3 times per week	PPA produced no significant change in BP or HR compared to placebo treatment.
Barrett et al. (1981)	DB Crossover	75 mg	75 mg of PPA, 12 mg CPM (SR), Triaminic	b.i.d. for 4 days	18	Healthy	Daily	Triaminic produced no change in BP (−4/+3 mm Hg) or HR (+4.2 bpm) compared to pretreatment values.
Renvall & Linquist (1979)	DB PC	100 mg	(SR) Monydrin Placebo	b.i.d. for 4 days	18 26	Chronic nonallergic rhinitis	Pretreatment and day 4	Monydrin twice daily for 4 days produced no significant change in BP (−4/−2 mm Hg) compared to pretreatment values.
Broms & Malm (1982)	DB PC Crossover	100 mg	(SR) Monydrin	b.i.d. for 10 days	19	Nonallergic rhinitis	NS	Monydrin produced no change in BP (+1/+1 mm Hg) or HR (−2 bpm) compared to pretreatment values.

TABLE 4.8. Continued.

Reference	Experimental Design	PPA Dose	Formulation/ Trade Name	Dosing Regimen	n[b]	Health Status	Frequency of Observation	Findings
				Special studies				
Cuthbert & Vere (1971)	Open study	0.9–20 mg	NS	Single dose, IV	3	Healthy	NS	IV PPA increased BP and decreased HR (no data presented).
Loman et al. (1939)	Open study	20–25 mg	NS	Single dose, IV	4	Healthy	NS	IV PPA produced an increase in BP (+16 to +28 mm Hg) and decrease in HR (−4 to −16 bpm).
		50 mg		Single dose, IV	8	Healthy	NS	IV PPA produced an increase in systolic BP (+44 to +82 mm Hg) and decrease in HR (−16 to −36 bpm) compared to pretreatment values.
Lorhan & Mosser (1947)	Open study	50 mg	NS	Single dose, IM	263	Surgical patient[i]	NS	IM PPA maintained the BP at preanesthetic level in 90% of patients; PPA did not change HR.

[a] ASA—aspirin; BA—belladonna alkaloids; BP—blood pressure; BPM—brompheniramine; caff—caffeine; CPM—chlorpheniramine; DB—double blind; GG—glycerol guaiacolate; HR—heart rate; IM—intramuscular; IR—immediate release; IV—intravenous; NS—not specified; OROS—osmotic release oral system; PC—placebo controlled; SB—single blind; SR—sustained release; TSG—theophylline sodium glycinate.

[b] Number of volunteers, or number who completed treatment/number who enrolled.

[c] Data read from graph.

[d] This study also investigated antagonism of PPA by propranolol; only the effects of PPA alone are reported here.

[e] The doses are not listed in the article. Currently, Triaminic tablets contain 12.5 mg of PPA and 2 mg of chlorpheniramine.

[f] Reviewed by Krakoff, 1985.

[g] Data on file at Thompson Medical Company.

[h] Data on file at Thompson Medical Company.

[i] Blood pressure results not reported for all patients.

[j] Spinal anesthesia

to 6 A.M.). Mean values were calculated for each 24-hr and each 2-hr period of recording. Subjects were seen four additional times during each study week for additional blood pressure determinations. Phenylpropanolamine had no effect on 24-hr systolic or diastolic blood pressures or heart rate during days 1 or 6. There were no statistical or clinical differences noted when the 2-hr periods on these days were compared individually. There was a trend toward increased heart rate noted at night during the final phenylpropanolamine monitoring. The authors concluded that the data supported the lack of any significant activity-related drug effects or diurnal variability of drug effects.

Pentel et al., (1985b) investigated propranolol antagonism of phenylpropanolamine-induced hypertension in normotensive subjects (3 males, 3 females, 18–40 years old). Propranolol given either PO as a pretreatment or IV after phenylpropanolamine antagonized the increase in blood pressure induced by oral phenylpropanolamine. Pretreatment with propranolol decreased the effect of 75 mg of phenylpropanolamine on systolic and diastolic pressures; at the lower dose of phenylpropanolamine (37.5 mg), propranolol affected only systolic pressure, perhaps because the effect of this dose of phenylpropanolamine alone on diastolic pressure was small. Left ventricular function studies showed that phenylpropanolamine increased stroke volume, ejection fraction, and cardiac output; propranolol IV reversed these effects. Systemic vascular resistance was increased by phenylpropanolamine, and further increased by propranolol. The authors concluded that phenylpropanolamine increased blood pressure by increasing systemic vascular resistance and cardiac output and that propranolol reversed the increased blood pressure by antagonizing phenylpropanolamine-mediated β_1-adrenergic cardiac stimulation.

The pressor effects of phenylpropanolamine (25 mg, PO) were investigated in nine patients with autonomic failure and orthostatic hypotension (Biaggioni et al., 1986). Blood pressure was measured every 5 min with the patients in sitting position. Phenylpropanolamine produced significant increases in systolic (32 mm Hg), diastolic (15 mm Hg), and mean (21 mm Hg) blood pressures. The pressor effect appeared within 60 min and was present 105 min after dosing. No changes in heart rate were noted. Patients with severe orthostatism (> 90 mm Hg drop in systolic blood pressure) had a greater pressor response than did patients with less severe disease (51 and 24 mm Hg, respectively).

The safety of a higher dose regimen in obese patients was also investigated (Noble, 1982). Phenylpropanolamine (50 mg, t.i.d.; twice the recommended daily dose) was administered to obese individuals for 12 weeks in a double-blind, placebo-controlled study. No significant increase in blood pressure occurred, even at this higher dose of phenylpropanolamine.

In a special safety and efficacy study, the effects of phenylpropanolamine in obese individuals with stable hypertension were investigated (Bradley & Raines, 1987). Seventy-two individuals, male and female, with ages ranging from 29 to 75 years were studied. All subjects had exogenous obesity and were 10–55% overweight. All had stable hypertension, with diastolic blood pressure at or below 94 mm Hg, with medication. Phenylpropanolamine (25 mg, t.i.d.) was given for 6 weeks in a controlled, randomized, double-blind, parallel-groups design. Vital signs, including supine and standing blood pressure and pulse, and body weight were recorded at biweekly intervals. In addition, supine and standing blood pressure and pulses were recorded at intervals ($^1/_2$, 1, 2, and 4 hr) following the initial dose.

Although there was a tendency for supine and standing blood pressures and pulse to decrease during the 6 weeks of the study, such decreases occurred in both the phenylpropanolamine and placebo groups and the magnitude of change was clinically insignificant. There were no statistically significant differences in vital signs between phenylpropanolamine and placebo groups at any time period during the study. No clinically significant effects of phenylpropanolamine on blood pressure or pulse rate were observed during the acute phase of the study. Administration of phenylpropanolamine produced no significant changes in laboratory values (hematology, blood chemistry, electrolytes, urinalysis).

The incidence of side effects during the study was low, and it was not possible to determine whether the occurrence of subjective side effects was related to administration of phenylpropanolamine. Twelve patients discontinued the study for various reasons, eight from the phenylpropanolamine group and four from the placebo group. The side effects reported in patients in the phenylpropanolamine group who dropped out of the study included insomnia, tingling hands, weakness, itchy scalp, allergic pruritus, urinary frequency, unstable angina, and dizziness (the incidence was 1/36 for each of these side effects).

In summary, no significant effects of phenylpropanolamine on blood pressure or pulse rate in obese hypertensive individuals were recorded. In addition, no effect of phenylpropanolamine on clinical laboratory values or body temperature were recorded; no subjective side effects were attributed to phenylpropanolamine administration. However, phenylpropanolamine did suppress hunger and increased weight loss in these patients; the efficacy data from this study are reviewed in greater detail in Chapter 5.

A series of studies was conducted to test the safety of phenylpropanolamine alone [reviewed by Bigelow (1985) and Krakoff (1985)]. These studies tested the effects of phenylpropanolamine on blood pressure, heart rate, and mood in normotensive healthy individuals. In addition, effects of phenylpropanolamine on normal weight, mildly overweight, and severely overweight individuals were compared. The doses employed were 25-mg phenylpropanolamine immediate-release formulation, t.i.d., and a single dose of a 75-mg sustained-release formulation. Table 4.9 summarizes the study design.

The effects of phenylpropanolamine on blood pressure, pulse, and mood in 150 healthy normotensive volunteers was conducted at the Behavioral Pharmacology Research Unit at the Johns Hopkins University School of Medicine. This study used a parallel-groups design. The study population consisted of 83 Caucasians, 63 blacks, 3 orientals, and 1 American Indian; the mean age was 25.9 years, and 58% of the subjects were men. Subjects were randomly assigned to one of three treatment groups. Group A received 75-mg phenylpropanolamine sustained-release capsules at 8:00 A.M. and placebo capsules at noon and 4:00 P.M.; group B received 25 mg of phenylpropanolamine at each of the three medication periods, and group C received placebo capsules at each medication period. Subjects were studied for a 12-hr testing session. Measurements of blood pressure (sitting, standing, and supine), pulse rate, and subjective drug effect ("mood") were determined nine times during the session—at baseline (before drug administration) and at 1/2, 1, 2, 4, 6, 8, 10, and 12 hr after initial dosing. Effects of phenylpropanolamine on mood were assessed by subjective rating of the individuals' responses.

No significant effects of drug treatment were observed on any of the measures. Differences in blood pressure between drug treatment groups were very small. No consistent pattern of differences between treatments was observed. On some measurement occasions, subjects receiving active treatments had higher mean blood pressures than did those receiving placebo treatment; on other occasions the situation was reversed. No statistically significant differences between drug treatments were found on any of the measurement occasions. Some statistically significant differences in blood pressure were found over the course of the daily sessions, which are expected normal circadian variations. In the dosage forms studied, phenylpropanolamine had no effect on subjective ratings of drug effect or drug liking. These findings indicate that, in the dosage forms studied, phenylpropanolamine had no adverse effects on blood pressure, pulse, or mood.

The effects of phenylpropanolamine on blood pressure, pulse rate, and mood were further investigated in 59 of the original 150 volunteers who participated in a double-blind crossover study. Fifty-nine subjects participated in two sessions, with the order randomly determined, one with placebo and the other with 75-mg phenylpropanolamine hydrochloride sustained-release capsules. The regimen of drug administration and determination of blood pressure, pulse rate, and mood were as described in the previous study.

Pulse rate tended to increase slightly during the session, showing a peak at about 6 hr postdosing with both placebo and active drug. Standing systolic blood pressure was relatively stable for both treatment groups. Standing diastolic pressure, sitting systolic and diastolic blood pressure, and supine sys-

TABLE 4.9. Clinical Studies of the Safety of Phenylpropanolamine

Study	PPA Dose (mg)	Patients				Design	Measurements
		n	Sex	Age (years)	Comments		
Parallel-groups	75 (SR)[a], 25 (t.i.d.)	150	M, F	$\bar{x}$ = 25.9	Normotensive volunteers	DB[b], PC[c]; parallel groups; repeated measures; 12-hr duration	Blood pressure (sitting, standing, supine); pulse; subjective drug effect (mood); ACRI[d], POMS[e]
Crossover	75 (SR)	59	M, F	$\bar{x}$ = 25.5	Normotensive volunteers	DB, PC; crossover; repeated measures; 12-hr duration	Blood pressure (sitting, standing, supine); pulse; subjective drug effect (mood); ACRI; POMS
Weight stratified	75 (SR), 25 (t.i.d.)	224	M, F	$\bar{x}$ = 31.6	Normotensive volunteers; normal weight (n = 46); mildly obese (n = 72); moderately obese (n = 71); severely obese (n = 35)	PC; parallel groups; repeated measures; 12-hr duration	Blood pressure (standing, supine); pulse; ARCI

Source: From reviews by Bigelow (1985) and Krakoff (1985).
[a]SR—sustained release.
[b]DB—double-blind.
[c]PC—placebo-controlled.
[d]Addiction Research Center Inventory.
[e]Profile of Mood States.

tolic and diastolic blood pressure all tended to peak at 4 and 12 hr after initial dosing and tended to be slightly higher following active drug treatment than following placebo. However, these differences were slight, with mean differences that ranged between 0.83 and 3.37 mm Hg and thus are clinically insignificant. The statistical significance of these slight differences is explicable in part by the fact that all the subjects served as their own individual controls, which would lower the overall error variance. As in the parallel groups study, there were the expected circadian effects on blood pressure related to time of day. There was no evidence of any differences of subjective ratings of drug effect or drug liking, with phenylpropanolamine not rated as any better or any worse than the placebo.

Although there were statistically reliable effects on blood pressure for the 75-mg phenylpropanolamine sustained-release form, these effects were extremely small and are not considered clinically relevant. No adverse effects were noted on pulse rate or mood.

The safety of phenylpropanolamine in individuals with various degrees of obesity was investigated in a multisite stratified parallel-groups study (Krakoff, 1985). At one of these sites a double-blind, placebo-controlled evaluation of the effects of phenylpropanolamine on blood pressure, pulse rate, and mood was conducted using 216 normotensive volunteers at the Cathedral Hill Obesity Clinic in San Francisco. Subjects had various degrees of overweight: normal weight ($n = 36$), mildly overweight ($n = 72$), moderately overweight ($n = 72$), and severely overweight ($n = 36$). Mild overweight was defined as 15–30% over ideal body weight, moderately overweight as 31–45% over ideal body weight, and severe overweight as greater than 46% above ideal body weight. The mean age was 32.3 years. Subjects in each weight category were randomly assigned to one of three groups. Group A received a 75-mg phenylpropanolamine sustained-release capsule at the first dose and placebo capsules at the other two dosing periods, group B received 25 mg of phenylpropanolamine hydrochloride at the three dosing periods, and group C received placebos at each of the three dosing periods. Measurements of blood pressure (standing and supine), pulse rate, and subjective drug effect using the Addiction Research Center Inventory (ARCI) were obtained 11 times during the session—at baseline before drug administration and from 1/2–12 hr after initial dosing.

No significant effects of drug treatment were observed on any of the measures. No statistically significant differences between drug treatments were found in blood pressure or pulse rate at any of the measurement periods. Subjects in the severely overweight categories consistently showed more rapid pulse rate, higher blood pressure, and higher peaks of mean diastolic blood pressure than did those in the normal weight or mildly overweight categories. These differences between weight categories were not affected by drug treatment. Some statistically significant but extremely small differences in systolic blood pressure, both standing and supine, were found during the 12-hr session that are attributed to normal circadian variation. There was no evidence of any subjective drug effect as measured by the ARCI drug inventory, and there were no statistically significant differences between drug treatments on any of the measures of drug effect, including euphoric effects. In general, subjects in all treatment groups reported feeling more energetic early in the session compared with later in the session.

In the dosage forms studied, phenylpropanolamine had no adverse effects on blood pressure, pulse rate, or subjective drug responses. In addition, there was no interaction between drug treatment and body weight.

At the second site of this multisite study, similar results were obtained in another stratified parallel-groups evaluation of the effect of phenylpropanolamine on blood pressure, pulse rate and mood done on 224 healthy normotensive volunteers performed at the Department of Medicine, University of Washington. Two dosage forms of phenylpropanolamine, 75-mg sustained-release and 25 mg t.i.d., were compared with placebo. Among the volunteers, weight categories were: normal ($n = 46$); mildly overweight, 15–30% ($n = 72$); moderately overweight, 31–45% ($n = 71$); and severely overweight, over 46% ($n = 35$). The mean age was 31.6 years. It was found that the degree of overweight was significantly related to blood pressure and pulse rate, with subjects in the heavier weight groups consistently showing higher blood pressure and more rapid pulse. All measures showed normal circadian effects during the 12-hr session that were unrelated to drug treatment. Subjects who received the 75-mg dose showed a small but statistically significant increase in supine blood pressure: supine systolic pressure was 4.5 mm Hg higher, and supine diastolic pressure was 3.7 mm Hg higher than in the placebo group. The group that received 25 mg t.i.d. had supine blood pressures approximately equal to the placebo group. There were no overall differences in standing blood pressure among the treatment groups, although the subjects who received the 75-mg dose showed larger increases of standing and supine blood pressure early in the session than did subjects in the other treatment groups.

Although there were some statistical differences in blood pressure of the subjects in the 75-mg group compared with placebo, these differences were small and not considered clinically significant. There was no evidence of any effect on subjective ratings of drug effect. The values for the two drug-treatment groups were not different from those for the placebo group, and there were no euphoric effects. There was no evidence that the drug is likely to be abused or is psychoactive. Phenylpropanolamine at dosages of 75 mg or 25 mg t.i.d. had no adverse effects on blood pressure, pulse rate, or subjective (mood) drug effects.

The effects of two dosage regimens of phenylpropanolamine—25-mg immediate-release tablets t.i.d. and 75-mg controlled-release capsules once a day—on blood pressure were compared in a crossover study of 14 normotensive, nonobese, male subjects aged 20–40 (average 27) years (Saltzman et al., 1983). In addition, plasma levels of phenylpropanolamine were measured. Subjects were given the test materials for 4 days, and blood pressure and plasma phenylpropanolamine levels were measured on day 4 at hourly intervals for 12 hr.

Mean values of systolic and diastolic blood pressures were the same for both drug regimens. Diastolic pressure rose above 90 mm Hg in only one subject on the t.i.d. regimen, 3 hr after the second 25-mg dose. No other subject's diastolic pressure rose above 90 mm Hg on day 4 in either dosage group. The 25-mg t.i.d. dose produced phenylpropanolamine plasma values with three peaks and the maximum level (138.3 ng/ml) at 10 hr after the first dose. The 75-mg controlled-release dosage produced phenylpropanolamine plasma values with only one peak and the maximum level (151.3 ng/ml) at 4–6 hr after dosing. Blood pressure did not rise in relation to plasma phenylpropanolamine levels on either regimen.

EFFECTS OF PHENYLPROPANOLAMINE ON SUBJECTIVE RATING OF DRUG EFFECT AND AFFECTIVE STATE

Effects of 75 mg of phenylpropanolamine (sustained-release, m.i.d.) and 25 mg of phenylpropanolamine (t.i.d.) on subjective rating of mood were evaluated in the parallel-groups study and in the crossover study [see the review by Bigelow (1985)]. The subjects rated their subjective responses on a visual analogue scale at various intervals after administration of phenylpropanolamine. The following questions were asked:

Are there any drug effects?
Are there good effects?
Are there any bad effects?
Do you like or dislike the effects?

In neither study were there significant effects of phenylpropanolamine on mood.

In two studies, effects of phenylpropanolamine on mood were rated by the Addiction Research Center Inventory (ARCI) and the Profile of Mood States (POMS) (Bigelow, 1985) (see also Table 4.9), standardized tests for measurement of drug effects on affective state. In the ARCI, the drug effects were compared to known psychotropic drugs. In the POMS, the subjective ratings on seven mood states were recorded and a composite score tabulated. In the parallel-groups study, there were no effects attributable to phenylpropanolamine in either the ARCI or the POMS. The crossover-design study employed a larger number of subjects per group, and a more powerful statistical analysis based on the repeated-measures design with the subjects as their own controls. By means of these more powerful statistical tests, several statistically significant differences between phenylpropanolamine and placebo were demonstrated. In each case, the rating for phenylpropanolamine was less than the rating for placebo. Thus, phenylpropanolamine was rated less like the pentobarbital-chlorpromazine-alcohol group and less like the LSD group of drugs in the ARCI. In the POMS, phenylpropanolamine was rated as producing less tension-anxiety, anger-hostility, and confusion-bewilderment than did placebo. Phenylpropanolamine may reduce the boredom and dissatisfaction involved in the participation in a drug evaluation study in a bland, unstimulating environment. This conclusion was based on the observation that the differences between phenylpropanolamine and placebo treatment tended to occur most frequently during the latter portion of the 12-hr testing period.

The lack of effect of phenylpropanolamine on affective state or mood is confirmed by the results of several clinical studies in which phenylpropanolamine did not produce CNS stimulation or excitement (Altschuler et al., 1982; Bigelow et al., 1984; Griboff et al., 1975; Hoebel et al., 1975; Schuster & Johanson, 1984; Seppala et al., 1981). The incidences of CNS-related side effects in clinical trials are summarized in Tables 5.9, 5.11, 5.12, 5.13, 5.20, and 5.26.

HIGH-DOSE STUDIES

The safety of phenylpropanolamine is further confirmed by clinical efficacy studies in which patients were given phenylpropanolamine at doses higher than currently recommended. In two early uncontrolled clinical case studies phenylpropanolamine was given at doses as high as 48 mg every 3 hr (Black, 1937; Boyer, 1938). No significant cardiovascular or CNS side effects were observed.

In patients with chronic nonallergic rhinitis, 100 mg of phenylpropanolamine (sustained-release formulation) produced no effect on blood pressure or heart rate (Broms & Malm, 1982).

In a randomized, double-blind, placebo-controlled clinical trial to test the efficacy of phenylpropanolamine in treatment of chronic nonallergic rhinitis, patients were given placebo, or 50 or 100 mg of phenylpropanolamine twice daily for 3 days (Renvall & Lindqvist, 1979). Even at the relatively high dose of 200 mg/day of phenylpropanolamine, no side effects such as CNS stimulation or elevation of blood pressure were noted.

In a steady-state bioavailability study, healthy volunteers were given either 75 mg of phenylpropanolamine plus 12 mg of chlorpheniramine (sustained-release formulation) twice daily or 25 mg of phenylpropanolamine plus 4 mg of chlorpheniramine (immediate-release formulation) every 4 hr for four consecutive days (Barrett et al., 1981). Neither treatment produced significant adverse effects on vital signs (body temperature, respiratory rate, standing blood pressure, and pulse), ECG parameters, or hematology, clinical chemistry, or urinalysis test results.

In a double-blind, crossover study, six obese, hyperglycemic patients were given 75 mg of phenylpropanolamine (sustained-release formulation) or placebo twice daily for 2 weeks (Krosnick et al., 1982). Phenylpropanolamine produced no significant change in blood pressure or heart rate.

SAFETY OF PHENYLPROPANOLAMINE IN COMBINATION WITH CAFFEINE

A controlled three-phase multisite study was conducted to determine the cardiovascular effects of orally administered 25 mg of phenylpropanolamine hydrochloride alone and in combination with 100 mg of caffeine (Silverman et al., 1980). In the first study, 15 healthy young men aged 17–24 years were given 25 mg of phenylpropanolamine hydrochloride in a single-blind acute study. Supine systolic and diastolic blood pressure did not significantly change during the 3-hr observation period. There was a slight decrease in pulse rate at 2 hr and at 3 hr, but not at 1 hr after drug administration. This was attributed to a decrease of anxiety following the initial examination.

In the second study, 12 healthy male volunteers ranging in age from 22 to 42 years participated in a double-blind crossover study in which they were administered a capsule containing 25 mg of phenylpropanolamine hydrochloride or a matching placebo capsule. Blood pressure and pulse rate were determined every 30 min for 4 hr after ingesting the capsule. After 48 hr the volunteers were administered the dosage form not previously taken; blood pressure and pulse rate were again measured. An analysis of variance (ANOVA) test revealed no significant differences in systolic or diastolic blood pressure or pulse rate at any time interval following drug administration compared with placebo.

Finally, 10 healthy young male volunteers aged 18–23 years each ingested one tablet containing 25 mg of phenylpropanolamine hydrochloride and 100 mg of caffeine. Supine blood pressure and pulse rates were determined every 30 min for 4 hr. There was no significant difference in systolic or diastolic blood pressure or pulse rate at any time interval after drug administration compared with the predrug determination.

The fact that no important effect on blood pressure or heart rate due to drug treatment was recorded in any of the three study groups leads to the conclusion that 25 mg of phenylpropanolamine hydrochloride alone or when combined with 100 mg of caffeine is not likely to adversely affect the myocardium or cause a significant vasopressor response.

In three double-blind studies (Altschuler et al., 1982), the effectiveness of the phenylpropanolamine-caffeine combination was compared to placebo, mazindol, or diethylpropion in producing weight loss in otherwise healthy adults. Subjects were obtained from three study areas: a general hospital, a Veterans Administration hospital, and a general practice. In study 1, 37.5 mg of phenylpropanolamine plus 140 mg of caffeine (sustained-release) or placebo was taken twice a day; in study 2, 50 mg of phenylpropanolamine plus 200 mg of caffeine (sustained-release) or 2 mg of mazindol was taken once a day; in study 3, 25 mg of phenylpropanolamine with 100 mg of caffeine and multivitamins or 25 mg of diethylpropion was taken three times a day. Each subject reported every 2 weeks during the study for interviewing, weighing, blood pressure and pulse rate measurement, and to report any side effects or adverse reactions.

None of the three dose regimens of phenylpropanolamine-caffeine used in this study had any significant effect on systolic or diastolic blood pressure or pulse rate (Table 4.10). Side effects were minimal, and the incidence of side effects was lower among subjects taking phenylpropanolamine-caffeine than among those taking either of the two comparative drugs.

The lack of cardiovascular side effects of a combination of phenylpropanolamine and caffeine was confirmed in one additional study (Noble, 1982). Phenylpropanolamine (50 mg) combined with caffeine (200 mg) in a controlled-release formulation was given to obese patients in a double-blind, placebo-controlled study. No significant effects on blood pressure were recorded.

SAFETY OF PHENYLPROPANOLAMINE COMBINED WITH BELLADONNA ALKALOIDS

Mitchell (1968) investigated the cardiovascular effects of the combination of phenylpropanolamine and belladonna alkaloids in humans. In this investigation 32 normotensive volunteers, 12 women and 20 men, 19–53 years old with a mean age of 24.5 years, were studied for 4 weeks. No drugs were given in the first week. In a 3-week blind crossover study the subjects received each of the following drugs for 5 days: (1) one placebo capsule b.i.d.; (2) 50 mg of phenylpropanolamine hydrochloride, sustained release, one capsule b.i.d.; and (3) 0.25 mg of belladonna alkaloids plus 50 mg of phenylpropanolamine hydrochloride, sustained release, one capsule b.i.d. Blood pressure and pulse rate in the sitting position were recorded daily on days 2–6. An electrocardiogram was recorded once each week on day 6. The mean arterial pressure (diastolic pressure plus one-third of the pulse pressure) was calculated for each recording of blood pressure.

There were no significant changes in the mean arterial pressure attributable to drug treatment. The pulse rate was significantly slowed only in those volunteers receiving phenylpropanolamine plus belladonna alkaloids.

TABLE 4.10. Effects of Phenylpropanolamine Plus Caffeine on Blood Pressure and Heart Rate in Humans

	Diastolic Pressure (mm Hg)		Systolic Pressure (mm Hg)		Pulse Rate (bpm)	
	Control	Treated	Control	Treated	Control	Treated
Study I (6-week evaluation)						
Phenylpropanolamine–caffeine b.i.d. (n = 28)						
Mean	78.9	78.1	124.4	124.4	73.4	72.9
Range	70–90	65–90	110–150	110–150	68–82	68–82
Placebo b.i.d. (n = 28)						
Mean	84.3	82.2	128.3	127.7	74.2	73.5
Range	65–90	70–100	110–150	110–150	64–88	70–88
Study II (6-week evaluation)						
Mazindol o.d. (n = 28)						
Mean	79.3	75.9	120.6	118.2	76.4	75.2
Range	58–94	54–88	108–146	102–138	64–90	66–96
Phenylpropanolamine–caffeine o.d. (n = 27)						
Mean	76.6	76.3	115.6	117.4	75.3	74.3
Range	60–90	62–86	90–142	96–150	60–90	60–86
Study III (8-week evaluation)						
Diethylpropion t.i.d. (n = 23)						
Mean	71.4	72.0	111.2	113.5	77.2	78.3
Range	60–80	60–82	94–130	100–140	62–88	72–100
Phenylpropanolamine–caffeine–vitamins t.i.d. (n = 25)						
Mean	69.9	70.1	110.8	112.8	78.1	78.8
Range	54–82	58–88	98–126	96–140	60–100	68–88

Source: Data from Altschuler et al. (1982).

The electrocardiograms showed no significant changes except for heart rate. Side effects were similar in the placebo and phenylpropanolamine groups but were significantly increased in the phenylpropanolamine-belladonna alkaloids group.

A substudy was done on six volunteers to determine whether a transient change in blood pressure or pulse rate could have occurred immediately after drug administration. These six normotensive volunteers who ranged in age from 21 to 27 years (mean 23 years) were studied on two occasions, each of 3-hr duration. In a blind crossover randomized design, each volunteer received either two capsules of placebo or two capsules containing phenylpropanolamine hydrochloride (50 mg) plus belladonna alkaloids (0.25 mg). Blood pressure and pulse rate were recorded at baseline and following drug administration, each 15 min for the first 90 min and each 30 min for the next 90 min. When compared with placebo, phenylpropanolamine plus belladonna alkaloids caused no statistically significant change in arterial pressure and pulse rate at any time interval.

In these studies, 50 mg of phenylpropanolamine hydrochloride plus 0.25 mg of belladonna alkaloids administered orally did not induce any pressor effect. The 50 mg dose of phenylpropanolamine hydrochloride used in this study was equivalent to or greater than that used in most proprietary preparations; consequently, these preparations can be considered extremely unlikely to have a hypertensive effect.

MISCELLANEOUS STUDIES

In more than 50 clinical efficacy trials reported to date, the incidence of reported side effects attributed to phenylpropanolamine taken at recommended doses has been consistently low; these results are reviewed in detail in Chapter 5. Additional evidence for the safety of phenylpropanolamine comes from analysis of poisoning cases reported to poison control centers (Ekins & Spoerke, 1983; Larson & Rogers, 1986) and two retrospective studies (Krupka & Vener, 1983; Aselton et al., 1985a).

Seventy cases of phenylpropanolamine-related poisonings were reported to a poison control center during a 5-month period (Ekins & Spoerke, 1983). There were more females (46/70, 65%) than males (24/70, 34%); their ages ranged from 9 months to 20 years for males and 1.5 to 54 years for females. Accidental poisonings in children and intentional use for either suicide or drug abuse in adults were analyzed.

Patients who took products that contained phenylpropanolamine alone either developed no symptoms or their symptoms were mild and brief. The estimated phenylpropanolamine dose for symptomatic patients was 17.5 mg/kg. For cases involving products that contained phenylpropanolamine and caffeine, all patients over 13 years old showed symptoms. The estimated doses of phenylpropanolamine and caffeine for patients less than 13 years old were 8.2–10.5 and 22–40 mg/kg, respectively; for patients 13 years or older, the doses were 5–8.8 and 15–26 mg/kg, respectively (235–575 and 680–1400 mg total dose, respectively). The symptoms most frequently observed were headache, nausea, vomiting, nervousness, and tachycardia.

Most patients required only supportive medical treatment. Only two patients (3%) required hospitalization; 20% of the patients were treated at an emergency department and released, and the remaining 77% of the patients were managed in the home with demulcents or emetics.

Thus, in this extensive series of cases from a poison control center there was a lack of serious side effects associated with products containing phenylpropanolamine with or without caffeine.

A prospective study analyzed 92 cases of phenylpropanolamine ingestion reported to a regional poison control center (Larson & Rogers, 1986). The criteria for treatment of phenylpropanolamine poisoning were: All patients who took >8 mg/kg and symptomatic patients who took <8 mg/kg were referred to a health care facility; patients who took 4–8 mg/kg were treated at home with ipecac. The symptoms most commonly associated with phenylpropanolamine ingestion were drowsiness (36% of patients), tachycardia (22%), hypertension (14%), vomiting (10%), nausea (8%), irritability (8%), ataxia (5%), and headache (2%). For patients reporting drowsiness, the mean phenylpropanolamine dose was 9.6 mg/kg (range 1.8–22.5 mg/kg). The mean dose for patients reporting hypertension was 13.6 mg/kg (range 1.7–60 mg/kg); 69% of these patients were 13 years old or older. In addition, mild blood pressure elevation occurred in five patients who took less than 8 mg/kg of phenylpropanolamine. Sustained-release phenylpropanolamine formulations were involved in 67% of the hypertensive cases. Two patients required medical treatment for hypertension; one was treated with nitroprusside and the other with hydralazine. Hypertensive episodes occurred most frequently in people who had taken at least 10 mg/kg of phenylpropanolamine (i.e., 650 mg total dose for a 65 kg person).

A retrospective study was conducted to evaluate whether ingestion of phenylpropanolamine was associated with subsequent hospitalization for malignant hypertension, cardiac arrhythmia, neuropsychiatric illness, or nonhemorrhagic stroke (Aselton et al., 1985a). This study evaluated the experiences of patients from the Group Health Cooperative of Puget Sound, Washington. Between 1977 and 1982, phenylpropanolamine-containing cough/cold remedies were prescribed 253,334 times. The relative risk for each specified illness was calculated (ratio of the incidence in the treated group/incidence in the untreated group). Phenylpropanolamine use produced no increase in the relative risk for malignant hypertension or arrhythmia. The relative risk for neuropsychiatric illness was only slightly increased (relative risk = 1.29; 95% confidence interval 0.2–4.8) and the relative risk for thrombotic or nonspecific cerebrovascular accident was actually reduced (relative risk = 0.25, 95% confidence interval 0.01–1.40). Thus, phenylpropanolamine was associated with a very low risk for these disorders.

In addition, one uncontrolled retrospective survey of the side effects of commercial diet products was reported (Krupka & Vener, 1983), using a self-administered questionnaire. This study surveyed 944 college undergraduates regarding their usage, perceived effectiveness and side effects of OTC diet pills containing phenylpropanolamine. There were 561 women and 383 men in the sample; 98% were between the ages of 18 and 21 years.

Approximately one out of three (30.1%) of the women and 3.7% of the men reported using appetite suppressants during the previous year; 19 different commercial diet products were used by the 169 women during the previous year. Of these 169 women, 83 took at least two different brands, 38 used three or more, and one woman took nine different products. In addition to phenylpropanolamine, many of these products also contained caffeine, with recommended dosages as high as 300 mg.

Forty-two women who had taken diet pills reported various side effects. The most frequently reported side effect was "nervousness," variously described as the condition of being "hyper," "shaky," "jumpy," tense, or anxious. Other reported symptoms were "feeling sick," upset stomach, dizziness, light-headedness, insomnia, and dry mouth. It should also be noted that 8 women and 4 of the 14 men took these compounds not as appetite suppressants but as stimulants.

The effects of phenylpropanolamine (50 mg, PO, b.i.d. for three doses) on psychomotor performance and subjective appraisal of sleep in human volunteers were investigated (Seppala et al., 1981). Psychomotor performance was evaluated by a battery of tests designed to evaluate the effects of drugs on safety for driving or operating machinery. Phenylpropanolamine was judged as not detrimental to competence for driving or operating machinery. Effects of phenylpropanolamine on sleep were assessed by subjective measures using a standardized sleep-evaluation questionnaire. Phenylpropanolamine increased the subjective rating of alertness during the day but had no effect on the subjective evaluation of sleep.

The effects of phenylpropanolamine on psychophysiologic performance were investigated in a placebo-controlled, double-blind, parallel-groups study (Nuotto & Seppala, 1984); interactions between phenylpropanolamine and diazepam were also investigated. The subjects were 239 healthy volunteers (135 females, 104 males; age 22.1 ± 2.5 years). The drug treatments were: phenylpropanolamine (80 mg), diazepam (10 and 20 mg), phenylpropanolamine plus diazepam, and placebo. A series of standard tests was used to evaluate psychophysiological performance (eye-to-hand coordination test, finger tapping speed, grip strength, critical flicker fusion, Maddox wing test for extraocular muscle function, digit/symbol substitution test for sensory recognition and concentration, letter-cancellation test for perceptual processing of sensory information, and body-sway test). Blood pressure, heart rate, and subjective assessments of drug effects (visual analog scales, questionnaire) were also evaluated.

Phenylpropanolamine alone and placebo treatment both improved psychophysiologic performance and diazepam impaired performance. Phenylpropanolamine antagonized some of the diazepam-induced performance impairment. Phenylpropanolamine increased systolic and diastolic blood pressure (mean increases ranged from 8 to 18 mm Hg) and decreased heart rate (decreases ranged from 12 to 17 bpm); diazepam antagonized these changes.

Only limited information is available regarding effects of phenylpropanolamine on reproduction and fertility. Effects of systemic administration of phenylpropanolamine on reproduction and fertility were not reported. Local application of norephedrine to the vas deferens in rats (Ratnasooriya et al., 1979) or rabbits (Ratnasooriya et al., 1981) produced infertility with reduced semen volume, sperm count, and sperm motility. Local application of norephedrine to the epididymis (Ratnasooriya et al., 1980) did not produce infertility. No clinical studies of effect of phenylpropanolamine on reproduction and fertility in humans have been reported. In one case, phenylpropanolamine was used to correct retrograde ejaculation, and during phenylpropanolamine treatment the patient conceived a child, suggesting that systemic phenylpropanolamine does not cause infertility (Proctor & Howards, 1983).

There have been no reports in the extensive literature searched that suggested phenylpropanolamine had mutagenic or carcinogenic effects in animals or humans.

TERATOLOGY

The prevalence of certain major congenital disorders among the infants of women who used a wide variety of drugs during the first trimester of pregnancy has been evaluated (Aselton et al., 1985b; Jick et al., 1981). The studies were carried out at Group Health Cooperative (GHC) of Puget Sound, which has approximately 280,000 members. Information on all GHC hospital discharges, including diagnosis of a congenital disorder, are recorded in computer files. In addition, prescriptions filled in regional outpatient pharmacies are computerized by GHC. It was thus possible to determine the prevalence of anomalies among the offspring of women and relate these congenital disorders to drug use just prior to or during pregnancy.

In the first study there were a total of 80 infants (1.2%) with 19 different congenital disorders among the 6837 pregnancies that terminated in a live birth (Jick et al., 1981). Among the 14 drugs most frequently prescribed during the first trimester of pregnancy, drugs used for the nausea and vomiting of pregnancy were prescribed most frequently (33% of women). The prevalence of congenital disorders among the users of these drugs was not significantly higher than among nonusers.

Of the 45 drugs prescribed during the first trimester of pregnancy, only one, Dimetapp (brompheniramine maleate, phenylephrine hydrochloride, and phenylpropanolamine hydrochloride), contained phenylpropanolamine. Of the 100–199 women who took Dimetapp during pregnancy, only one gave birth to an infant with a congenital disorder; thus, the incidence of birth defects among infants born to women who took Dimetapp was similar to the overall incidence (1.2%). These findings indicate that phenylpropanolamine was not a factor in congenital disorders in infants from these 6837 pregnancies (Jick, et al., 1981).

In a follow-up study, there were 6509 pregnancies that resulted in live births; 105 infants (1.6%) had congenital abnormalities (Aselton et al., 1985b). Analysis of the first-trimester drug use by these women showed no strong association between any drug and the occurrence of congenital disorders. There was a slightly higher incidence of congenital disorders among infants born to women who took Dimetapp (relative risk = 1.8; 95% confidence interval 0.8–4.4); no other phenylpropanolamine-containing product was associated with increased risk of congenital disorders. The significance of the observation with Dimetapp was questioned by the authors because there was no increased risk with Dimetapp in their previous study (Jick et al., 1981).

Between 1958 and 1965, the Collaborative Perinatal Project conducted a prospective study of drug use during pregnancy and birth defects (Heinonen et al., 1977). Maternal drug use during early pregnancy was tabulated; several hundreds of drugs were evaluated. The standardized relative risk (SRR) was calculated as the ratio of the incidence of malformations for drug users/ incidence for nonusers. An SRR higher than unity indicated some increased risk of congenital malformations. A total of 50,282 pregnancies were studied; 2277 of the infants had birth defects, for an overall incidence of 45.3/1000. While the SRR for phenylpropanolamine was statistically significantly higher than unity, the authors pointed out that the increased risk may be unrelated to phenylpropanolamine per se. Sympathomimetic drugs frequently are taken for symptomatic treatment of viral upper respiratory infections. It is possible that viral infections, rather than the medications, were responsible for the birth defects; due to limitations in the experimental design, it was impossible to assess this possibility.

A prospective study was conducted to determine whether drug use or smoking during early pregnancy is associated with birth defects in infants (Sandahl, 1985). A total of 2436 pregnant women were evaluated at the General Hospital of Malmo, Sweden, in 1979 and 1980. During the 17th week of pregnancy the fetuses were evaluated by ultrasound techniques and the mothers were questioned regarding exposure to contraceptives, x-rays, cigarette smoking, and drugs. At the time of delivery, birth defects, infant survival, birth weight, and duration of pregnancy were recorded. There were no birth defects associated with ingestion of phenylpropanolamine during early pregnancy.

The effects of maternal allergy medications on the fetus were reviewed by Hill and Tennyson (1985). The authors stated that "There are no adverse effects reported in fetuses due to phenylpropanolamine...." However, they advised close monitoring of phenylpropanolamine use in pregnancy because the sympathomimetic drug phenylephrine has been shown to decrease uterine blood flow, decrease fetal arterial pO_2 and pH, and increase fetal arterial pCO_2.

DRUG ABUSE LIABILITY

Although phenylpropanolamine had been linked with drug abuse in association with the so-called amphetamine look-alikes and pseudospeed (Wesson & Morgan, 1982; see also Chapter 1), several experimental studies in both humans and animals indicate that phenylpropanolamine alone has low drug abuse liability. Abuse liability in humans can be assessed by subjective rating scales in which the subjects are asked to rate the drug-induced effects on mood or to compare the drug to other drugs of abuse. Studies of the effects of phenylpropanolamine on subjective mood in humans are reviewed here. Studies of drug abuse liability testing in experimental animals were reviewed in Chapter 3 and support the conclusion that phenylpropanolamine has low drug abuse liability.

Effects of phenylpropanolamine on mood were investigated [reviewed by Bigelow (1985)]. In a parallel-groups design, 150 normal volunteers received 25 mg of phenylpropanolamine hydrochloride t.i.d., 75 mg of phenylpropanolamine hydrochloride sustained-release form once daily, or placebo. In a second phase of the study, 59 of these volunteers were administered 75 mg of phenylpropanolamine sustained-release form and placebo on separate occasions in a double-blind, crossover design. In both studies phenylpropanolamine was found to have minimal to no effect on blood pressure, pulse rate, or subjective rating of drug effect and drug liking over a 12-hr experimental session.

These same subjects filled out two standardized test forms at each measurement occasion in order to compare subjective effects of phenylpropanolamine with those of other CNS-active drugs and to more rigorously evaluate the effects of phenylpropanolamine on affective state or mood. The first test used was the Addiction Research Center Inventory (ARCI), which scored clusters of items to reflect patterns of five major drug categories: amphetamine, benzedrine, morphine-benzedrine, pentobarbital-chlorpromazine-alcohol, and LSD. The second test was the Profile of Mood States (POMS), which measures six identifiable moods and overall mood.

In the parallel-groups study, the effects of phenylpropanolamine were not different from those of placebo in any of the measures studied. Subjects in all groups tended to feel more sedated or tired as the session progressed, with lessening of the sedative effect just before the conclusion of the study; this effect was not related to drug treatment.

In the crossover study there were some statistically significant differences between the 75-mg phenylpropanolamine sustained-release treatment and placebo administration. On the ARCI test, the phenylpropanolamine treatment resulted in less sedation-fatigue and less dysphoria compared with placebo. However, no evidence of amphetaminelike effect or euphoria was found. In general, subjects felt better earlier in the course of the study. The POMS test results confirmed these effects—subjects felt less tense or anxious, less hostile, and less confused after taking phenylpropanolamine as compared with placebo.

Overall no euphoric effects were noted for phenylpropanolamine, although there is some evidence that phenylpropanolamine reduced dysphoria and boredom associated with a 12-hr session in a restricted and relatively bland environment. Phenylpropanolamine showed no pattern of subjective effects indicative of abuse liability and no amphetaminelike or euphoric effects.

A second method for assessing the abuse liability of drugs in humans is clinical drug self-administration studies (Bigelow, 1985). In these studies, volunteers are given two or more drugs on separate occasions; in subsequent tests the subjects are given the choice of taking either (or any) of the previously administered drugs. A drug that is selected more frequently than placebo is considered to have abuse potential. Three separate clinical self-administration studies revealed that phenylpropanolamine does not have abuse potential. In normal human volunteers ($n = 12$), 12.5-, 25-, or 50-mg doses of phenylpropanolamine were not chosen more frequently than placebo (Chait et al., 1984; Schuster & Johanson, 1985). In this study, subjective rating tests showed that phenylpropanolamine increased ratings of anxiety, depression, and CNS stimulation but had no effect on hunger. In two studies, phenylpropanolamine (75 mg, sustained-release) was not selected more frequently than placebo by obese women (Bigelow et al., 1984, 1985). Phenylpropanolamine produced significantly greater weight loss than placebo, and subjective rating scales (POMS) showed decreases in fatigue-inertia and depression-rejection and increases in rigor-activity (Bigelow et al., 1984). These subjective effects were recorded after 1 week of phenylpropanolamine treatment; no subjective effects were recorded after a single day of phenylpropanolamine treatment.

Another method used to evaluate drug abuse liability is the drug discrimination test. The general concept of drug discrimination testing was described in Chapter 3; in brief, animals or humans can be trained to discriminate between a known drug of abuse and a placebo. A test drug is then substituted for the drug of abuse to determine whether the test drug will maintain drug discrimination. Twenty healthy volunteers (8 males and 12 females) enrolled in a drug-discrimination test (Chait et al., 1986). During an initial training phase, the volunteers were given 10 mg of amphetamine and placebo on separate occasions in a randomized, single-blind procedure; the Profile of Mood States (POMS) and the Addiction Research Center Inventory (ARCI) were used to rate subjective drug effects on mood. After analysis of the results from the training phase, 12 volunteers were selected because they could reliably discriminate amphetamine from placebo. During the subsequent testing phase, the volunteers were given a single dose of a test drug but were not told the identity of the drug. At 1, 3, and 6 hr after taking the drug, each subject was asked to identify the drug as "active drug" (i.e., amphetamine-like) or "inactive drug" (i.e., placebo). Each subject was given a test drug on eight separate days. The test drugs were 25 and 75 mg of phenylpropanolamine and 0.5 and 2.0 mg of mazindol. For both phenylpropanolamine and mazindol, the drug discrimination properties were dose-related. The subjects rated the low dose of either drug as placebo-like and the high dose as amphetamine-like. In subjective ratings of drug effects, 25 mg of phenylpropanolamine was rated as sedative-like and 75 mg of phenylpropanolamine was rated as similar to, but weaker than, amphetamine; either dose of mazindol produced minimal changes in mood.

ADVERSE EFFECTS

There are always some individuals who have adverse reactions to any drug or combination medication. This is evidenced by the adverse reaction warning section in the *Physicians' Desk Reference* (PDR) and the constant monitoring of all marketed drugs and combination medications for adverse reactions. Caution must be used in singling out any one drug as the causative agent of an adverse reaction in a combination product.

In this review of all reported adverse reactions attributed to phenylpropanolamine, the majority of these reactions seem not justifiably attributable to phenylpropanolamine. Morgan's analysis (1986) concurs with this view. It is remarkable, furthermore, that there have been so few adverse reactions to phenylpropanolamine in view of its wide marketing and use throughout the world for over 40 years.

In this context, an adverse drug reaction will be defined as an unwanted drug reaction that occurs when the drug is taken at recommended dosages. Overdose cases, which occur when substantially higher than recommended dosages are consumed, are reviewed in the following section. There are some cases in which the definitions of adverse reaction and overdose tend to overlap—for example, in cases when individuals take two or three pills rather than the recommended one pill. In reality, these cases are simply drug reactions that occur at various parts of the dose-response curve and represent a spectrum of activity ranging from therapeutic to mild overdose to frank overdose and toxic levels.

A total of 64 published reports have listed 108 cases of adverse drug reactions and overdoses (Table 4.11). Adverse drug reactions constitute slightly more than half of these cases. The predominant adverse effects reported are cardiovascular and CNS effects. As will be demonstrated in the following analysis, there appears to be little or no dose separation between the effects on the cardiovascular and central nervous systems. This is somewhat surprising in light of the limited penetration of phenylpropanolamine into the brain rela-

TABLE 4.11. Summary of Adverse Drug Reaction Reports to Phenylpropanolamine-Containing Products[a]

	Recommended Dose	Overdose	Total
Publications	38	26	64
Cases	63	45	108
Effects			
Cardiovascular	42	32	74
CNS	43	21	64
Renal	1	2	3
Other	4	4	8
Preparations			
Decongestant	20	13	33
Diet	42	13	55
Street drugs	4	16	20
Sex			
Male	11	21	32
Female	55	21	76
Preexisting conditions	13	10	23
Deaths	2	7	9

[a]Comparison of therapeutic dose versus overdose cases. Reports involving drug interactions are not included in this table.

tive to the rest of the body (see Chapter 3). Perhaps this simply reflects the common misconception that phenylpropanolamine is an "amphetaminelike" drug, which may bias the observations of the individuals who report the adverse reactions.

Historically, the first reports of adverse drug reactions to phenylpropanolamine containing products were published in the 1960s (Kane & Green, 1966; Ostern & Dodson, 1965). Since that time, there has been an escalation of reported phenylpropanolamine-related adverse reactions. During 1960–1969, five adverse reaction reports were published; during 1970–1979, 14 reports were published; and from 1980 to 1986 (only 6 years), 47 reports have appeared. This increase may result from several factors. One factor undoubtedly is the increase in the consumption of phenylpropanolamine-containing products that occurred following the restriction of the manufacture and sale of amphetamines in the 1970s. Another factor may be an increased awareness among both the medical community and the general population of the importance of postmarketing surveillance of drug safety. However, the increase in reporting of adverse drug reactions may also be a form of "bandwagonning" wherein publication of one adverse reaction report stimulates publication of additional reports and may not reflect a bona fide increase in the incidence of adverse reactions in the general population. Indeed, the series of adverse drug reaction reports based on the Australian drug Trimolets (Frewin et al., 1978; Horowitz et al., 1979; King, 1979) appear to have provided just such a stimulus. This is especially unfortunate since the pharmaceutical formulation of Trimolets was significantly different from the formulations manufactured in the United States and other countries (see Chapter 1).

The adverse drug reactions and overdose cases are discussed according to the following pharmaceutical categories: decongestant preparations, appetite suppressants, and "street drugs" (amphetamine look-alikes, pseudospeed, etc.). The reason for this is that the formulations of the three categories are significantly different: the decongestant preparations frequently contain antihistamines and/or anticholinergics, the appetite suppressants formerly contained caffeine, and the street drugs typically contain caffeine and ephedrine. Thus it is likely that the adverse reactions would be different for these three categories.

In general, the syndromes of adverse drug reactions can be characterized on the basis of the intensity of the reaction. In the case of the phenylpropanolamine-containing preparations, a mild reaction consists of headache, nausea, vomiting, and sometimes blurred vision. In moderate cases, increased blood pressure and heart rate and confusion or other mild CNS signs occur. In severe cases, psychosis, hallucinations, and/or seizures have been reported.

In addition to case reports, another source of information is surveys of adverse reactions in larger, defined populations. Such surveys can provide more balanced information regarding the risk factors involved in drug usage, since the incidence of adverse reactions as a proportion of the total drug use can be evaluated.

The experience of the Puget Sound GHC relative to the use of cough-cold preparations containing phenylpropanolamine and development of cerebral hemorrhage was reviewed by the Boston Collaborative Drug Surveillance Program (Jick et al., 1984). At local GHC pharmacies from 1977 to 1981 there were 216,189 prescriptions filled for products containing phenylpropanolamine for members less than 65 years of age. These patients were considered at risk for 30 days after having the prescription filled. Among users of phenylpropanolamine, one person was admitted to the hospital for cerebral hemorrhage; among nonusers, there were 113.

ADVERSE DRUG REACTIONS: DECONGESTANT PREPARATIONS CONTAINING PHENYLPROPANOLAMINE

PREPARATIONS CONTAINING PHENYLPROPANOLAMINE ALONE

In Scandinavia, several decongestant preparations that contain phenylpropanolamine without other drugs are available, whereas in the rest of the world the decongestant preparations are combination products. From a pharmacological point of view, this is convenient since the phenylpropanolamine-only preparations can be compared to combination products in an attempt to factor out the contribution of phenylpropanolamine to the combination effect. Three cases of adverse drug reactions to decongestants that contain phenylpropanolamine alone were reported (Norvenius et al., 1979) (see Table 4.12). Two young boys and one woman had mild CNS effects after taking these products. Unfortunately, the dosages and amounts of drug taken were not reported. Cardiovascular effects were not specifically mentioned. The CNS effects remitted within a few hours to a day, apparently without therapy.

COMBINATION DECONGESTANT PRODUCTS

Sixteen adverse drug reactions to phenylpropanolamine-containing combination decongestants have been reported (Table 4.12). The dosages of phenylpropanolamine ranged from 10–12.5 mg to 100–200 mg, with most reactions reported at a 50-mg dose. In addition, responses to ingestion of one, two, three, or four capsules of Ornade were reported (Duvernoy, 1969; Kane & Green, 1966; Ostern & Dodson, 1965). Thus in this case the dose-response relationship can be evaluated. The following case reports demonstrate representative experiences.

> CASE 1.   An 18-year-old obese woman had a severe frontal headache, nausea, epigastric pain, blurred vision, and shakiness 2¹/₂ hr after taking two Comtrex tablets

TABLE 4.12. Case Histories of Adverse Drug Reactions to Phenylpropanolamine-Containing Products[a,b]

Product	Form/Contents	Dose	Age	Sex	Preexisting Conditions	Adverse Effects	Treatment	Clinical Outcome	Reference
A. Decongestants: PPA alone									
Rinexin	PPA	NS	3	M	NS	Confusion	NS	Resolved in a few hours	Norvenius et al. (1979)
Rinexin	PPA	NS	8	M	NS	Confusion	NS	Resolved in a few hours	Norvenius et al. (1979)
Monydrin	PPA	NS	25	F	NS	Excitement; sleep disturbance; muscle twitching; paranoia	NS	Resolved in 24 hr	Norvenius et al. (1979)
NS	25 mg PPA	Single dose	32	F	NS	Throbbing headache Vasospasm of cerebral vessels	NS	Headache persisted for >10 days; abated without treatment	Travnelis & Brick (1986)
B. Decongestants: Combination products									
Dimetapp elixir	5 mg PPA/5 ml + brompheniramine + phenylephrine	10 ml per night	8	F	Mild recurrent bronchospasm	Spasmodic torticollis	Haloperidol	Symptoms disappeared after stopping medications	Lewith & Davidson (1981)
Anahist	12.5 mg PPA + thorsylamine + phenyltoxolamine + phenacetin + caffeine + aspirin + vitamin C	30 tablets in 8 days	37	M	None	Paranoid psychosis	Chlorpromazine	Asymptomatic after 1 week	Wharton (1970)
Comtrex	12.5 mg PPA + acetaminophen + chlorpheniramine + dextromethorphan	2 tablets	18	F	None	Headache, nausea, blurred vision, shakiness, grand mal seizures	Hydralazine, diazepam	Asymptomatic after 16 days	Bernstein & Diskant (1982)

TABLE 4.12. Continued.

Product	Form/Contents	Dose	Age	Sex	Preexisting Conditions	Adverse Effects	Treatment	Clinical Outcome	Reference
Vicks Cold-Care	12.5 mg PPA + NS	6 pills in 18 hr	37	F	Hypermetropy	Bilateral acute glaucoma, mydriasis	Acetazolamide, pilocarpine	Vision normalized after treatment	James & Price (1984)
Ornade DM	15 mg PPA + chlorpheniramine + dextromethorphan	5 ml 3–4 times per day (double the recommended dose)	4	F	None	Visual hallucinations, restlessness, agitation, sleep disturbances	Sponge baths for fever; antibiotics for urinary tract infection	Resolved after 3 days	Dungal & Griffiths (1984)
NS	25 mg PPA + chlorpheniramine + acetaminophen	2 tablets	23	F	None	Severe headache, erratic behavior, hemiparesis, cerebral hemorrhage	NS	Pronounced improvement; recovery from hemorrhage	McDowell & LeBlanc (1985)
Contac	50 mg PPA + chlorpheniramine + belladonna alkaloids	1 capsule	24	F	None	Headache, blurred vision, nausea, chest pain	Nitroprusside	Blood pressure stabilized after 48 hr; follow-up study revealed unrecognized autonomic dysfunction	Pentel et al. (1982) Pentel & Mikell (1982)
Contac 500	50 mg PPA + belladonna alkaloids	2 capsules	23	M	None	Weakness, nausea, pounding sensation in chest	None	Symptoms subsided within a few hours	Teh (1979)
Ornade	50 mg PPA + chlorpheniramine + isopropamide	As recommended	68	F	None	Acute psychotic syndrome: delusions, hallucinations, confusion, disorientation, delirium	Chlorpromazine	Recovery	Kane & Green (1966)
Ornade	50 mg PPA + chlorpheniramine + isopropamide	3 spansules	21	M	NS	Abdominal pain, nausea, headache, increased BP	Phenobarbital, codeine, phentolamine, chlorpromazine	Recovery in 2 hr	Duvernoy (1969)

Product	Formulation	Dose	Age	Sex	Prior condition	Acute schizophrenia / adverse reaction	Treatment	Outcome	Reference
Ornade	50 mg PPA + isopropamide + chlorpheniramine	1 spansule a day for 2 days + 2 a day the third day	36	F	None	None	Chlorpromazine	Asymptomatic within 11 days	Kane & Green (1966)
Ornade	50 mg PPA + isopropamide + chlorpheniramine	4 spansules	20	M	None	Increased BP, agitation	Reserpine	Blood pressure returned to normal after 18 hr	Ostern & Dodson (1965)
Lunerin	PPA + brompheniramine	NS	4	F	NS	Hallucinations, grand mal seizures	NS	NS	Norvenius et al. (1979)
Decongestant	50 mg PPA + antihistamine	Unknown	35	M	None	Paranoid schizophrenia	Chlorpromazine, Cogentin	Recovery	Kane & Green (1966)
Propadrine	PPA	As recommended	35	M	None	None		(Symptomatic relief of sinusitis while hospitalized; no adverse reaction?)	
Decongestant	"Proprietary"	Two bottles in one week	35	M	None	Recurrence of paranoid schizophrenia	Chlorpromazine, trihexyphenidyl Avoidance of PPA	Recovery	Speer et al. (1978)
Triaminic Contac Listerine Cold Tablets Dimetapp	(All contain PPA)	NS	24	F	Hayfever, asthma	Dyspnea, wheezing, coughing, hives, facial swelling		No reaction in 7 years	
Triaminic Sineoff Sinutab	(All contain PPA)	One dose each (separate occasions)	48	F	Hives	Urticaria, purpuritis, wheezing, chest tightness, fatigue	NS	NS	Speer et al. (1978)
C. Appetite suppressants: PPA alone									
NS	50 mg PPA	Single tablet	17	F	None	Agitation, dizziness, tachypnea, increased HR	None	Effects subsided in 2–4 hr	Dietz (1981)
NS	50 mg PPA	2 tablets	45	F	Chronic depression; treatment with phenylzine	Headache, coma, increased BP, apnea, cerebral hemorrhage	NS	Death	McDowell & LeBlanc (1985)

TABLE 4.12. Continued.

Product	Form/Contents	Dose	Age	Sex	Preexisting Conditions	Adverse Effects	Treatment	Clinical Outcome	Reference
Trim-Tabs	60 mg PPA	1 tablet	22	F	None	Headache, nausea, increased BP	NS	NS	McEwen (1983)
Dexatrim	65 mg PPA [sic]	1–2 capsules daily for 3 years; 3–4 capsules daily for 2 months	45	F	None	Abdominal pain, bloody diarrhea, fever, dehydration, ischemic bowel infarction	Surgical resection of bowel	No recurrence for 1 year	Johnson et al. (1985)
NS	75 mg PPA	Single tablet	20	F	None	Anxiety, agitation, dizziness, tachypnea, increased HR	None	Effects subsided in 2–4 hr	Dietz (1981)
NS	75 mg PPA	Single tablet	22	F	None	Agitation, dizziness, tachypnea, increased HR	None	Effects subsided in 2–4 hr	Dietz (1981)
NS	75 mg PPA	Single tablet	24	F	Previous history of reaction to PPA	Anxiety, agitation, dizziness, tachypnea, increased HR	None	Effects subsided in 2–4 hr	Dietz (1981)
Diadax	75 mg PPA + grapefruit extract + vitamins C, E	As recommended	44	F	History of convulsion after taking "cold medication" as a child	Headache; blurred vision; cold, clammy sweats; grand mal seizures	Diazepam, phenytoin	No seizures after 4 hr	Deocampo (1979)
Control	75 mg PPA	NS	52	F	Psychiatric disorder	Violent behavior; irritable mood	NS	NS	Achor & Extein (1981)

Product	Dose	Dosage	Age	Sex	History	Symptoms	Treatment	Outcome	Reference
Dietgard	75 mg PPA	1 capsule a day for 2 days	54	F	Adult-onset diabetes	Headache, confusion, cerebral hemorrhage	Undescribed "conservative treatment"	Death	Elliott & Whyte (1981)
Dexatrim	75 mg PPA	Recommended dosage	20	F	Prior psychiatric treatment, drug abuse	Sleep disturbance, confused thinking, affective disorder, auditory hallucinations	Lithium carbonate Thiothixene	Normalized after 4 weeks of treatment; maintained on lithium	Grigg & Gover (1986)
Acutrim	75 mg PPA	Single daily dose for 1 week	13	F	Obesity	Throbbing headache, numbness, paresthesias, increased BP	None	Asymptomatic	Higgins et al. (1985)
D. Appetite suppressants: Trimolets[c]									
Trimolets	85 mg PPA + ferrous gluconate + various vitamins	1 capsule	21	F	None	Headache, vomiting, increased BP	None	Blood pressure returned to normal a few hours later	Frewin et al. (1978)
Trimolets	85 mg PPA + ferrous gluconate + various vitamins	1 capsule twice daily	17	F	NS	Headache, dizziness, palpitations, increased BP	NS	NS	Horowitz et al. (1979)
		6 capsules on day of admission (Same person)					Bed rest	Blood pressure returned to normal in 48 hr	
Trimolets	85 mg PPA + ferrous gluconate + various vitamins	1 tablet	29	F	NS	Tightness in chest, dyspnea, palpitations, neck pain, high BP, irregular HR	NS	NS	King (1979)
Trimolets	85 mg PPA + ferrous gluconate + various vitamins	2 tablets	37	F	None	Headache, nausea, vomiting, slurred speech, hemiparesis, dysphasia	NS	Asymptomatic after 2 weeks	King (1979)
Trimolets	85 mg PPA	1 capsule	32	F	None	Severe headache, decreased HR, increased BP, profuse sweating	Pentazocine	Recovery	McEwen (1983)

243

TABLE 4.12. Continued.

Product	Form/Contents	Dose	Age	Sex	Preexisting Conditions	Adverse Effects	Treatment	Clinical Outcome	Reference
Trimolets	85 mg PPA	1 capsule	28	F	None	Severe headache, increased BP	None	Recovery	McEwen (1983)
Trimolets	85 mg PPA	1 capsule	38	F	None	Increased BP	None	NS	McEwen (1983)
Trimolets	85 mg PPA	2 capsules	41	F	None	Severe headache, increased BP, delerium	None	Recovery	McEwen (1983)
Trimolets	85 mg PPA	2 capsules	19	F	None	Increased BP, headache, paresthesias, vomiting	None	Recovery	McEwen (1983)
Trimolets	85 mg PPA	2 capsules	34	F	None	Severe headache, dizziness, chest pain	NS	NS	McEwen (1983)
Trimolets	50 mg PPA[d]	1 capsule per day for 8 days	49	F	Hay fever	Increased BP, headache, paresthesias, vertigo	Bendrofluazide	Recovery	McEwen (1983)
E. Appetite suppressants: PPA + caffeine									
Diet pills (brand not stated)	25 mg PPA + caffeine + methylcellulose + assorted vitamins	3 tablets per day for 5 weeks	15	F	Obesity	Increased BP, cardiac arrhythmia	Atropine, lidocaine, reserpine	Asymptomatic after 20 hr	Peterson & Vasquez (1973)
Dexatrim	50 mg PPA + caffeine	NS	19	M	Psychiatric disorder	Hyperactivity, irritability	NS	NS	Achor & Extein (1981)
NS	50 mg PPA + caffeine	Single tablet	45	F	NS	Agitation, hallucinations, tachypnea, increased HR, acute psychosis	Hospitalization	Resolved over several days	Dietz (1981)

Product	Dose	Usage	Age	Sex	History	Symptoms	Treatment	Outcome	Reference
NS	50 mg PPA + caffeine	Single tablet	45	F	None	Agitation, hallucinations, tachypnea, increased HR	None	Effects subsided in 2–4 hr	Dietz (1981)
Diet pills	50 mg PPA + caffeine	1 pill + 2 glasses of wine	13	F	NS	Headache, vomiting, grand mal seizure, increased BP, increased HR	Diazepam, phenytoin, dexamethasone, phenobarbital	Improved over 2 days	Bale et al. (1984)
Dexatrim	50 mg PPA + caffeine	1 tablet daily for 1 month; 2 tablets daily for 5 months	20	F	Obesity	Headache, increased BP, mild hemiparesis, nystagmus, cerebral hemorrhage, cerebral vasculitis	Furosemide Diazoxide	Recovery	Fallis & Fisher (1985)
Dexatrim	50 mg PPA + caffeine	Intermittent use for 2–3 months; 1 capsule with coffee and aspirin	48	F	Controlled hypertension; mitral valve prolapse	Loss of vision in one eye, central retinal vein occlusion	NS	Recovery in 3 months	Gilmer et al. (1986)
Dexatrim	50 mg PPA + caffeine	Single capsule	45	F	None	Severe headache, nausea, vomiting	NS	Partial resolution in 10 days	Kikta et al. (1985)
Dexatrim Prolamine	50 mg PPA + caffeine 37.5 mg PPA + caffeine	2 Dexatrim one day alternating with two Prolamine the next day for 3 weeks	23	M	Family history of hypertension	Jitteriness, excessive sweating, nausea	NS	Recovery	Mueller et al. (1985)
Dexatrim	NS	1 capsule	36	F	NS	Irritability, restlessness, sleeplessness	NS	Recovery	Mueller et al. (1985)
Dexatrim Extra Strength	75 mg PPA + caffeine	NS	32	F	Psychiatric disorder	Uncontrollable behavior, delusional thinking	NS	NS	Achor & Extein (1981)
NS	75 mg PPA + caffeine	Single tablet	27	F	None	Agitation, anxiety, hallucinations, dizziness, tachypnea, increased HR	None	Effects subsided in 2–4 hr	Dietz (1981)

245

TABLE 4.12. Continued.

Product	Form/Contents	Dose	Age	Sex	Preexisting Conditions	Adverse Effects	Treatment	Clinical Outcome	Reference
Thera-Trim	75 mg PPA + caffeine	2 pills	56	F	None	Severe headache, vomiting, hemiparesis, increased BP, cerebral hemorrhage (bilateral)	NS	Recovery in 3 months	Kikta et al. (1985)
Dexatrim Extra Strength	75 mg PPA + caffeine	1 tablet daily for 5 days	36	F	None	Acute memory loss, nominal aphasia	None	Recovery in 36 hours	Puar (1984)
Diet pills (brand not stated)	75 mg PPA + 200 mg caffeine	Unspecified amount	43	F	Hypertension	Palpitations, shortness of breath, inability to stand, tachycardia	Clonidine	Asymptomatic after a few days	Clark & Simon (1983)
Fullstop diet pills	Formula not stated	Unspecified amount in 3 weeks	28	F	None	Acute renal failure (multisystem toxic reaction)	Ampicillin	NS	Swenson et al. (1982)

F. Street Drugs

Product	Form/Contents	Dose	Age	Sex	Preexisting Conditions	Adverse Effects	Treatment	Clinical Outcome	Reference
"Pick-me-up" pill	PPA + caffeine + pseudoephedrine (doses not specified)	1 pill	17	F	2 weeks postpartum	Headache, seizures	Phenobarbital	Discharged a few days later	Mueller & Solow (1982)
"Black beauty"	PPA + pseudo-ephedrine + caffeine + barbiturate	Single pill	23	F	None	Headache, nausea, vomiting, aphasia, hemiparesis, increased BP, hemianopsia, cerebral hemorrhage	"Managed conservatively"	Modest improvement	Stoessl et al. (1985)
"Amphetamine look-alike"	PPA + ephedrine + caffeine	2 capsules	20	F	None	Severe headache, nausea, hemiparesis, aphasia, hemianopsia, cerebral hemorrhage	"Managed conservatively"	Slow and incomplete recovery	Stoessl et al. (1985)

G. Formulation Unknown

NS	NS	NS	16	F	None	Initial hospitalization: headache, diaphoresis, abdominal pain, nervousness, fatigue, grand mal seizure, increased BP	Hydralazine	Normotensive	Hyams et al. (1985)
						Second day: increased BP, generalized seizure, apneic, cardiac arrest	Phenytoin		
						Next 3 months: episodic hypertension, tremulousness, agitation, apnea, cardiac arrest, (PPA identified in serum and urine)	Carbamazepine Phentolamine	Recovery; no further hypertensive episodes	

[a] This table contains reports of adverse reactions occurring at recommended doses of phenylpropanolamine-containing products. In a few instances, reports of reactions to multiple doses (usually two doses) are included for comparison. Abbreviations: BP, blood pressure; HR, heart rate.

[b] NS—not specified; BP—blood pressure; HR—heart rate; F—female; M—male.

[c] Trimolets was reported to contain "D-Phenylpropanolamine" (SIC).

[d] The formulation of Trimolets was changed from 85 mg to 50 mg phenylpropanolamine.

247

for "congestion" (Bernstein & Diskant, 1982). (Each tablet contained 325 mg of acetaminophen, 12.5 mg of phenylpropanolamine hydrochloride, 1 mg of chlorpheniramine maleate, and 10 mg of dextromethorphan hydrobromide.) Initial examination revealed blood pressure, 210/130 mm Hg; pulse rate, 120/min; respiration rate, 24/min; and temperature, 37°C. She was oriented but tremulous, anxious, and restless. Hydralazine 10 mg was administered IM. En route to a local hospital the patient had a grand mal seizure. On arrival the patient was disoriented and lethargic and shortly thereafter had a second grand mal seizure. After diazepam 10 mg was administered IV, seizure activity ceased. Her blood pressure was 148/98 mm Hg, pulse rate 134/min, respiratory rate 24/min, and temperature 37.1°C. Her electrocardiogram showed sinus tachycardia at a rate of 120/min. Four hours after admission her blood pressure was 118/80 mm Hg. The day following admission, the electroencephalogram was abnormal, with a basic dysrhythmia of sagittal origin. An electrocardiogram 48 hours after admission was within normal limits. The patient required no further medication and was discharged from the hospital free of neurological deficit.

CASE 2.   A paranoid psychosis resulting from use of a nasal decongestant, Anahist by a 37-year-old general duties officer in the British Royal Air Force has been reported (Wharton, 1970). The subject ingested 30 tablets in 8 days for treatment of nasal stuffiness. Each tablet of Anahist contains 6.25 mg of thorsylamine hydrochloride; 6.25 mg of phenyltoxamine citrate; 12.5 mg of phenylpropanolamine hydrochloride; 97.2 mg of phenacetin; and unspecified amounts of caffeine, aspirin, and ascorbic acid. The wife of the subject noted that he showed increased physical activity and garrulousness. He became bewildered, anxious, and increasingly paranoid, believing that he was excluded from some kind of plot to overthrow the government. After some embarrassing scenes he was admitted to a mental hospital in an apprehensive and excited state. He was treated with 100 mg of chlorpromazine t.i.d. and within 2 days was free of his paranoid convictions. A second, less florid paranoid outburst occurred 8 weeks later, possibly as a result of justified fear for his future. With further treatment this paranoid episode disappeared. Six months after first taking Anahist, he had good insight and no evidence of paranoid attitudes. The author attributed this episode to phenylpropanolamine as a "potential psychotomimetic drug" despite the presence of antihistamines, analgesics, and caffeine.

CASE 3.   A 23-year-old male took two Contac 500 capsules for a head cold (Teh, 1979). Each Contac 500 capsule contains 50 mg of phenylpropanolamine and 0.2 mg of belladonna alkaloids. Three hours later the subject felt faint, had generalized weakness, some nausea, a pounding sensation in the chest, and a gradually increasing frontal headache. He had a supine blood pressure of 160/110 mm Hg and a pulse rate of 54/min. His symptoms subsided over the next few hours without treatment. Within 3 hr his blood pressure was 130/80 mm Hg, and by the next morning his pulse rate was 80/min.

CASE 4. A few hours after taking three Ornade spansules, a 21-year-old black military corpsman had a sudden onset of diffuse abdominal pain, nausea, and a throbbing right-sided headache (Duvernoy, 1969). Ornade contains chlorpheniramine maleate, 8 mg; phenylpropanolamine hydrochloride, 50 mg; and isopropamide iodide, 2.5 mg. The patient's blood pressure was 240/120 mm Hg. After 330 mg of phenobarbital and 32 mg of codeine were administered, his blood pressure decreased to 170/120 mm Hg. On admission to the hospital, the patient was in acute distress, complaining of a throbbing right-sided headache; his blood pressure was 180/130 mm Hg and fundoscopic examination revealed arteriolar spasm.

After IV administration of 5 mg of phentolamine the blood pressure was 120/60 mm Hg at 30 sec, 112/65 at 3 min, 134/90 at 5 min, and 170/116 at 10 min; the headache subsided. Chlorpromazine, 50 mg IM, was given for sedation. Two hours later the blood pressure was 120/85 mm Hg and remained within normal range.

These case reports demonstrate that a wide range of both cardiovascular and CNS effects has been attributed to phenylpropanolamine or phenylpropanolamine-containing products. They also demonstrate that the effects were not dose related. These and other reports indicate that phenylpropanolamine-containing products frequently are associated with effects on vision. Effects of phenylpropanolamine-containing products were especially pronounced in a 37-year-old woman in England who was hypermetropic and had episodes of blurred vision and headache for 9 months (James & Price, 1984). After she took six Vicks Cold-Care capsules (each containing 12.5 mg of phenylpropanolamine) over 18 hr, she awoke the next morning with bilateral acute-angle-closure glaucoma and widely dilated pupils. Vision normalized with acetazolamide and pilocarpine. The author suggests that the timing and the bilaterality point to phenylpropanolamine as the precipitating factor. He also points out that even if sales of products containing phenylpropanolamine were limited to maximum recommended dosages of 75 mg daily, such a restriction would not have prevented this episode.

One report indicated that a phenylpropanolamine-containing decongestant was involved in two separate episodes of paranoid schizophrenia in a man with no previous psychiatric history (Kane & Green, 1966).

CASE 5. A 35-year-old tobacco farmer had an attack of perennial allergic rhinitis for which he took an unknown quantity of an antihistaminic-decongestant combination drug containing 50 mg of phenylpropanolamine. He became restless and then gradually developed a classic paranoid-schizophrenic episode and was hospitalized. His illness was treated with Cogentin (benztropine mesylate) and 1650 mg of chlorpromazine daily for management of behavior and agitation. Unaware of this patient's history of taking "hay fever pills," the physician ordered the administration of Propadrine (phenylpropanolamine hydrochloride) for symptomatic treatment of nasal allergy or sinusitis, apparently without adverse effect. He was discharged on a regimen of 300 mg of chlorpromazine daily. One month later he was virtually normal after a week off all medication. In the autumn he again developed upper respiratory allergic symptoms and took two bottles of an unnamed nasal decongestant. He again became restless, followed by a repetition of the acute paranoid-schizophrenic behavior, which necessitated his readmission to the hospital. It was then that the use of the medication for hay fever was revealed. His neurological symptoms were managed with Artane (trihexyphenidyl hydrochloride) and chlorpromazine, and the nasal congestion was treated with nose drops alone. He improved steadily and was discharged virtually asymptomatic on a regimen of 600 mg of chlorpromazine daily.

Although the author did not comment specifically, it appears that the subject did not have an adverse reaction to Propadrine, which contains phenylpropanolamine alone. If so, it is questionable that phenylpropanolamine was the causative factor in these episodes of acute schizophrenia. Other components of the decongestants, not specified in the article, may have been the cause of the CNS adverse reaction.

Establishment of a particular drug as the source of an atopic reaction is often very difficult. Skin tests and other objective methods of diagnosis can be applied to only a few drugs, and challenging a patient with a suspected agent may be dangerous. Therefore, etiologic diagnosis usually must depend on the clinical history. Two cases of suspected allergic response to phenylpropanolamine have been reported (Speer et al., 1978).

CASE 6. A female was first seen by an allergist when she was 17 years old because of hay fever and asthma. She was found to be sensitive to molds, house dust, ragaweeds, grasses, and chocolate. An unusual feature was her violent reaction to four different medications: Triaminic Tablets, Contac, Listerine Cold Tablets, and Dimetapp, all with the one common ingredient of phenylpropanolamine. Exposure to these medications was followed by dyspnea, wheezing, coughing, hives, and facial swelling. By carefully avoiding phenylpropanolamine, she had no similar reactions for the next 7 years.

CASE 7. A 48-year-old female was seen by an allergist because of hives. The lesions were urticarial with purpuric involvement, limited to the lower extremities, particularly the inner aspects of the thighs. She related having a similar reaction on two previous occasions, both starting about 10 days after beginning a course of Triaminic tablets. She had also developed chest tightness, wheezing, and marked fatigue after taking Sineoff, Sinutab, and Sinutab II. In each instance the reaction was so marked that she took only one dose.

Phenylpropanolamine was included in the eight preparations to which these two subjects (Cases 6 and 7) reacted. Neither subject knew the constituents of these preparations or was aware that they contained phenylpropanolamine, and neither had known reactions to other drugs.

Spasmodic torticollis was reported as an adverse drug reaction in a single case (Lewith & Davidson, 1981) (see Table 4.12).

CASE 8.   An 8-year-old girl had been treated for 6 years for mild recurrent bronchospasm, for which she had received Salbutamol (albuterol) and antibiotics intermittently. She developed a cough at night for which Dimetapp elixir, 5 ml at night, was prescribed. Dimetapp elixir contains 5 mg of phenylpropanolamine hydrochloride, 4 mg of brompheniramine maleate, and 5 mg of phenylephrine hydrochloride per 5 ml. The Dimetapp was only partially effective in suppressing the cough and thus was increased to 10 mg per night. Immediately thereafter she began to have increasingly severe episodes of spasmodic torticollis and finally an oculogyric crisis. The day before she had been given one dose of 1.5 mg of haloperidol. Both drugs were withdrawn and the child had no further dystonic reactions. The author stated that a variety of dystonic reactions to antihistamines have been reported to the Committee of Safety of Medicines in Great Britain. It would appear that this dystonic reaction is attributable to the antihistamine brompheniramine. The safety and effectiveness of Dimetapp when used by adults is well established and attested to by the author who stated, "Dimetapp is a commonly used drug and was prescribed, or continued, at 761 consultations in our practice of 8000 patients over the last year (University of Southampton, 1980)." This particular adverse effect was not reported in any of the other 70 adverse reaction cases.

In one case a child developed acute drug-induced esophagitis after taking one cough/cold tablet without drinking fluids.

CASE 9.   A 10-year-old boy was given a single Rinasal tablet (250 mg acetaminophen, 25 mg norephedrine, 100 mg thiazinium methylsulfate) without fluids before going to bed (Rives et al., 1985). The next morning he awoke with severe pain in the throat. Fibroscopic examination 22 hr after the drug ingestion showed very serious esophagitis with necrotic mucosa and hemorrhagic ulcer. A repeat fibroscopic examination 3 days later showed clear improvement of the esophagitis.

ADVERSE DRUG REACTIONS: APPETITE SUPPRESSANTS

APPETITE SUPPRESSANTS CONTAINING PHENYLPROPANOLAMINE ALONE

Twelve cases of adverse drug reactions to appetite suppressants that contain phenylpropanolamine alone were reported (see Table 4.12). The dosages of phenylpropanolamine ranged from 50 to 75 mg. Both cardiovascular and CNS effects were cited.

One individual had grand mal seizures after taking Diadax at the recommended dosage, but she also had experienced a convulsion after taking "cold medication" as a child (Deocampo, 1979).

CASE 10.   A 44-year-old moderately obese housewife took one Diadax capsule for her obesity. One hour later she entered a hospital emergency room because of sudden onset of severe headache, blurred vision followed by transient loss of vision, and "cold, clammy sweats." Shortly thereafter she had a grand mal seizure. Her blood pressure was 180/90 mm Hg, she had mild right-gaze palsy, and deep tendon reflexes were exaggerated bilaterally without any Babinski toe reflex. All other physical signs, clinical laboratory tests, chest and skull x-rays, and electrocardiogram were normal. The patient had three episodes of grand mal seizures in the ensuing 4 hr, each terminated by IV diazepam. On spinal fluid examination the opening pressure was over 260 mm of water with grossly bloody fluid. Bilateral transcervical angiography was normal. Supportive medical measures were utilized together with 100 mg of phenytoin IV q. 6h. A brain scan, computerized tomography (CT) of the brain, and electroencephalogram were all normal. This patient had no additional seizures and was discharged from the hospital on the seventh day. The patient verified ingestion of Diadax. It was also substantiated that she had a convulsive seizure when 5 years old after taking a "cold medication."

In a retrospective study based on hospital emergency room records, seven cases of "amphetaminelike reactions to phenylpropanolamine" occurred in a 6-month period (Dietz, 1981). All were women 17–45 years of age, and all had side effects that appeared within 1–2 hr after ingestion of a single tablet. The tablets were anorectic agents containing 50 or 75 mg of phenylpropanolamine with or without caffeine. Each of these subjects had hyperventilation and tachypnea. Respiratory rates ranged from 20 to 34 (mean 26.6) per minute and pulse rates, from 95 to 120 (mean 106) per minute. Other common side effects were dizziness, tremor, agitation, anxiety, and nausea. With the exception of one patient, side effects subsided in 2–4 hr without treatment, and all the subjects were discharged from the hospital without sequelae. One patient had an acute psychosis with severe hallucinations that resolved over several days. Another patient had had a similar episode 1 year earlier after ingesting a similar agent. No blood or urine samples were analyzed for the presence of phenylpropanolamine; thus the ingestion of phenylpropanolamine-containing products could not be verified (Morgan, 1984).

One individual with a history of psychiatric disorders experienced violent behavior and irritable moods after ingesting an unspecified amount of Control tablets containing 75 mg of phenylpropanolamine (Achor & Extein, 1981).

One death associated with ingestion of phenylpropanolamine-containing diet pills was reported (Elliott & Whyte, 1981). This was a woman with adult-onset diabetes but no history of hypertension. After taking phenylpropanol-amine-containing diet pills for 2 days, she experienced headache, vomiting, and confusion, rapidly progressing to coma. On admission to the hospital she showed elevated blood pressure (160/100 mm Hg), coma, and quadriparesis. A CT scan revealed a left occipital hematoma. She was "treated conservatively" (the details were not reported) but died on the following day.

One woman developed ischemic bowel infarction following long-term use of phenylpropanolamine-containing appetite suppressants (Johnson et al., 1985). This woman had been taking Dexatrim [65 mg phenylpropanolamine (sic)] for 3 years; initially she took one or two capsules/day but for approximately 2 months before hospitalization she had been taking 3 or 4 capsules/day. Thus, this may be a case of misuse of phenylpropanolamine rather than a true adverse reaction because the woman had been taking phenylpropanolamine longer than recommended and at higher than recommended doses.

CASE 11.   This 45 year-old woman had a history of abdominal cramps and blood diarrhea for 24 hr. The initial physical examination showed that she had fever, was dehydrated, had hypoactive bowel sounds, abdominal tenderness, and bloody stools. During 12 hr after admission the patient became hemodynamically unstable and developed peritonitis. An exploratory laparotomy revealed an ischemic proximal colon with necrosis of the midtransverse colon. There was no evidence of arterial or venous obstruction. The colon was repaired surgically. The patient recovered, was advised to avoid using appetite suppressants, and had no recurrence of abdominal complaints during a 1-year followup.

APPETITE SUPPRESSANTS: TRIMOLETS

In 1979 three articles were published reporting four cases of adverse drug reactions to the Australian drug Trimolets (Frewin et al., 1978; Horowitz et al., 1979; King, 1979) (see Table 4.12). One additional article reported seven adverse reactions to Trimolets (McEwen, 1983). Furthermore, two clinical trials of the safety of the Trimolets preparation were reported (Horowitz et al., 1979, 1980). These reports collectively are frequently cited as evidence that phenylpropanolamine can produce cardiovascular side effects, including hypertensive crisis. However, several factors limit the interpretation of these studies. Trimolets was an immediate-release formulation which, according to the packaging information, contained 85 mg of "D-phenylpropanolamine," 15 mg of ferrous gluconate, and various vitamins including 15 mg of nicotinamine. This dose is higher than the recommended dose of phenylpropanolamine for immediate-release formulations. Of primary importance, however, is the fact that in some formulations of Trimolets the active ingredient was D-phenylpropanolamine. It is well established that the D form is considerably more toxic in animals than the L form (Table 4.5)—thus one would expect it to elicit more responses in humans. In the United States only the racemic form is used. Use of the *D* form of phenylpropanolamine may well explain why more side effects attributed to phenylpropanolamine have been reported from Australia than elsewhere. Also, the symptoms of headache, nausea, lassitude, tingling feelings in the head, headache, dizziness, rash, tinnitus, and a "hot feeling" may have been caused by ingredients other than phenylpropanolamine.

The four case histories of adverse drug reactions to Trimolets are summarized below.

CASE 12.   Thirty minutes after taking a Trimolets tablet, a 29-year-old Cuban woman complained of tightness in the chest, dyspnea, palpitations, and neck pain. She had "high blood pressure and irregular heart beat." No results of any measurements were provided. The next day her blood pressure was 130/90 mm Hg (King, 1979).

CASE 13.   A 37-year-old woman took two Trimolets before going to bed (King, 1979). She awoke during the night with a mild bilateral occipital headache, chest pain, fever, and sweating. As the headache became more severe, she felt nauseated and vomited. Half an hour later she developed weakness of the right arm and leg, facial weakness, and slurred speech. The following morning her speech was still slurred and she had right hemiparesis. When examined 36 hr after ingestion of the tablets, she had a mild dysphasia with right hemiparesis; her blood pressure was 120/80 mm Hg. A CT scan showed several small hemorrhages in the region of the left internal capsule; apart from a slight mass effect, the left carotid angiogram was normal. After 2 weeks the patient's blood pressure remained normal and her signs had essentially resolved.

CASE 14.   A 21-year-old female student nurse had a severe headache that started about 1½ hr after ingestion of a Trimolets tablet (Frewin et al., 1978). The headache was throbbing and generalized and the patient vomited four or five times. On a recent physical examination her blood pressure had been 90–110/50 mm Hg, although she had a family history of hypertension. At this time her blood pressure was 190/120 mm Hg, but she had no visual disturbances, vertigo, or other neurological symptoms. When she was hospitalized (4½ hr after onset of the headache) her blood pressure was 140/100 mm Hg and her pulse rate was 56/min. The electrocardiogram showed a sinus bradycardia, but all other physical and laboratory determinations were within normal limits. No therapy was administered. Within 5½ hr of the onset of the headache, the patient had a blood pressure of 120/70 mm Hg standing and 110/60 mm Hg lying down; the headache abated more slowly. She was carefully monitored for 3 days and her blood pressure stabilized at 95–120/60–70 mm Hg. This patient had previously had an idiosyncratic reaction or side effects to oral contraceptive agents.

CASE 15.   A 17-year-old girl had taken Trimolets capsules b.i.d. for 3 weeks with some episodes of dizziness and palpitations (Horowitz et al., 1979). She then took six Trimolets (total dose 510 mg, in an immediate-release formulation) and 3 hr later had a bifrontal headache and some nausea; her blood pressure was 200/130 mm Hg. When admitted to the hospital she had a supine blood pressure of 150/95 mm Hg and pulse rate of 62/min; her standing blood pressure and pulse rates were 95/60 mm Hg and 98/min, respectively. On physical examination, no other abnormalities were found; electroencephalogram, serum electrolyte, serum glucose, and 24-hour urinary catecholamines were within normal limits.

When the patient was rechallenged with Trimolets (85 mg) 3 weeks later there was no change of pulse rate, but there was a rise of blood pressure to a maximum of 175/120 mm Hg, supine, 90 min after ingestion of the drug; on standing, the mean blood pressure dropped to 38 mm Hg. Ephedrine (30 mg) induced a less marked hypertensive response with little postural hypotension and an increase of pulse rate of up to 15 bpm.

The hypertensive and postural hypotensive responses of this patient appear to be evidence of drug overdose, evidenced by the fact that she took six Trimolets capsules, each containing 85 mg of phenylpropanolamine, or a total dose of 510 mg, which is 10.2 times the maximum dose recommended by U.S. manufacturers. Because of the evidence of increased blood pressure on rechallenge with phenylpropanolamine (85 mg) and a less marked hypertensive response and an increased pulse rate following rechallenge with ephedrine (30 mg), it is probable that this patient had an idiosyncratic response. The author's theory that such a hypertensive response was mediated by increased catecholamines is unsupported by three 24-hr urinary catecholamine determinations on this patient that were within normal limits.

In addition to these case reports, two clinical trials of the Trimolets preparation were reported. The first study was a double-blind crossover study, in which six normotensive medical students (four male, two female) 22–24 years of age and weighing 59–79 kg each received one Trimolets capsule (containing 85 mg of phenylpropanolamine) and one matching placebo capsule on different days (Horowitz et al., 1979). Blood pressure and heart rate were measured at half-hourly, then hourly, intervals for 6 hr. Results were analyzed by the Student's t-test.

In all six volunteers, there was a significant rise of both systolic and diastolic blood pressure after ingestion of the Trimolets capsule, which persisted through the 6 hours of the study. The peak mean supine blood pressure was 151/100 mm Hg 3 hr after drug ingestion; two subjects had diastolic pressures higher than 110 mm Hg. There was a less marked but statistically significant rise in blood pressure when the subjects were standing. Two hours after drug ingestion, supine pulse rate fell from 71 $\pm$ 4.6 to 55.2 $\pm$ 3.2/min. Five of the six subjects complained of malaise, headache, or tightness in the chest.

In the second clinical trial, a group of medical students 21–28 years old and in apparent good health participated in a double-blind study in which they ingested either Trimolets, Contac 500, or matching placebos (Horowitz et al., 1980). In one phase of the study, 37 subjects took Trimolets, and 35 subjects took placebo. During the control period, mean supine diastolic blood pressure was 70 ± 1.4 mm Hg for the Trimolets group and 74 ± 1.4 mm Hg for the placebo group. After ingestion of either a Trimolets or a matching placebo, supine and erect blood pressure and pulse rate were determined every $1/2$ hr for 3 hr. Blood pressure reached a peak at $1^{1}/_2$–3 hr; mean peak diastolic pressure was 94 ± 2.6 mm Hg for the Trimolets group and 77 ± 1.6 mm Hg for the placebo group. Symptoms reported by subjects who took Trimolets were: tingling feeling in head, six; dizziness (not postural), five; dizziness (postural), four; palpitations, five; headache, six; chest tightness, three; rash, three; tremor, two; nausea, two; lassitude, one; and tinnitus, one; no symptoms were reported by seventeen subjects.

In the other phase of this study, 34 subjects took Contac 500, and 35 took a matching placebo. Control period mean supine diastolic pressure was 78 ± 1.9 mm Hg for the drug group and 77 ± 2.2 mm Hg for the placebo group. After drug ingestion, mean peak supine diastolic pressure was 83 ± 1.5 mm Hg and after placebo, 77 ± 1.4 mm Hg. Four subjects taking Contac had supine diastolic pressure of 100 mm Hg or more, and one subject had a maximum supine blood pressure of 145/110 mm Hg. No subjects taking the active drug or placebo reported any symptoms.

This study has frequently been referred to in the literature as evidence of an increase of blood pressure in 141 medical students following ingestion of phenylpropanolamine. In fact, 37 subjects took Trimolets (fewer than half of these had blood pressure increases greater than those in the placebo group), and 35 subjects took a matching placebo; 34 subjects took Contac 500 (with a mean supine blood pressure increase of 3–4 mm Hg), and 35 subjects ingested a matching placebo. Thus blood pressure was measured following phenylpropanolamine ingestion in 71 subjects and following placebo ingestion in 70 subjects.

APPETITE SUPPRESSANTS CONTAINING PHENYLPROPANOLAMINE AND CAFFEINE

Nineteen cases of adverse drug reactions to appetite suppressants containing phenylpropanolamine and caffeine have been reported (Table 4.12). The effects reported include both cardiovascular and CNS effects similar to the effects just described for decongestant products and appetite suppressants containing phenylpropanolamine alone. In addition, it must be remembered that caffeine also has cardiovascular and CNS stimulant effects that undoubtedly contribute to the adverse reactions to these combination products.

CASE 16.   A 43-year-old black woman was hospitalized following two episodes of palpitations associated with shortness of breath, tinnitus, dizziness, diaphoresis, and inability to stand. The patient reportedly had ingested diet capsules containing 75 mg of phenylpropanolamine and 200 mg of caffeine, but neither the brand nor the number of capsules ingested was reported (Clark & Simon, 1983) (see Table 4.12). The patient had a history of hypertension controlled without medication. On admission her blood pressure was 180/120 mm Hg. Within 2 hr after 50 mg of hydrochlorothiazide and 0.1 mg of clonidine PO, her blood pressure decreased to 140/110 mm Hg. The optic fundi showed some arteriolar narrowing, serum lactic dehydrogenase was 262 mU/ml, and the electrocardiogram showed paroxysmal atrial tachycardia. All other physical and clinical laboratory determinations were within normal limits. The patient's blood pressure was 160/110 mm Hg, and her pulse rate 100/min and respiratory rate 20/min. A second dose of clonidine (0.1 mg) was administered. Two days later the electrocardiogram showed normal sinus rhythm and the patient was discharged free of symptoms.

CASE 17.   A 48-year-old woman with controlled systemic hypertension and mitral valve prolapse had been taking Dexatrim (50 mg of phenylpropanolamine and 200 mg of caffeine) for 2–3 months (Gilmer et al., 1986). She experienced a sudden onset of visual loss 6–8 hr after ingestion of one Dexatrim and three 500-mg aspirin tablets along with a cup of coffee. Ophthalmic examination 13 days later showed a nonischemic occlusion of the central retinal vein in the right eye. By 3 months her vision was only 20/100 due to persistent disc and macular edema.

CASE 18.   A 36-year-old obese woman took one Extra Strength Dexatrim (75 mg of phenylpropanolamine and 200 mg of caffeine) daily for 5 days (Puar, 1984). Two hr after the last dose she experienced sudden onset of memory loss, difficulty with speech, and clumsiness. A physical examination showed that she was normotensive, had a heart rate of 80/min, and was afebrile. A neurologic examination showed that she had nominal aphasia, selective memory loss, slightly slurred speech, normal affect and attention, and no hallucinations or paranoia. The patient's symptoms resolved within 36 hr without medical treatment.

STREET DRUGS CONTAINING PHENYLPROPANOLAMINE

In the case of street drugs, the definition of adverse drug reaction is questionable because it is difficult to determine "desired" versus "undesired" effects and to determine the "recommended" dosages. Presuming that a single pill is the recommended dose, and that mild CNS stimulation or relief from fatigue is the desired effect, four case reports could be interpreted as adverse drug reactions (see Table 4.12).

CASE 19.   A 17-year-old woman who was 2 weeks postpartum took a "pick-me-up" pill she believed to be an amphetamine compound (Mueller & Solow, 1982) (see Table 4.10). About a $1/2$ hr later she became tense, developed a severe generalized headache, stiffened, and rocked backward. Then her head and eyes deviated to the left, she choked and bit her lip, and she had tonic-clonic movements of both arms that lasted 4–5 min, followed 10 min later by a similar episode. Later she complained of a severe right temporo-occipital headache. An electroencephalogram showed focal, low-amplitude, irregular theta activity over the right cerebral hemisphere interpreted as compatible with a focal structural lesion. No further seizures occurred, and 2 months later her EEG and CT scan were normal. Analysis of the "pick-me-ups" or "look-alikes" taken by this patient showed they contained a large amount of caffeine and lesser amounts of phenylpropanolamine and pseudoephedrine—although the precise amounts were not indicated.

Several other reports of frank overdoses of phenylpropanolamine-containing street drugs are reviewed in the following section.

ADVERSE DRUG REACTIONS: OTHER REPORTED EFFECTS

RHABDOMYOLYSIS

Rhabdomyolysis has been reported to occur following ingestion of phenylpropanolamine (Bennett, 1979; Swenson et al., 1982) or D-norpseudoephedrine (Rumpf et al., 1983). The details of these four cases are discussed below. First, however, the pathophysiology of rhabdomyolysis is briefly reviewed. Although numerous clinical case reports (Hampel et al., 1983; Koffler et al., 1976; Penn et al., 1972; Perkoff et al., 1967; Richter et al., 1971; Schrier et al., 1967) and experimental studies (Knochel & Carter, 1976; Knochel et al., 1974) have been published, the mechanisms by which muscle damage resulting in myoglobinemia and myoglobinuria can cause rhabdomyolysis and acute renal failure are not clearly defined. It is well established, however, that this entity is associated primarily with severe exercise during heat stress, especially in the obese or those with a large unconditioned muscle mass. Common physical symptoms are muscle stiffness, tenderness, swelling, and weakness, often accompanied by ischemia, anoxia, hypotension, and hypothermia, although fever and anuria are sometimes present. Biochemical abnormalities include a diminished rise in lactic acid in response to ischemic exercise, myoglobinemia and myoglobinuria, and markedly elevated enzyme levels of serum glutamic oxalacetic transaminase, creatine phosphokinase, aldolase, and lactic dehydrogenase. In addition, there is hyperuricemia, hypokalemia, and usually hypocalcemia and hypophosphatemia as well as high serum creatinine relative to the blood urea nitrogen level.

After intense physical exercise in a hot environment, normal subjects have myoglobin in serum and urine with an increase of creatine phosphokinase and creatinuria (Knochel et al., 1974). The myoglobinuria results from necrosis of skeletal muscle with release of intracellular constituents—primarily pigment, enzymes, and potassium—into the bloodstream. It is postulated that the hypercatabolism affects the membrane transport mechanism and cellular energy production, causing both morphological and biochemical changes. With exercise and the increased demand for glycogen, a depletion of potassium—the regulator of glycogen synthesis—occurs. There is an increased demand for ATP and depletion of cellular stores of ATP as well as release of purine precursors into the circulation, resulting in an overproduction of uric acid that appears to be related to the myoglobinemia, myoglobinuria, and rhabdomyolysis. When renal failure occurs, it is usually secondary to exercise and heat stress and the overproduction of uric acid in the presence of an acid urine.

Apart from strenuous exercise during heat stress, the only other known cases of rhabdomyolysis are in chronic alcoholics after a severe drinking bout (Koffler et al., 1976; Perkoff et al., 1967), street drug addicts after using heroin contaminated with quinine (Koffler et al., 1976; Richter et al., 1971), and in prescription drug addicts after taking very large doses of depressant drugs—usually barbiturates (Hampel et al., 1983; Koffler et al., 1976; Penn et al., 1972).

There have been a few unconvincing reports in the literature that attribute rhabdomyolysis to the use of phenylpropanolamine.

One subject, a 28-year-old woman (Bennett, 1979), appears to have had some symptoms and clinical laboratory results indicative of rhabdomyolysis, but the key diagnostic clinical laboratory determinations of creatine phosphokinase, aldolase, and serum and urine concentrations of myoglobin were not done. She had been taking an appetite suppressant (Fullstop) for 3 weeks. There was no evidence of any relationship between the subject's symptoms and biochemical changes and the ingestion of phenylpropanolamine.

Two other alleged cases of rhabdomyolysis associated with ingestion of phenylpropanolamine were reported (Swenson et al., 1982). One, a 28-year-old woman, was said to have symptoms, signs, and laboratory evidence of rhabdomyolysis, but these were not reported (see Table 4.12). In addition, she was diagnosed as having acute interstitial nephritis "which could have been due to drug ingestion (including an antibiotic) or pyelonephritis." The second case was a 21-year-old man with a history of binge drinking who consumed 9 1/2 quarts of malted beverages the previous week together with 30–50 appetite suppressants containing phenylpropanolamine (see Table 4.12). His reported symptoms and clinical laboratory results would seem to indicate some evidence of rhabdomyolysis, possibly attributable to alcoholism, one of the substantiated causes of rhabdomyolysis.

The authors postulated a mechanism of action by which phenylpropanolamine exerts a direct toxic effect on muscle cells or perhaps acts on muscle cells indirectly through sympathomimetic effects that increase muscle cell metabolic demands. There is no evidence to substantiate these hypotheses. The authors state that "proof of a cause-and-effect relationship with phenyl-propanolamine is not definitive."

A 46-year-old male member of an antialcohol society presented biochemical changes and clinical laboratory results suggestive of rhabdomyolysis after taking 20 pills of "Antiadipositum X-112" (Rumpf et al., 1983). These pills each contain 15 mg of cathine hydrochloride (*D*-norpseudoephedrine—an isomer of phenylpropanolamine), 8 mg nikethamide, 10 mg of caffeine, 10 mg of salicylate sodium, and 19 herbal ingredients. In addition, the subject's regular self-medication included 600 mg of carbromal, 30 mg of di-phenhydramine, and 150 mg of secobarbital. Alcohol and drug abuse are known causes of rhabdomyolysis. This subject appears to have been an abuser of alcohol and obviously used a myriad of drugs.

RAYNAUD'S PHENOMENON

A relationship between Raynaud's phenomenon and phenylpropanolamine ingestion has been reported (Caperton, 1983). The author simply stated that he had observed three young women with "significant complications" of Raynaud's phenomenon that promptly disappeared when they discontinued using phenylpropanolamine. One of these women had "suffered a stroke" and had diagnostic evidence (a positive antinuclear antibody test) of lupus erythematosus. Like other peripheral vascular syndromes, the cause of Raynaud's phenomenon is unknown, and one of its primary characteristics is its cyclic, transient, and variable symptoms. There are no other reports in the literature and no evidence to indicate any relationship between phenylpropanolamine and Raynaud's phenomenon.

ADVERSE DRUG REACTIONS: SUMMARY

The experience gained from this review (presented in this chapter) of adverse drug reaction reports involving phenylpropanolamine-containing products indicates that there are some individuals who will display either cardiovascular or CNS effects in response to therapeutic or "recommended" doses. This review does not, however, consider one critical factor in determining the safety or risk of phenylpropanolamine-containing products, specifically an evaluation of the incidence of adverse reactions in proportion to the total consumption of phenylpropanolamine. In this country alone, billions of doses of phenylpropanolamine-containing products are consumed yearly. Nonetheless, the review of adverse reactions does reveal certain general patterns of reactions to phenylpropanolamine.

First, the duration of the adverse effects is generally relatively brief. In most instances, the adverse reactions lasted no more than a few hours, and rarely more than 24–48 hr. In fact, considering the rapid elimination of phenylpropanolamine in both experimental animals and humans, the brief duration of the adverse reactions is not surprising. In the few instances when the adverse reaction was either prolonged or delayed for several days, it must be questioned whether phenylpropanolamine was indeed the causative agent involved.

Second, a wide range of therapeutic maneuvers were used to treat the adverse reactions. In most cases, no therapy was required and the drug effects disappeared spontaneously. The CNS adverse effects were treated with anticonvulsants for seizures and in some cases with phenothiazines for severe behavioral disorders. Antihypertensive medication used to treat cardiovascular effects included clonidine, nitroprusside, reserpine, and phentolamine. It is rather surprising, since the cardiovascular effects of phenylpropanolamine are probably mediated via a mixture of indirect and direct adrenergic activities, that an α-blocker was used in only one case to treat cardiovascular reactions to phenylpropanolamine.

It appears that some individuals are especially sensitive to the adverse effects of phenylpropanolamine. In 13 cases, preexisting conditions were noted (see Table 4.11), although such observations do not necessarily indicate a causative relationship. In two cases, the history revealed that the individual had previously experienced adverse reactions to phenylpropanolamine-containing products (Deocampo, 1979; Dietz, 1981). In one case, a single individual experienced adverse reactions to phenylpropanolamine-containing products on at least two occasions (Kane & Green, 1966). Two cases of drug allergy to phenylpropanolamine were documented (Speer et al., 1978). Several cases suggest that individuals with a history of psychiatric disturbances may be at risk for adverse drug reactions to phenylpropanolamine (Achor & Extein, 1981; Grigg & Goyer, 1986; Kane & Green, 1966).

In several cases, ingestion of a phenylpropanolamine-containing product was temporally associated with a cerebrovascular hemorrhage (Elliott & Whyte, 1981; Fallis & Fisher, 1985; Kikta et al., 1985; McDowell & LeBlanc, 1985; Stoessl et al., 1985), although a temporal correlation does not necessarily indicate a causal relationship.

It is interesting to note that the ratio of adverse drug reactions among females and males was 5:1 (Table 4.11). Although it could indicate a true sex-linked difference in drug response, the observation that males and females were involved in overdose cases in equal proportions argues against this explanation. The sex ratio in adverse drug reactions may simply reflect the fact that more females than males take phenylpropanolamine-containing products; this seems likely to be the case for diet pills since society seems to place more importance on the undesirability of excess body weight for females than for males.

OVERDOSE CASES

In some instances, it is difficult to classify a particular case as either adverse drug reaction or overdose. In the strictest sense, adverse reactions occur at therapeutic or recommended dosages, and thus overdose reactions occur at doses above the recommended levels. There is a gray area, however, between these two categories. Some individuals may experience untoward reactions after taking only slightly higher than recommended dosages. In the previous section, a few of the adverse drug reactions were cases in which individuals had allegedly taken only two or three phenylpropanolamine-containing pills rather than the recommended one pill per dose. In the present section, cases are presented in which individuals took 2 to as many as an estimated 30–50 phenylpropanolamine-containing pills. Although the latter is obviously an extreme overdose case, the former is only marginally "overdose." In actuality, these cases merely represent a spectrum of activity covering a large portion of the phenylpropanolamine dose-response curve. The important point is not to attempt a rigid classification of these cases, but rather to estimate the separation between therapeutic and toxic dose levels and to estimate the probability that a given individual will experience an adverse reaction at a given dose level. On both of these counts, phenylpropanolamine can be rated a "safe" drug: its margin of safety is high, and the incidence of adverse reactions at therapeutic dosages is low.

Twenty-six publications documenting 45 cases of overdose reactions have been published (see Table 4.13). The estimated doses of phenylpropanolamine range from 30 to 3500 mg, but these doses should be interpreted with caution. In almost all overdose cases, with any drug, the documentation of dosage consumed is based on the history. This history is rarely substantiated by witnesses. For obvious reasons, such estimates of dosages consumed are prone to error, since many individuals are unwilling or unable to report accurately the circumstances surrounding the overdose. The most objective and reliable measures of the severity of the overdose are measurement of drug levels in biological fluids (stomach contents, blood, urine, etc.). Such documentation is lacking in most of the phenylpropanolamine overdose cases reported. In fact, the safe and toxic blood levels of phenylpropanolamine have not been defined.

One additional factor must be considered in evaluating these phenylpropanolamine overdose cases. In almost all cases, other drugs in addition to phenylpropanolamine are involved in the overdose, raising the question of drug interactions. Most commercial OTC phenylpropanolamine-containing products are combinations containing one or more drugs in addition to phenylpropanolamine. Illicit phenylpropanolamine-containing drugs likewise are frequently combination products, and in these cases the formulation of the particular product is questionable. Also, drug abuse commonly involves polydrug use, and in several cases phenylpropanolamine-containing products were taken in conjunction with alcohol, marijuana, or other drugs of abuse.

Finally, preexisting factors are involved in several of the overdose cases. In several cases, the individuals had histories of neuropsychiatric disturbances or chronic drug or alcohol abuse. Such preexisting factors must be considered in evaluation of the reactions.

OVERDOSE CASES: DECONGESTANT PREPARATIONS CONTAINING PHENYLPROPANOLAMINE

In all cases, overdoses of phenylpropanolamine-containing decongestants involved combination products (see Table 4.13). These products were either cough syrup (one case) or pills containing antihistamines, anticholinergics, antitussives, sympathomimetics, or other drugs.

The overdose reactions were similar to the adverse drug reactions described above but in some cases more severe. Both cardiovascular and CNS syndromes are described, and there seems to be no particular dose-response relationship. Mild reactions of headache, tachycardia, increased blood pressure, and nonspecific CNS signs were reported at dosages ranging from four to eight pills containing 50 mg of phenylpropanolamine plus other components; cardiovascular effects were reported at high doses also. Severe CNS effects (paranoia, seizures, hallucinations, etc.) were reported at both low and high doses. The following case reports illustrate the range of overdose reactions reported.

CASE 20. A 13-year-old girl deliberately ingested eight capsules, each containing 50 mg of phenylpropanolamine, 8 mg of chlorpheniramine, and 2.5 mg of isopropamide (Pentel et al., 1982). Two hours later she had a headache, her blood pressure was 190/110 mm Hg, and her pulse was 120 bpm. Over the next hour her diastolic blood pressure rose to 150 mm Hg, and then returned to normal within an hour on treatment with IV hydralazine. The subsequent course was uneventful, and she remained asymptomatic and normotensive. Phenylpropanolamine and chlorpheniramine were found on analysis of the urine.

CASE 21. Three and one-half hours after ingesting 15–20 Ornade Spansules, a 17-year-old white male was hospitalized (Rumack et al., 1974). Despite IV therapy and gastric lavage, he had incessant vomiting, marked excitation, and hallucinations; his blood pressure was 230/130 mm Hg, pulse rate 96/min, and temperature 36.9°C. He was transferred to another hospital; on arrival his blood pressure was 280/140 mm Hg, pulse 84/min, and respiration 16/min, and his electrocardiogram showed a bigeminal ventricular ectopic arrhythmia. After 1 mg of physo-

TABLE 4.13. Case Histories of Overdoses to Phenylpropanolamine-Containing Products[a,b]

Product	Form/Contents	Dose	Age	Sex	Preexisting Conditions	Adverse Effects	Treatment	Clinical Outcome	Reference
					A. Decongestant products				
Triaminicol cough syrup	12.5 mg PPA/5 ml + pyrilamine + dextromethorphan + ammonium Cl + pheniramine	12 oz	28	F	Borderline personality disorder; suicidal tendencies	Paranoia, homicidal behavior, seizures	Diazepam	Recovery (a 50-mg challenge dose of PPA produced clinical temporal lobe seizures)	Cornelius et al. (1984)
Vicks Cold-Care	12.5 mg PPA + ?	6 pills in 18 hr	37	F	Hypermetropy	Acute glaucoma, extreme mydriasis	Acetazolamide, pilocarpine	Vision normalized after treatment	James & Price (1984)
Triaminicin	25 mg PPA + chlorpheniramine + aspirin + caffeine	13 capsules	13	F	None	Lightheadedness, increased BP, irregular HR, decreased HR, ECG showed sinus bradycardia and AV block	Ipecac Activated charcoal Magnesium citrate	Recovery	Woo et al. (1985)
Ornade	50 mg PPA + isopropamide + chlorpheniramine	4	20	M	None	Increased BP, agitation	Reserpine	BP returned to normal in 18 hr	Ostern & Dodson (1965)
Not stated	50 mg PPA + chlorpheniramine + isopropamide	8	13	F	None	Headache	Hydralazine	No sequelae	Pentel et al. (1982)
Eskornade	50 mg PPA + isopropamide + diphenylpyraline	8	16	M	None	Tachycardia, increased BP	NS	Recovery	Salmon (1965)
Contac	50 mg PPA + belladonna (SR)	8-9 capsules	15	F	None	Initially: drowsy, increased BP, increased HR, after 30 hr: breathlessness, hemoptysis,	Furosemide Metoprolol Dobutamine Methylprednisolone	Death	Logie & Scott (1984)

Product	Composition	Dose	Age	Sex	History	Clinical effects	Treatment	Outcome	Reference
Ru-Tuss	50 mg PPA + phenylephrine + chlorpheniramine + hyoscyamine + atropine + scopolamine	10–12	19	F	None	Chest pain, labored respiration, cardiopulmonary arrest	"Keflex," meperidine, antibiotics, propranolol, calcium Cl, epinephrine, digoxin, metarminol, lidocaine, dopamine, atropine, Plasminate	Death 5 days after poisoning	Patterson (1980)
Ornade	50 mg PPA + isopropamide + chlorpheniramine	15–20	17	M	None	Increased BP, cardiac arrhythmia, hallucinations	Physostigmine	Disappearance of adverse effects	Rumack et al. (1974)
Ornade	50 mg PPA + isopropamide + chlorpheniramine	15–30	23	F	None	Tachycardia, respiratory distress, high fever	Supportive therapy	Death	Rumack et al. (1974)
Danbade + Drixoral	75 mg PPA + chlorpheniramine; Pseudoephedrine + dexbrompheniramine	40–50 capsules; Up to 20 capsules	24	M	Previous suicide attempt; Type I diabetes mellitus	Vomiting, somnolent, increased BP, decreased HR, sweating. After 24 hr: disorientation, meningismus, intracerebral hematoma	Ipecac, Activated charcoal, Magnesium citrate	Complete recovery	Kizer (1984)
Rinexin + Rinomar	PPA; PPA + brompheniramine	"Large quantities"; "Large quantities"	17	M	NS	Motor excitement, aggressive behavior, psychosis (mania), hallucinations, confusion	NS	NS	Norvenius et al. (1979)
Decontabs	PPA + phenylephrine + chlorpheniramine + phenyltoloxamine	30–40 tablets	24	M	None	Increased BP, decreased HR, ECG showed nearly complete AV block, headache	Ipecac, Activated charcoal, Acetaminophen, Codeine	Recovery	Burton et al. (1985)

TABLE 4.13. Continued.

Product	Form/Contents	Dose	Age	Sex	Preexisting Conditions	Adverse Effects	Treatment	Clinical Outcome	Reference
B. Appetite suppressants: PPA without caffeine									
NS	NS	5 times the recommended dose	25	M	None	Severe headache, increased BP, decreased HR 5 days later: unremitting headache, stiff neck, subarachnoid hemorrhage	None (against medical advice) Bed rest Dexamethasone	Recovery	Mesnard & Ginn (1984)
NS	75 mg PPA	7 pills	16	F	None	Increased BP, decreased HR, ECG showed sinus bradycardia and AV block	Activated charcoal Magnesium citrate	Recovery	Woo et al. (1985)
Trimolets	85 mg PPA + ferrous gluconate + various vitamins	6	17	F	NS	Increased BP	Bed rest	BP returned to normal in 48 hr	Horowitz et al. (1979)
		1 (b.i.d.) (same person)	17	F	NS	Headache, dizziness, palpitations	NS	NS	
C. Appetite suppressants: PPA with caffeine									
Dex-a-diet II	75 mg PPA + caffeine	1 per day for 2 weeks; 2 on day of admission	13	F	None	Headache, nausea, vomiting, seizures	Phenytoin	No sequelae	Howrie & Wolfson (1983)
Dietac	37.5 mg PPA (+ other substances?)	3–8 pills daily for 4 months	34	M	None	Lethargy, right-sided hemiparesis	Heparin therapy; coumarin	Asymptomatic 10 months later	Johnson et al. (1983)
NS	50 mg PPA + caffeine	1 tablet per day for 8 days; then 5 tablets at once	45	M	Recurrent major depression; treated with doxepin and fluphenazine	Confusion, lack of sleep, slurred speech, social withdrawal, catatonia, stereotypy, increased BP, increased HR	Benztropine	Recovery	Castellani (1985)

Product	Composition	Dose	Age	Sex	History	Symptoms	Treatment	Outcome	Reference
NS	50 mg PPA + caffeine	8 pills	18	F	None	Increased BP, decreased HR, generalized convulsion. After 24 hr: deterioration of mental state, loss of brain stem reflexes, cerebral hemorrhage, death	Atropine sulfate Gastric lavage	Death	McDowell & LeBlanc (1985)
Dexatrim	50 mg PPA + caffeine	8-10 pills daily for 3 months	24	M	None	Hemiplegia, decreased motor & sensory functions	NS	Asymptomatic 1 year after incident	Johnson et al. (1983)
Dexatrim + Permathene	50 mg PPA + caffeine 75 mg PPA + caffeine	3-5 pills a day from each for a few days	23	F	No psychiatric history	Psychosis, paranoia	No medication	Recovered after 3 days	Schaffer & Pauli (1980)
Dexatrim (type NS) and "Speckled pups" (look-alike diet pills)	PPA + caffeine NS	3 capsules 6 pills	15	F	None	Increased BP	NS	Recovery	Mueller et al. (1985)
Dexatrim (type NS)	PPA + caffeine	17 capsules	19	F	None	Increased BP	NS	Recovery	Mueller et al. (1985)
Dexatrim Extra Strength	75 mg PPA + caffeine	Up to 5 capsules daily for 5 months	44	F	NS	Increased BP	NS	Recovery	Mueller et al. (1985)
Diet pills (brand not stated)	35 mg PPA + caffeine	34	25	M	None	Acute renal failure	NS	Recovery in 12 days	Duffy et al. (1981)
Dexatrim	50 mg PPA + caffeine	30-50 (5 days prior to admission)	21	M	History of binge drinking	Weakness, sore muscles, GI tract bleeding, rhabdomyolysis, acute renal failure	IV fluids; peritoneal dialysis	Discharged 4 days later	Swenson et al. (1982)

TABLE 4.13. Continued.

Product	Form/Contents	Dose	Age	Sex	Preexisting Conditions	Adverse Effects	Treatment	Clinical Outcome	Reference
Not stated	50 mg PPA + caffeine	40	31	F	Schizophrenia	Agitation, hypertension	Urecholine Chloride, trifluoperazine	No sequelae	Pentel et al. (1982)
Dex-a-Diet II	75 mg PPA + caffeine	22 capsules	22	M	Drug abuse	Dizziness, giddiness, vomiting, severe headache, coma, increased BP, increased HR, muscle spasm, cerebral hemorrhage	NS	Death	Lai & Lai (1982)
					D. Street Drugs				
"Black pick-me-ups"	50 mg PPA + ephedrine + caffeine	2 capsules	17	M	None	Agitation, confusion, coma, grand mal seizures, respiratory arrest	Diazepam, phenobarbital	Death (massive intracerebral hemorrhage)	Bernstein & Diskant (1982)
"Black legal stimulants"	50 mg PPA + caffeine + ephedrine	2 capsules + 3–6 oz whiskey	26	M	NS	Vomiting, difficult breathing, subarachnoid and intraventricular hemorrhage	Naloxone	Death	Bernstein & Diskant (1982)
"Black beauties"	50 mg PPA + caffeine + ephedrine	4	21	M	Genetic predisposition, alcohol, & drug binges	Palpitations, hyperactivity, aberrant behavior, bipolar affective disorder, mania	Thioridazine	NS	Lake et al. (1983)
RJ8 ("look-alike" pills)	50 mg PPA + ephedrine + caffeine	15–18	14	F	None	Cardiac arrhythmias, palpitations, blurred vision	Lidocaine (IV), propranolol	Uneventful recovery	Weesner et al. (1982)

Street name	Drug	Dose	Age	Sex	History	Symptoms		Outcome	Reference
"Pick-me-up" pills	50 mg PPA + caffeine + pseudoephedrine	1	17	F	None	Seizures	NS	NS	Mueller (1983)
"Pseudospeed"	50 mg PPA + caffeine + ephedrine	1	27	F	None	Seizures	NS	NS	Mueller (1983)
"Pseudospeed"	PPA + ?	2	37	M	None	Headache, vomiting	NS	NS	Mueller (1983)
"Black beauties"	PPA + caffeine	2	21	M	None	Headache, tremor, diaphoresis, nausea, vomiting	NS	NS	Mueller (1983)
"Black beauties"	PPA ? + 2 joints	At least 2	29	M	None	Bizarre behavior	NS	NS	Mueller (1983)
"Black beauties"	PPA + ?	3	22	M	None	Headache, abnormal ECG	NS	NS	Mueller (1983)
"Pseudospeed"	PPA + unidentified substance	5-6	38	M	None	Headache, tremulousness	NS	NS	Mueller (1983)
"Pink ladies" + "Speckled pups"	PPA + caffeine + Unidentified substances	"Some" 15	19	F	None	Headache, diaphoresis, vomiting, abnormal ECG	NS	NS	Mueller (1983)
"Black beauties"	PPA + ?	"Several"	17	F	None	Neuropsychiatric symptoms	NS	NS	Mueller (1983)
NS	PPA + ?	NS	13	M	None	Attempted suicide	NS	NS	Mueller (1983)
Unidentified white pill	PPA + ?	"Overdose"	25	F	Chronic undifferentiated schizophrenia	Acute psychosis	NS	NS	Mueller (1983)
"Crank"	PPA + caffeine + unidentified amine	Approximately 250 mg total dose, IV	24	F	IV Drug abuse	Feeling grumpy, epigastric pain, increased HR, leukocytosis	IV antibiotics	Recovery	Paulman et al. (1986)

[a]Within each subsection, the case reports are arranged in order of ascending total dose of phenylpropanolamine, where this can be determined. In Mueller (1983), phenylpropanolamine and other drugs were determined from urine samples and not from the actual drug (except where noted).

[b]NS—not specified; HR—heart rate; BP—blood pressure; M—male; F—female.

269

stigmine was given IV, the electrocardiogram showed an atrial ectopic pacemaker; after a second dose of physostigmine, there was conversion to normal sinus rhythm. After a total of five doses of 1 mg of physostigmine within a 3½-hr period, his blood pressure was normal. The patient was monitored for 96 hr and showed no evidence of arrhythmias, elevation of blood pressure, hallucinations, or other adverse effects.

CASE 22.   Following an argument with her boyfriend, a 23-year-old white female ingested 15–30 Ornade Spansules (Rumack et al., 1974). Shortly thereafter she was agitated and had tachycardia and hyperpnea; her pulse was 150/min, respiratory rate 32/min, and blood pressure 110/70 mm Hg. She was given ipecac with emesis resulting. She was admitted to the hospital 14 hr later because she was agitated, cyanotic, and in severe respiratory distress. Her temperature was higher than 41.5°C (maximum temperature on the thermometer used). Her respiratory rate was 60/min and blood pressure 90/78 mm Hg, and she had fine rales throughout both lungs. The electrocardiogram revealed large Q waves in leads II, III, AVF, and V_{1-4}. Laboratory data showed an increased hematocrit, increased white blood count, a serum glutamic oxalacetic transaminase of 120 units, a pO_2 of 46 mm Hg, a pCO_2 of 18 mm Hg, and a pH of 7.41. Within 4 hr after admission her temperature was reduced to 39°C by ice water immersion. Endotracheal intubation was done and assisted ventilation provided, followed by a 6-hr hemodialysis.

On the second and third days of hospitalization, her chest x-ray showed improvement and her blood pressure stabilized. Her platelet count was slightly reduced, prothrombin time slightly increased, and partial thromboplastin time markedly increased, although the tests for fibrin split products and fibrinogen were normal. On the fourth day this patient was less responsive to stimuli, was hypotensive, and had upper GI bleeding, although her hematocrit, electrolytes, arterial blood gases, and cerebrospinal fluid were normal and blood cultures were negative. On the fifth day she was unresponsive to stimuli and was bleeding spontaneously from venipuncture sites. Coagulation studies showed fibrinogen 75 mg%, platelets 24,000/mm³, prothrombin time 37 sec (control 13 sec), and fibrin split products positive at a dilution of 1:128. The following day cerebral angiography revealed no filling of the anterior cerebral vessels. Cerebral edema and an infarcted right cerebral hemisphere were seen at craniotomy. She died shortly thereafter. Death was attributed to diffuse small vessel thrombosis, disseminated intravascular coagulation, and cerebral and myocardial infarctions. These appeared to be sequelae of the hyperthermia.

This patient was reported to have taken 15–30 Ornade capsules; 30 capsules contain 240 mg of chlorpheniramine maleate, 1500 mg of phenylpropanolamine hydrochloride, and 75 mg of isopropamide. With this combination of an antihistamine that would cause drying of the mucous membranes, a weak sympathomimetic amine that can cause vasoconstriction and arrhythmias at excessive dose levels, and an anticholinergic that would reduce sweating and decrease heat dissipation and could cause mild hypertension, it is not surprising that hyperthermia resulted. The sequelae to marked hyperthermia of coagulopathy, renal failure, and diffuse organ hemorrhage have been documented. It is possible that this patient had a preexisting condition that contributed to the sequence of events. This was a case of frank abuse of a combination drug product.

CASE 23.   One case of delayed fatal outcome attributed to a phenylpropanolamine-containing decongestant was reported (Patterson, 1980). A 19-year-old white female, in a depression, intentionally ingested 10–12 Ru-Tuss prolonged-action tablets. These each contain 25 mg of phenylephrine hydrochloride, 50 mg of phenylpropanolamine hydrochloride, 8 mg of chlorpheniramine maleate, 0.1936 mg of hyoscyamine sulfate, 0.0362 mg of atropine sulfate, and 0.0121 mg of scopolamine hydrobromide. When she was seen in the emergency room an hour later the patient complained of drowsiness. She was given ipecac and vomited a large quantity of yellow material, but no pills were seen. She was admitted to the hospital and given a saline cathartic and IV saline and glucose. Vital signs and electrocardiogram were normal. The patient remained drowsy and slept intermittently on the first day of hospitalization; she was afebrile and more alert on the second day, but her white blood count was somewhat elevated, and a chest x-ray showed a right lower lobe infiltrate. Keflex was administered IV and she was recovering, alert, and ambulatory. On the third day she complained of shortness of breath and pleuritic-type chest pain; bilateral wet rales and labored respiration developed that progressed rapidly in the next 4 hr to cardiopulmonary arrest. Supportive and emergency measures were utilized and she was transferred, on a respirator, to a university hospital. There she was diagnosed as having respiratory distress or "shock lung"; she had sinus bradycardia and bilateral rales; blood gases and pH indicated metabolic acidosis. She was given "appropriate" therapy. Twenty-two hours after arrival she had an episode of ventricular tachycardia; she was unresponsive to all measures and died about 5 days after consumption of the tablets.

Autopsy showed evidence of disseminated intravascular coagulation with left ventricular mural thrombosis formation and nonbacterial thrombotic endocarditis. During the course of treatment, at least ten different drugs were used in attempts to treat this overdose (see Table 4.13).

One unusual case demonstrates a severe reaction to chronic abuse of a phenylpropanolamine-containing decongestant in an individual with a history of psychiatric disturbance.

CASE 24.   A 28-year-old woman with borderline personality disorder and a history of multiple suicide attempts and polysubstance abuse had exclusively abused Triaminicol during the previous 2 years (Cornelius et al., 1984). This cough syrup, available OTC contains phenylpropanolamine hydrochloride 12.5 mg, pheniramine maleate 6.25 mg, pyrilamine maleate 6.25 mg, dextromethorphan hydrobromide 15 mg, and ammonium chloride 90 mg. The subject had a day-long binge in which she drank about 12 oz of the cough syrup following which she "sat perfectly still, staring straight ahead, as if in a trance." The next day, believing that her mother was sadistically sabotaging her life, she drove to her parents' home and, without warning, repeatedly stabbed the mother in the chest and arms with a kitchen knife. The woman then drove to the psychiatric hospital where she had previously been a patient. She was disheveled, confused, tearful, mute, and fearful. She huddled almost motionless in her bed for the next 2 days. On the third day she had a 50-sec grand mal seizure with loss of consciousness, tonic-clonic seizures, tongue biting, and a marked postictal increase of fear and confusion. She was given 10 mg of diazepam IV. An EEG the next day showed very frequent slow-wave transients that occurred independently over the right and left midtemporal regions. Within days she improved markedly and an EEG a week later was normal.

This patient had had two grand mal seizures within the previous 6 months, both occurring while she was in psychiatric hospitals after the surreptitious ingestion of large amounts of Triaminicol. Both were accompanied by similar behavior patterns and EEG findings. When this patient was challenged with 50 mg of phenylpropanolamine, she displayed clinical evidence of a temporal lobe seizure: chewing movements, fright, and focal EEG abnormality that lasted 4 min.

This subject was obviously an habitual abuser of the Triaminicol cough syrup, and it appears that she had an adverse or hypersensitivity reaction to some of the ingredients. Sensitivity to phenylpropanolamine was demonstrated by the challenge dose of this ingredient. A rechallenge with any of the other ingredients was not reported; such tests would be necessary to pinpoint the causative agent with certainty.

OVERDOSE CASES: APPETITE SUPPRESSANTS

APPETITE SUPPRESSANTS CONTAINING PHENYLPROPANOLAMINE WITHOUT CAFFEINE

Three cases of overdose reactions to appetite suppressants containing phenylpropanolamine without caffeine have been reported (Table 4.13). Two of these cases involved appetite suppressants available in the United States and one involved the Australian product Trimolets. In all three cases only cardiovascular reactions were described and no CNS reactions occurred. In contrast, overdoses of appetite suppressants containing both phenylpropanolamine and caffeine were associated with both CNS and cardiovascular effects.

In one case, a man experienced unremitting headache for 5 days following ingestion of five times the recommended dose of a liquid diet preparation containing phenylpropanolamine (Mesnard & Ginn, 1984). Subsequent medical evaluation showed that he had a subarachnoid hemorrhage. In another case, a woman took seven pills containing 75 mg of phenylpropanolamine each to get "high." She was admitted to an emergency department where she was found to have elevated blood pressure (180/90 mm Hg) and bradycardia (40 bpm). Analysis of the ECG showed a sinus bradycardia with atrioventricular blockade (Wenckebach pattern). She was given supportive medical treatment and her symptoms subsided within 6 hr.

One case involved the Australian product Trimolets, which, as described in a previous section (on adverse drug reactions) is different in several important respects from phenylpropanolamine-containing appetite suppressants sold in the United States and other parts of the world. Consequently, the effects reported in this case cannot be directly compared to other overdose cases involving phenylpropanolamine-containing appetite suppressants. A 17-year-old girl had an adverse reaction to ingestion of Trimolets on two separate occasions (Horowitz et al., 1979) (see Table 4.13). On one occasion she took one tablet twice daily (i.e, at recommended doses) and experienced headache, dizziness, and palpitations. On another occasion she took six tablets simultaneously and experienced increased blood pressure that required bed rest. Her blood pressure returned to normal in 48 hours, with no pharmacological intervention.

APPETITE SUPPRESSANTS CONTAINING PHENYLPROPANOLAMINE AND CAFFEINE

Thirteen cases of overdose reactions to appetite suppressants containing phenylpropanolamine and caffeine were reported. Seven were acute cases in which individuals took up to 50 appetite suppressants. In four cases, the individuals had been taking moderate overdoses for up to 5 months. In two cases, the individual had been taking the appetite suppressant at recomended doses for 1–2 weeks, and then took an overdose.

Given such a wide range of doses and dosing schedules, it is difficult to generalize about these overdose cases. Consequently, several cases will be briefly summarized.

CASE 25. A 31-year-old schizophrenic woman ingested approximately 40 tablets containing 50 mg of phenylpropanolamine and 200 mg of caffeine (Pentel et al., 1982). Her medications were Urecholine Chloride (bethanecol chloride) and trifluoperazine. About an hour after ingesting the tablets she began vomiting and was agitated, her blood pressure was 180/126 mm Hg, and her pulse was 90/min. Her blood pressure returned to normal within 3 hr without medication. Total creatine kinase and its MB isoenzyme fraction were normal on admission, were increased at 12 and 24 hr and were normal at 36 hr. No further rhythm disturbance occurred, and she remained normotensive and asymptomatic.

Two acute overdose cases involved acute renal failure. One of these also involved rhabdomyolysis and other severe reactions (Swenson et al., 1982) (see Table 4.13) and is described in detail in the section on rhabdomyolysis (see above).

CASE 26. A 25-year-old man was admitted to a hospital emergency room 12 hr after ingesting 34 "diet pills" as a suicide gesture. Each tablet contained 35 mg of phenylpropanolamine and 140 mg of caffeine (Duffy et al., 1981). Examination revealed no abnormalities; blood pressure was 120/76 mm Hg, and blood urea nitrogen was 8 mg/dl. Twenty-four hours later the patient had low-back pain and decreased urine output. He became progressively ill with anorexia, malaise, and fatigue during the next 18 hr. His blood pressure was 160/100 mm Hg, his blood urea nitrogen was 52, and his creatinine was 13.8 mg/dl. Renal ultrasound revealed normal-sized kidneys without evidence of obstruction. Five days after drug ingestion, a percutaneous renal biopsy showed normal-appearing glomeruli, marked degenerative changes, and areas of overt tubular necrosis in the proximal tubules and mild interstitial edema. During the next 7 days, urine output increased and serum creatinine decreased to 2.1 mg/dl. This patient consumed 1190 mg of phenylpropanolamine and 4780 mg of caffeine, obvious drug abuse. It is probable that the effects on the kidneys are attributable to the massive intake of caffeine because it is known to cause vasoconstriction.

One case involved acute overdose following a brief course of drug intake at recommended doses.

CASE 27. A 13-year-old girl had been taking Dex-A-Diet II (75 mg of phenylpropanolamine, and 200 mg of caffeine in a timed-release capsule) daily for 2 weeks, and that morning had taken two capsules, following which she complained of light-headedness, severe headache, and nausea; her blood pressure was 210/100 mm Hg (Howrie & Wolfson, 1983). She vomited and then had a 2-min generalized seizure, followed by a 15-min period of confusion and combativeness. Blood pressure readings before and following the seizure were 200/100 and 150/80 mm Hg, respectively. Twenty minutes later in the hospital emergency room, she was alert and oriented but complained of dizziness and headache; her blood pressure was 170/100 mm Hg. Four hours after the first seizure, she had a second generalized seizure that lasted 30 sec. Phenytoin 500 mg was administered IV. The patient had no further seizures and remained normotensive.

Three cases involved moderate overdoses of phenylpropanolamine-containing appetite suppressants for durations ranging from 8 days to 4 months.

CASE 28. A 23-year-old married woman and mother was taken to a psychiatric emergency service because of her bizarre behavior after taking too many "diet pills" (Schaffer & Pauli, 1980). About 5 days before, she began taking three to five pills daily of both Permathene and Dexatrim and about 3 days before admission began taking "copious amounts" of the drugs. During that time she slept less, made bizarre statements, and exhibited paranoid behavior. When admitted to the hospital, the patient was alert but agitated, hyperactive, and disoriented, with disorganized thoughts and inappropriate verbal responses. The patient returned to normal, without any medication, after 3 days. When taking five pills per day of each appetite suppressant, this patient consumed 625 mg of phenylpropanolamine and 1700 mg of caffeine; when the patient took "copious amounts" of both "diet pills" the total amount of each drug consumed is unknown.

CASE 29.   A 24-year-old previously healthy man was hospitalized for evaluation of right-sided hemiparesis after being found on the floor of his navy barracks with marked right-sided weakness (Johnson et al., 1983). The only abnormal physical findings were right-sided hemiplegia with right central facial involvement and decreased motor and sensory function. On the sixth day, a CT scan showed a lesion in the left front parietal area suggestive of an evolving infarct. Brain scan was consistent with a cerebral vascular accident involving the left middle cerebral artery. The patient then admitted to taking 8–10 "diet pills" a day for over 3 months, each Dexatrim tablet containing 50 mg of phenylpropanolamine and 200 mg of caffeine. Motor function slowly improved, and the patient had no neurological relapses. At ten Dexatrim tablets per day he was consuming 500 mg of phenylpropanolamine and 2 g of caffeine each day. To this may presumably be added the amount of coffee an enlisted navy man usually drinks each day, and it is quite apparent this man had been consuming toxic amounts of caffeine daily for at least 3 months.

CASE 30.   A 34-year-old man was hospitalized because of lethargy and right-sided hemiparesis, including the face, and right hemihypesthesia and an expressive aphasia (Johnson et al., 1983). The neurological deficit resolved in 7 hr but returned twice very briefly. He was given heparin therapy; CT scan, EEG, echocardiogram, and cerebral arteriogram were normal. It was revealed that this subject had been taking three to eight Dietac tablets per day (37.5 mg of phenylpropanolamine per tablet) for over 4 months. At eight Dietac tablets a day he was consuming 300 mg of phenylpropanolamine each day.

OVERDOSE CASES: ILLICIT DRUGS
CONTAINING PHENYLPROPANOLAMINE

Sixteen cases of drug overdose attributed to phenylpropanolamine-containing illicit drugs have been reported (see Table 4.13). Street drug abuse of these amphetamine look-alike or pseudospeed drugs is a relatively recent phenomenon, and all the overdose cases were reported since 1982. Of the 16 cases, 11 were reported in a single publication (Mueller, 1983).

Documentation of the drug, dose, and formulation involved in overdoses of street drugs is tenuous at best. The most frequently abused illicit preparation is the triple combination of phenylpropanolamine, ephedrine, and caffeine. Because of the illicit nature of the experience, many overdose patients are unwilling or unable to provide details of their experiences. Moreover, many drug abusers are polydrug users, and drug interactions are likely to affect the total drug response. Definitive identification of the presence of phenylpropanolamine in biofluids in overdose cases was presented in only one of the overdose reports and no quantitative data were given (Mueller, 1983).

As might be expected, the most frequently mentioned signs of overdose were referable to CNS stimulation (see Table 4.13). Several factors undoubtedly contribute to the preponderance of CNS signs in these cases compared to overdose with decongestant or appetite-supressant products. One factor is that many of the illicit products have contained ephedrine, which is known to have potent CNS stimulating effects. Also, since the individuals took the illicit products either thinking them to be amphetamines or simply "pick-me-ups," they were probably anticipating amphetaminelike effects. The health care practitioners and investigators reporting the overdose cases might likewise have a bias toward identification of CNS effects if they suspect that the individual took amphetamine look-alikes or pseudospeed. Cardiovascular effects have also been reported in a few cases (see Table 4.13).

Four of the most severe and best documented overdose cases are presented below (Cases 31–34). Three of the cases involved relatively low doses of two or four capsules. In one case, two capsules alone were taken, and in two cases, two capsules were taken along with large amounts of alcohol. Two individuals died following overdoses. It is remarkable that these two individuals took the lowest doses among the cases reported. One individual who took a dose reported to be seven to nine times higher recovered from the overdose. Also, individuals have consumed licit OTC products containing as much as 1000–1500 mg of phenylpropanolamine and survived. It seems highly likely that in the cases of the two individuals who died after reportedly taking only two illicit triple combination pills, either the dosages were severely underestimated or other factors were involved.

CASE 31.   Shortly after a 17-year-old man ingested two "black capsules," he became tremulous, agitated, and unable to sleep but was oriented and alert (Bernstein & Diskant, 1982). The capsules identified as pick-me-ups contained 200 mg of caffeine, 25 mg of ephedrine, and 50 mg of phenylpropanolamine. There was an abrupt change about 6 hr later. He became agitated, confused, and disoriented, with incomprehensible, slurred speech. His brother repeatedly stated that the subject was "just crashing from speed." He was drowsy, slept 2–3 hr at a time, and was disoriented when aroused. He was taken to the hospital emergency room about 17 hr after taking the capsules. His blood pressure was 120/60 mm Hg, pulse rate 60/min, respiratory rate 12/min, and temperature 37°C. His speech was slurred, and he made inappropriate responses to verbal or painful stimuli; however, fundoscopic and neurological findings were unremarkable. Urinary ephedrine level was 2 μg/ml; no ethanol, opiates, methaqualone, or amphetamines were detected; phenylpropanolamine was not determined.

Approximately 15 hr after admission, the patient became deeply comatose and had decerebrate posturing, and shortly thereafter had a grand mal seizure followed by respiratory arrest. Seizures were controlled with 10 mg of diazepam IV, and 60 mg of phenobarbital was given IM. Mechanical ventilatory support was required. A CT scan showed a large intracerebral hemorrhage in the left parietooccipital area with a moderate mass effect and midline shift. The next day there was evidence of bilateral brainstem dysfunction. On the fourth day of hospitalization it was determined that brain death had occurred. Mechanical ventilatory support was discontinued; shortly thereafter the patient died. A massive intracerebral hemorrhage in the left parietooccipital and intraventricular hemorrhage on the left side were found at autopsy, but no abnormalities of the intracranial vessels were seen.

CASE 32.   About 3–4 hr before admission to the hospital emergency room, a 26-year-old man had taken two "black capsules," and 8 hr before admission he drank 3–6 oz of whiskey (Bernstein & Diskant, 1982). The capsules were "legal stimulants," each containing 200 mg of caffeine, 25 mg of ephedrine, and 50 mg of phenylpropanolamine. About an hour after ingestion of the capsules he appeared to be sober, was without somatic complaints, and went to sleep. About 2 hr later he vomited and had trouble breathing, presumably because of an upper airway obstruction that was cleared manually by a friend who then took him to the emergency room. On arrival, the patient was in obvious respiratory distress, was slightly cyanotic, and was unresponsive to stimuli. His blood pressure was 134/78 mm Hg, pulse rate 60/min, and respiratory rate 40/min with stridor. His pupils were symmetrically dilated and unreactive to light; a large subhyaloid hemorrhage on the right and splinter hemorrhages on the left were seen at fundoscopic examination, and the oculocephalic reflex was absent. The muscles were flaccid. Blood alcohol was 5 mg % and serum ephedrine 3 μg/ml; screening tests for tricyclic antidepressants, opiates, glutethimide, and amphetamine were negative; phenylpropanolamine was not determined.

In the intensive care unit naloxone was administered without apparent effect, a nasotracheal airway was inserted, and IV solution was started. The blood pressure rose to 156/110 mm Hg and later to 208/148 mm Hg; several hours later it dropped to 80 mm Hg systolic and dopamine was administered. Approximately 11 hr after admission, the patient developed ventricular fibrillation and died. Extensive subarachnoid and intraventricular hemorrhage was found at autopsy, although the origin of the hemorrhage could not be localized.

CASE 33.   A stimulant-induced mania in a genetically predisposed patient was reported (Lake et al., 1983). A 21-year-old single man ingested four street "black beauties." These were alleged to contain 100–200 mg of caffeine, 50 mg of phenylpropanolamine, and 25 mg of ephedrine. Within 30 min he experienced palpitations, diaphoresis, flushing, and hyperactive behavior which lasted over 4 hr. For the next 4 days his behavior became increasingly aberrant. On hospitalization he was diagnosed as having major bipolar affective disorder.

This patient had no previous manic episodes but had been hospitalized 2 years earlier because he was withdrawn and depressed and had contemplated suicide. Two of his four older brothers had been hospitalized several times with mania, both with major bipolar affective disorder. The patient had a history of alcohol abuse and had abused other drugs such as marijuana and LSD, although he had not taken LSD for about 7 months. At the time of this hospitalization he denied taking any additional drugs during the 4 previous days with the exception of "a couple of joints" and two or three beers a day. With this patient's history of alcohol and drug abuse, together with a family history of mania, he conceivably might have been predisposed to psychotic behavior from stimulants. The black beauties contain CNS stimulants, primarily caffeine, of which he took 400–800 mg. As the authors point out, CNS stimulants, including caffeine, appear to increase noradrenergic neurotransmission, which is thought to be associated with mania.

CASE 34. A 14-year-old white female ingested 15–18 capsules called "RJ8" in a suicide gesture following expulsion from school (Weesner et al., 1982). Each capsule contained 25 mg of of ephedrine, 50 mg of phenylpropanolamine and 200 mg of caffeine. About 1 1/2 hr after ingesting the capsules, the subject complained of blurred vision, nervousness, tremor, and inability to walk. On hospitalization her blood pressure was 104/62 mm Hg, with a heart rate of 180/min and frequent aberrant beats. She was given ipecac and activated charcoal. An electrocardiogram showed premature ventricular contractions, functional ectopic beats, and premature arterial contractions as well as short periods of ventricular tachycardia. Intravenous lidocaine therapy was started without effect on the arrhythmias. When transferred to a university hospital, the girl was alert and responsive but complained of palpitations, nervousness, and blurred vision. Her blood pressure was 135/68 mm Hg and pulse 140 beats/min. When the patient was given 1 mg of propanolol IV over a 3-min period, her heart rate converted to a normal sinus rhythm with a rate of 86/min. The patient's recovery was uneventful.

In addition, Mueller reported that between 1980 and 1982, 11 subjects, 6 male and 5 female, 13 to 38 years old, had acute-onset of headache, psychiatric symptoms, or seizures, related to the ingestion of look-alike pills (Mueller, 1983).

Five patients had headache and elevated blood pressure of $175 \pm 10/92 \pm 4$ mm Hg. Of these patients, three vomited, two were diaphoretic, two were tremulous, one had dilated pupils, and two had ECG abnormalities—one with sinus arrhythmia and multifocal premature ventricular complexes, and the other with transiently prolonged QTU segments that had resolved 3 days later. Four patients had disturbances of thought processes. One with chronic undifferentiated schizophrenia appeared to be acutely psychotic with auditory and visual hallucinations, one attempted suicide by hanging, one acted in a bizarre fashion by taking off his clothes at the airport, and the fourth alleged sexual assault in the absence of any evidence of assault. Two subjects had generalized convulsive seizures; in one, the first seizure occurred 20 min after ingestion of "a pill," and a second convulsion followed 10 min later. The EEG showed focal, low-amplitude, irregular theta activity over the right temporal region interpreted as compatible with a structural defect that subsequently resolved. The other subject had a single seizure 12 hr after ingesting a look-alike pill.

All of these subjects took look-alike pills—namely, "pink ladies," "black beauties," or "speckled pups," which are illicit or illegal drugs of unknown content, concentration, and purity. Most of the subjects thought they had taken "speed" and reported taking up to six pills, although the author has stated that "patients are reluctant to give physicians information concerning ingestion of street drugs." These subjects may well have taken much higher doses than admitted to. Some of these pills were known to contain caffeine in unknown concentrations; thus, the possibility of a caffeine overdosage exists. Some of these pills contained unidentified substances, and some contained caffeine and pseudoephedrine, or caffeine and ephedrine together with phenylpropanolamine—a combination that the FDA has declared to be an unapproved new drug and has removed from the legal marketplace.

A rather unusual overdose case occurred in a man who regularly abused a variety of drugs including pentazocine and tripelennamine, OTC diet pills, cocaine, and marijuana (Jackson et al., 1985). Pentazocine is an orally active opiate analgesic with mixed agonist-antagonist activity; tripelennamine is an antihistamine. The combination of pentazocine and tripelennamine frequently is abused; this combination is known as "T's and Blues" ("T" for Talwin, the tradename for pentazocine, and "blues" for the color of the tripelennamine tablet). Apparently, tripelennamine enhances the psychogenic activity of pentazocine.

This man developed neurologic symptoms after taking several IV doses of pentazocine and tripelennamine over 6 hr; after he went into a coma he was taken to an emergency department. Physical examination showed elevated blood pressure (200/120 mm Hg) and supraventricular tachycardia (200 bpm); neurologic examination showed multiple neurologic symptoms. Computerized tomography (CT) of the brain at the time of admission showed no abnormalities. His neurologic status continued to deteriorate and a second CT scan the morning after admission showed intraparenchymal cerebral hemorrhage. The man was pronounced brain dead 48 hr later.

The authors of the report stated "A case of fatal intracranial hemorrhage following overdose with phenylpropanolamine, pentazocine, and tripelennamine is presented." The man had taken an Extra Strength Dexatrim capsule (75 mg of phenylpropanolamine and 200 mg of caffeine) 20 hr before the onset of neurologic symptoms. A urine sample taken at the time of admission tested positive for amphetamine and negative for opiates by an EMIT test (EMIT does not detect pentazocine and cannot distinguish phenylpropanolamine from amphetamine without a confirmatory test).

Another unusual overdose case involved possible IV abuse of phenylpropanolamine in an illicit street drug. A 24-year-old woman took 250 mg of what she thought was "crank" (methamphetamine) IV (Paulman et al., 1986). Twelve to 14 hr later she entered an emergency department with complaints of "feeling jumpy" and midepigastric pain. Cardiac examination was normal except for tachycardia (124 bpm). Hematology tests showed the white cell count was 52,000/mm^3. This peripheral leukocytosis gradually resolved over 5 days. A toxicology screen showed the presence of phenylpropanolamine, caffeine, and an unidentified amine (neither D-amphetamine nor methamphetamine; the report does not specify whether this was a plasma or urine test).

ADVERSE DRUG INTERACTIONS

Numerous reports of adverse drug interactions with phenylpropanolamine-containing preparations have been published. These adverse interaction reports are reviewed here. All these reports were individual case studies, and in only a few cases were studies conducted to verify the drug interaction. Few preclinical or clinical trials have been reported in which these drug interactions were specifically tested. These few reports are reviewed in Chapter 3 and earlier in this chapter ("Animal Studies, Drug Combinations").

MONOAMINE OXIDASE INHIBITORS

Adverse drug interactions between phenylpropanolamine and monoamine oxidase inhibitors were investigated in one controlled clinical case study (Cuthbert et al., 1969). Baseline studies were conducted in which three normotensive adult male subjects were given 50 mg of phenylpropanolamine in gelatin capsules. This treatment produced a modest rise (18–26 mm Hg) in systolic blood pressure, but no change in diastolic pressure or pulse rate. When 100 mg of phenylpropanolamine was given orally there was a more pronounced rise in systolic blood pressure and some rise in diastolic pressure, but no change in pulse rate. When 50 mg of phenylpropanolamine was given in a slow-release form combined with an atropinelike compound, there was no significant change in systolic or diastolic blood pressure.

Two subjects were given 100 mg of phenylpropanolamine together with 12.5 mg of trimeprazine, a phenothiazine with weak α-receptor blocking properties. There was no significant change in the pressor response to phenylpropanolamine. One subject was given 50 mg of phenylpropanolamine while taking the monamine oxidase inhibitor tranylcypromine (30 mg daily for 20–30 days). There was a rapid rise of blood pressure to 210/140 mm Hg at 2 hr with an associated bradycardia and throbbing headache. A similar response resulted when the same dose of phenylpropanolamine was given as Vallex linctus. In both instances, phentolamine was administered IM to reduce the blood pressure. When a Procol capsule (50 mg of phenylpropanolamine and 2.5 mg of isopropamide in a slow-release form) was given immediately after tranylcypromine, there was a gradual rise of blood pressure to a maximum of 160/100 mm Hg at 90 min. The subjective symptoms were not severe, and blood pressure returned to normal after about 2 hr.

In general, pressor responses to indirect-acting sympathomimetic amines are potentiated by monoamine oxidase inhibitors. Two mechanisms have been proposed for such interactions. The exogenous amines may be degraded by monoamine oxidase, and thus the inhibitors decrease the metabolism of the amines. Alternatively, the exogenous amines produce pressor responses by releasing endogenous stores of catecholamines. Since catecholamines are metabolized by monoamine oxidase, MAO inhibitors potentiate the effects of the catecholamines. Ephedrine displaces noradrenaline from tissue stores, and this pressor response is potentiated by monoamine oxidase inhibitors. Phenylephrine is a substrate for monoamine oxidase; when taken orally after an MAO inhibitor, it can cause a rapid, marked rise of blood pressure. However, phenylpropanolamine is a poor substrate for MAO.

It is important to note, however, that the slow-release form of phenylpropanolamine induces a much less rapid and less marked hypertensive response in the presence of an MAO inhibitor than the immediate-release phenylpropanolamine.

CASE 35.   Another patient who had been taking an MAO inhibitor and had a hypertensive crisis after ingesting an appetite suppressant has been reported (Smookler & Bermudez, 1982). A 28-year-old man with chronic depression had been treated with phenelzine sulfate 15 mg q.i.d. for 2 years. Within 1 hr after taking two capsules of Control containing 75 mg of phenylpropanolamine, he developed diaphoresis and an excruciating occipital headache radiating to the top of his head. At a local care facility his blood pressure was measured as 220/115 mm Hg; he was given meperidine IM for the headache. Soon thereafter he was observed to be very diaphoretic, agitated, and in acute distress from a severe headache; his blood pressure was 180/120 mm Hg. A thorough medical history, physical examination, and clinical laboratory data were all negative. The patient was administered oxygen at 5 liters/min and 5 mg of phentolamine mesylate IV; his blood pressure decreased to 170/90 mm Hg with no relief of the headache. After 2 mg of propanolol was given IV the headache began to subside. He was then given 500 mg of methyldopa IV and 50 mg of meperidine IM. After 24 hr of observation his blood pressure was 124/78 mm Hg and he was discharged from the hospital.

CASE 36.   A 24-year-old female had been treated for depression for 1 year with 45 mg/day of phenelzine and then took one Sinutab (without codeine) for sinusitis

(Terry et al., 1975). After $1/2$ hr she noticed palpitation and an irregular pulse. At the emergency room, she had a pulse rate of 40/min and an atrioventricular Wenckebach phenomenon. Her heart rate spontaneously reverted to sinus brady-cardia (50/min) and then to normal sinus rhythm over the next 6 hr.

CASE 37.   A healthy 28-year-old man was reported to have taken two Mucron tab-lets (each containing 32 mg of phenylpropanolamine) for relief of nasal deconges-tion (Gibson & Warrell, 1972). After 10 min he had an excruciating headache, a sensation of colored lights, a feeling of lightness in the chest, and a pounding heart. Then 20 min later his blood pressure was 180/100 mm Hg, 1 hr later it was 160/90 mm Hg, and 12 hr later it was 140/80 mm Hg; there were no other abnor-mal signs. It was learned that the subject had ingested a meal containing cheese before taking the tablets. The authors speculated that the hypertensive episode may have been precipitated by the synergistic action of the tyramine in the cheese and ingestion of phenylpropanolamine.

Each year many hundreds of idiosyncratic or hypersensitivity reactions are reported in individuals ingesting a combination of foods, a combination of food and drugs, or a combination of drugs. It would appear that this individ-ual had a hypersensitivity or an idiosyncratic reaction to the combination of cheese and phenylpropanolamine. There have been no other clinical reports of such reactions and no preclinical studies have tested the interaction be-tween phenylpropanolamine and tyramine.

BETA BLOCKERS

CASE 38.   McLaren (1976) reported on a 31-year-old male who had acute glo-merulonephritis when he was 14 years old. A year before the reported episode he had a blood pressure of 200/120 mm Hg and a blood urea nitrogen of 133 mg/dl. Methyldopa, 250 mg b.i.d., and oxprenolol, 160 mg t.i.d., apparently stabilized his blood pressure at 140/80 mm Hg. However, his renal function continued to deteriorate; he had a blood urea nitrogen level of 183 mg/dl.

Three months later he was prescribed Triogesic (12.5 mg of phenylpropa-nolamine and 500 mg of acetaminophen) at a dosage of two tablets t.i.d. for a cold. Two days later the patient complained of decreasing energy, occasional head-aches, and increasing nausea "over the preceding few weeks" and paresthesia of his hands and feet "since the onset of his cold." At that time his blood pressure was 200/150 mm Hg, his pulse rate was 90/min, and his blood urea nitrogen was 253 mg/dl. There were no objective signs of peripheral neuropathy, hypertensive retinopathy, or cardiac failure. The Triogesic was discontinued, but the usual doses of methyldopa and oxprenolol were continued. The following day his blood pressure was 140/110 mm Hg and the paresthesia had disappeared. Because he continued to vomit, peritoneal dialysis was initiated. Thereafter the patient contin-ued to take oxprenolol, 80 mg t.i.d., without methyldopa, and his blood pressure stabilized at 140/90 mm Hg.

The author postulated that there may be potentiation of the pressor effects of sympathomimetic drugs with methyldopa and β-adrenergic receptor blockers or the β-blockade may allow an unopposed α-constrictor response to adrenergic stimulation. However, the β-blocker propranolol blocked phenylpropanolamine-induced cardiovascular responses (Pentel et al., 1985b).

It must be pointed out that after peritoneal dialysis the patient's blood pressure was stabilized on oxprenolol at one-half the previous dose and without methyldopa. The patient had decreasing energy, occasional headaches, increasing nausea, and paresthesia of the hands and feet over the weeks preceding the ingestion of Triogesic. It was also apparent that his renal function had continued to deteriorate. Acetaminophen (3000 mg/day was taken) is known to cause renal tubular necrosis and decreased renal function; the plasma acetaminophen concentration would increase and cause further renal damage, which, in turn, would exacerbate the hypertension. This patient's renal failure alone could have exacerbated the hypertension because methyldopa is largely excreted by the kidney, and it is known that metabolites of methyldopa with possible pressor effects are increased in uremia.

NONSTEROIDAL ANTIINFLAMMATORY DRUGS

CASE 39.   A patient who had a severe headache and hypertension after ingestion of indomethacin with phenylpropanolamine has been reported (Lee et al., 1980). The 27-year-old woman had been taking one capsule a day of the appetite suppressant Trimolets (85 mg of D-phenylpropanolamine) for some months; within 15 min after taking 25 mg of indomethacin for tendonitis, she had a severe, throbbing, bifrontal headache. Within the next few hours her systolic blood pressure ranged from 210 to 150 mm Hg, diastolic from 110 to 80 mm Hg, and pulse from 72 to 56/min. When hospitalized, she was given 10 mg of morphine IV. Her headache continued intermittently. Cardiac and renal tests were normal; urinary catecholamines and 3-methoxy-4-hydroxymandelic acid were normal the day of admission and 3 weeks later.

Under careful hospital supervision, she was later challenged with indomethacin alone (slight increase of blood pressure), Trimolets alone (no change), and the combination of indomethacin and placebo (no change). When 25 mg of indomethacin was given 40 min after a Trimolets capsule, within 30 min the patient had a severe, throbbing, bifrontal headache; systolic and diastolic pressures rose to 200 and 150 mm Hg, respectively, "associated with bradycardia." Intravenous diazepam had no effect on blood pressure; phentolamine rapidly reduced her blood pressure and the severity of headache.

The authors have theorized about this interaction, suggesting that phenylpropanolamine directly stimulates α-adrenergic receptors in blood vessels and releases noradrenaline from sympathetic nerve endings to constrict arterioles. Because indomethacin inhibits prostaglandin synthesis, it could reduce prostaglandin-controlled negative feedback acting on catecholamine release at sympathetic nerve endings; within the vessel wall, synthesis of vasodilator prostaglandins could be suppressed, causing more severe vasoconstriction.

In view of the number of doses of phenylpropanolamine taken by millions of subjects each year in various OTC and prescription products as well as the millions of doses of indomethacin prescribed each year for arthritis, tendonitis, and bursitis, it would be reasonable to assume that hundreds of people each year would at some time take indomethacin and phenylpropanolamine together. Nevertheless, this is the only case reported in the literature of an adverse effect resulting from the interaction of phenylpropanolamine and indomethacin, and is presumably an individual idiosyncratic reaction.

One can further question this reported reaction because it occurred in Australia after the subject ingested Trimolets and the pharmaceutical formulation of this preparation is unclear. Many more hypertensive reactions have been reported in Australia in individuals taking Trimolets than reported in the United States in individuals taking other *dl*-phenylpropanolamine-containing products.

The lack of adverse drug interactions between phenylpropanolamine and another nonsteroidal antiinflammatory drug (NSAID), aspirin, was confirmed in a 30-day clinical safety study (P.T. Pugliese, unpublished data reviewed in the Federal Register, 1976). In a randomized, placebo-controlled study, 65 adult males and 3 adult females were assigned to one of four treatment groups. The four treatments were 50 mg of phenylpropanolamine plus 10 gr of aspirin, 50 mg of phenylpropanolamine alone, 10 gr of aspirin alone, and placebo. The subjects took these doses four times per day for a total of up to 30 days. Vital signs were measured and clinical observations were made on days 0 (the day before beginning treatment), 7, 15, 22, and 30; laboratory tests were conducted on days 0, 30, and 37 (one week after the end of treatment). Fifteen volunteers were withdrawn from the study for various reasons; none of these volunteers withdrew because of adverse reactions. There were no significant differences among the treatment groups in vital signs (oral temperature, body weight, pulse rate, blood pressure) or clinical laboratory test results (clinical chemistry, hematology, and urinalysis tests) for any of the observation times. In this study, 50 mg of phenylpropanolamine, with or without aspirin, taken four times daily for up to 30 days produced no significant elevation of blood pressure and no change in pulse rate compared to placebo treatment. The results of this study substantiate the lack of adverse drug interactions between phenylpropanolamine and NSAIDs.

IMIPRAMINE

CASE 40. A 13-year-old white male had a 6-week history of sustained systemic hypertension and tachycardia (Rumack et al., 1974). The patient had been taking

Tofranil (50 mg of imipramine hydrochloride) for enuresis together with Ornade Spansules, for chronic allergic rhinitis. Reserpine and phenoxybenzamine hydrochloride were ineffective in controlling the hypertension and tachycardia. When admitted to the hospital, his blood pressure was 144/90 mm Hg and sleeping pulse rate 110/min. His urinary vanillylmandelic acid (VMA) was 40 mg/liter. Otherwise his physical examination and clinical laboratory data were within normal limits. There was no family history of hypertension. Even though all medication was discontinued, the hypertension and tachycardia persisted for 7 days. After discharge from the hospital, 4 weeks after discontinuing the drugs, he had a blood pressure of 114/74 mm Hg, sleeping pulse rate of 86/min, and urinary VMA of 1.3 mg/liter. At that time, 50 mg of imipramine hydrochloride and one spansule of 8 mg of chlorpheniramine hydrochloride and 50 mg of phenylpropanolamine hydrochloride, each once per day, were reinstituted. After 3 weeks, the hypertension and tachycardia returned, so the drugs were discontinued immediately. These drugs singly or in combination were avoided, and neither hypertension nor tachycardia recurred in the subsequent 3 years.

THIORIDAZINE

A death attributed to ventricular arrhythmia induced by thioridazine in combination with a single Contac.C capsule has been reported (Chouinard et al., 1978).

CASE 41. A 27-year-old woman in good physical health had been hospitalized four times since first diagnosed as schizophrenic at the age of 17. Previous therapy included first trifluoperazine, then electroconvulsive treatment, followed by levomepromazine with perphenazine and trihexyphenidyl. Later when she was prescribed chlorpromazine and procyclidine, she developed a photosensitivity reaction. At that time her electrocardiogram showed sinus tachycardia with a heart rate of 110/min. Then 12 weeks later her ECG showed sinus tachycardia (heart rate 115/min) and a grade 1 T-wave abnormality with decreased amplitude in leads V_4, V_5, and V_6.

When she exhibited agitation and bizarre behavior 5 months later, she was given haloperidol, levomepromazine, and methyprylon. A month later, because of apparent akathisia, other medications were discontinued and she was prescribed thioridazine and procyclidine. A month later, at the time of her last follow-up, she was taking 100 mg of thioridazine and 2.5 mg of procyclidine b.i.d. Two days later she was given the usual dose of thioridazine and, because she was complaining of nasal congestion, a single capsule of Contac.C (4 mg of chlorpheniramine maleate and 50 mg of phenylpropanolamine hydrochloride). Approximately 2 hr later she was found dead in bed. Autopsy showed evidence of respiratory insufficiency, pulmonary congestion and edema, and pulmonary aspiration. Thioridazine concentrations were 0.5 mg/dl in blood and 1.1 mg/100g in liver. Death was attributed to ventricular fibrillation.

There are many factors involved in this case, and the cause of death may be attributed to any one of, or a combination of, several factors. Although the author attributed this death to ventricular arrhythmia induced by thioridazine in combination with a single capsule of Contac.C, the relationship appears dubious. In fact, Wendkos (1979) reported that repeat doses of Ornade (the same ingredients as in Contac.C) in psychiatric patients receiving 600–800 mg/day of thioridazine did not result in untoward effects. The blood and liver levels of thioridazine in this patient were within the toxic range, and it is possible that this patient had surreptitiously taken additional thioridazine tablets, resulting in death due to a drug overdose. Finally, it is possible that the death of this patient, who had a history of cardiac abnormalities, was due to spontaneous ventricular fibrillation unrelated to any medication.

AMPHETAMINE

CASE 42.   A 12-year-old boy in good physical health and no known allergy was included in a double-blind crossover study to compare the effects of two stimulant drugs in the treatment of hyperkinetic children (Huestis & Arnold, 1974). Levoamphetamine, placebo, and dextroamphetamine were each administered for 4 weeks. Levoamphetamine, to which he had an excellent response, was judged best by parents, teacher, and clinician; therefore, levoamphetamine succinate, 42 mg/day, was prescribed for maintenance therapy.

The boy's father had observed that for 2 days the drug seemed to be ineffective; it was revealed that he had taken five Contac cold capsules in those 2 days. Later the boy's grandmother noted that he had 3 difficult days during a long visit with her. He had been given nine Allerest tablets during those 3 days for an upper respiratory inflammation. On both occasions, the boy returned to his previous level of improved behavior after the other medications were discontinued.

The two common ingredients of these two medications are phenylpropanolamine and chlorpheniramine maleate. The authors stated that one or both of these agents might have been responsible for the unexpected neutralization of the amphetamine-induced behavioral improvement. Phenylpropanolamine, although in the same general class of drugs as amphetamine, has more decongestant activity and much weaker CNS activity than levoamphetamine and may have competitively inhibited the absorption or action of levoamphetamine. Chloropheniramine belongs to the same drug class (antihistamines) as diphenhydramine, which has been reported beneficial in the treatment of hyperkinetic children. However, diphenhydramine is an ethanolamine, while chlorpheniramine is an alkylamine. The alkylamines are not so prone to induce drowsiness, but side effects involving CNS stimulation are more common in this group of antihistamines. The chlorpheniramine side effects may have neutralized the levoamphetamine activity.

CASE 43.   A 24-year-old obese, female black college student was taken to a psychiatric clinic because of bizarre behavior (Tornatore & Gilderman, 1982). Over the previous 2 days she had stopped eating and would not leave her bedroom even to use the bathroom. The subject was suspicious, frightened, and delusional, although her orientation, memory, and intellectual functions were intact. She was diagnosed as schizophrenic, hospitalized, and given 10 mg of haloperidol t.i.d. There was no history of psychiatric treatment or family history of mental illness. She was discharged after 4 days and referred to an outpatient clinic for follow-up, where she discussed troublesome side effects from the haloperidol. On further questioning she revealed that she had been taking a prescription amphetamine and a nonprescription phenylpropanolamine-containing appetite suppressant, both taken until 2 weeks before her hospitalization. Her diagnosis was changed from schizophrenia to drug-induced organic mental disorder, and the dosage of haloperidol was reduced without any futher side effects. When seen 8 months later the patient had no further symptoms.

THEOPHYLLINE

In one report, ingestion of a combination product containing phenylpropanolamine and caffeine plus illicit drugs containing barbiturates and amphetamine was associated with elevation of serum theophylline levels in an asthmatic patient, leading to theophylline toxicity. It is impossible to determine which of these drugs was responsible for the interaction with theophylline.

CASE 44.   A 17-year-old girl was hospitalized for management of severe steroid-dependent asthma (Szefler et al., 1984). Her asthma medications were theophylline, prednisone, beclomethasone (by inhaler), metaproterenol (by respiratory nebulizer), atropine, and cromolyn. During her hospitalization she experienced an episode of headache, abdominal pain, and emesis. A blood sample was taken and the serum theophylline level was 63 μg/ml (the therapeutic range is 5–20 μg/ml); the prior theophylline dose had been administered 12 hr previously. She was treated with activated charcoal which induced vomiting. The elimination of theophylline was determined from serial blood samples; the level fell below 10 μg/ml approximately 20 hr after administration of the activated charcoal. The terminal elimination half-life was calculated to be 5.5 hr; this was similar to the theophylline half-life measured for this patient in a previous evaluation.

Several potential causes of the elevated theophylline levels were considered. Drug interaction with her other therapeutic medications was unlikely because none of them inhibits theophylline metabolism. There was no evidence of impaired liver function. The patient denied taking additional theophylline doses or an intentional overdose.

The patient admitted she had been taking Extra Strength Dexatrim (75 mg of phenylpropanolamine and 200 mg of caffeine) during the previous week. She also admitted taking illicit drugs ("black beauties" and "yellow jackets" possibly containing barbiturates and amphetamines) 48 hr prior to the onset of theophylline toxicity. No analysis of the illicit drugs was performed. No analysis for barbiturates or amphetamine in the patient's serum was performed; no caffeine was present in the serum.

MISCELLANEOUS DRUG INTERACTIONS

Table 4.14 shows a list of potential drug interactions with phenylpropanolamine listed in the reference book *Evaluations of Drug Interactions* (Shinn et al., 1985). Of these drug interactions, only two—tranylcypromine and indomethacin—are rated as clinically significant. Most of the other drugs listed are included not because interactions with phenylpropanolamine per se have been demonstrated, but because of similarities between phenylpropanolamine and drugs known to interact with the compounds listed in Table 4.14.

TABLE 4.14. Potential Drug Interactions With Phenylpropanolamine

Category	Drug
Highly clinically significant	Tranylcypromine
Clinically significant	Indomethacin
Not specified	Bethanidine
	Chlorpromazine
	Dicumarol
	Fenoprofen
	Furazolidone
	Halothane
	Hydrochlorothiazide
	Ibuprofen
	Insulin
	Isocarboxazid
	Lithium carbonate
	Meclofenamate
	Mefenamic acid
	Methyldopa
	Methyldopa, oxprenolol, acetaminophen
	Maproxen
	Nonsteroidal antiinflammatory agents
	Phenylbutazone
	Pargyline
	Phenelzine
	Phenylbutazone
	Piroxicam
	Procarbazine
	Propoxyphene
	Reserpine
	Sulindac
	Tolmetin

Source: From Shinn et al. (1985).

OVERVIEW OF PHENYLPROPANOLAMINE SAFETY

Safety evaluation inevitably involves estimating risk, and assessing risk requires the identification of adverse effects or toxicity. Responsible safety evaluation requires quantitative estimates of toxicity, for, as Paracelsus (1493–1541) noted, "All substances are poisons; there is none which is not a poison. The right dose differentiates a poison and a remedy."

From the foregoing data review, two kinds of adverse effects emerge as important in the evaluation of phenylpropanolamine safety: those involving the cardiovascular system and those involving the central nervous system (CNS). The following sections aim at synthesizing the data and, from those data, estimating the risk involved when phenylpropanolamine is ingested. Morgan's book (1986) provides a more extensive critique of adverse reactions and overdoses involving phenylpropanolamine.

CARDIOVASCULAR TOXICITY

Phenylpropanolamine was originally developed as a phenylethylamine derivative. Two principal actions of phenylethylamines are elevating blood pressure and accelerating heart rate. Thus, phenylpropanolamine, as a phenylethylamine derivative, can be predicted, *as a function of the dose,* to act on the cardiovascular system. The questions that need to be addressed are: What is the (minimum) dose of phenylpropanolamine that produces a clinically significant elevation of blood pressure? What is the relationship between therapeutic dose and toxic dose? How frequently do people experience toxicity?

Clinical trials provide the most compelling and scientifically reliable evidence regarding the potential cardiovascular toxicity of phenylpropanolamine. More than 50 clinical trials involving approximately 3000 volunteers have tested the cardiovascular effects of phenylpropanolamine; Table 4.8 summarizes the published studies. The dose of phenylpropanolamine in these trials ranged from 25 to 250 mg given as single doses, and from 75 to 200 mg/day in repeated-dose studies. In these controlled studies, single doses greater than 50 mg of phenylpropanolamine as an immediate-release formulation produced moderate increases in blood pressure (e.g., 100 mg of phenylpropanolamine increased blood pressure approximately 15 to 25 mm Hg). On the other hand, repeated daily dosing with as much as 200 mg/day of phenylpropanolamine in sustained-release formulation produced no clinically significant increase in blood pressure. Furthermore, in uncontrolled studies, patients were given phenylpropanolamine doses as high as 48 mg every 3 hr for 2 days; no significant increase in blood pressure was observed. It appears that phenylpropanolamine, taken at recommended doses for up to 2 months, is unlikely to produce significant cardiovascular toxicity. Even at higher-than-recommended doses, sustained-release phenyl-propanolamine formulations produced no significant elevation of blood pressure.

Additional evidence regarding the cardiovascular toxicity of phenylpropanolamine comes from case reports of adverse drug reactions and overdoses. One-hundred-eight such case reports have been published: 63 cases of adverse reactions and 45 overdose cases.[a] Most of these cases were reported after 1965. Cardiovascular effects were involved in 74/107 cases. These effects ranged from subjective report of palpitations and headache, to clinically confirmed elevation of blood pressure with either increased or decreased heart rate, cardiac arrhythmia, cardiac arrest, or cerebrovascular hemorrhage. In acute adverse reactions and overdoses, the dose of phenylpropanolamine ranged from 25 to more than 3000 mg; no relationship between the dose and intensity of the cardiovascular responses can be discerned. Undoubtedly, some adverse reactions to phenylpropanolamine at recommended doses were idiosyncratic responses (i.e., rare and peculiar individual reactions) such as may occur with any drug. In addition, many of these cases involved combination drug products and, therefore, it is impossible to attribute the effects solely to phenylpropanolamine (or any other of the drugs in the formulation). Furthermore, in most of the cases no tests were conducted to confirm the presence of phenylpropanolamine in blood or urine.

In most of the cases, the cardiovascular reactions were relatively mild and brief. Most patients required no medical treatment, and the symptoms resolved within a few hours.

However, a few of the reported cardiovascular adverse reactions and overdose effects were severe. Thirteen cases of cerebrovascular hemorrhage and nine fatalities have been reported. Products containing phenylpropanolamine alone were involved in only three cases: One person had diabetes, one was taking a prescription MAO inhibitor for a preexisting psychiatric disturbance, and one took an overdose (five appetite suppressant capsules, dose not specified). The other cases involved ingestion of combination products (phenylpropanolamine and caffeine, decongestant products, look-alike stimulants; four cases each); thus the toxicity cannot be attributed solely to phenylpropanolamine. The dose of phenylpropanolamine appears to be unrelated to the clinical outcome in these cases. One fatality occurred in a woman (a diabetic) who reportedly took one 75-mg phenylpropanolamine capsule a day for 2 days; at the other extreme, in a suicide attempt one man took an estimated 3000–3750 mg of phenylpropanolamine plus pseudoephedrine and an-

---

[a]These figures do not include the adverse drug reactions to the Australian drug Trimolets because Trimolets most likely was formulated with a phenylpropanolamine isomer rather than phenylpropanolamine itself.

tihistamines, developed an intracerebral hematoma, but survived and recovered completely. These examples demonstrate the extreme variability in the case reports.

Finally, the number of adverse drug reactions and overdose cases must be balanced against the total phenylpropanolamine consumption by the general public. It has been estimated that approximately 3–5 billion doses of phenylpropanolamine are consumed annually in the United States. By comparison, only 108 adverse reactions and overdose cases have been reported in over 20 years. It is impossible to estimate how many adverse reactions are unreported. Nonetheless, the number of adverse reactions must be a very small fraction of the total number of doses consumed.

Thus, the results of extensive clinical trials demonstrate that phenylpropanolamine is unlikely to produce clinically significant cardiovascular toxicity when administered at recommended doses. In rare instances cardiovascular adverse reactions occur even at recommended doses, and cardiovascular reactions do occur in overdose cases.

Are there, then, other factors that influence an individual's susceptibility to phenylpropanolamine toxicity? Certainly, simultaneous ingestion of other medications, especially MAO inhibitors, can increase the cardiovascular response to phenylpropanolamine. Preexisting disease conditions such as cardiovascular disease may increase the risk of phenylpropanolamine toxicity. However, in a controlled clinical trial phenylpropanolamine produced no significant elevation of blood pressure in patients with controlled, stable hypertension. Finally, the pattern of use and the pharmaceutical formulation also influence the cardiovascular toxicity of phenylpropanolamine.

CNS TOXICITY

Another important issue to consider is the potential central nervous system (CNS) toxicity of phenylpropanolamine. Phenylpropanolamine is often described in the medical literature as an "amphetamine-like" CNS stimulant. This is a mistake. While it is true that phenylpropanolamine and amphetamine have similar chemical structures, the pharmacologic properties of the two drugs are quite different. Both phenylpropanolamine and amphetamine are phenylethylamine derivatives. Some phenylethylamines stimulate the CNS; others do not. For orally administered phenylethylamines, the CNS-stimulating potency depends largely on drug distribution: If a drug is to act on the CNS it must first cross the blood-brain barrier and enter the brain. Blood-brain barrier transport depends largely on the drug's lipid solubility. Since phenylpropanolamine is highly water soluble but poorly lipid soluble it is unlikely to cross the blood-brain barrier. Furthermore, in animal studies phenylpropanolamine has low potency for CNS stimulation, producing CNS effects only at very high, near-lethal doses.

Thus, there is reason to question whether phenylpropanolamine produces CNS toxicity. *As a function of the dose,* will phenylpropanolamine stimulate the CNS? As with cardiovascular toxicity, the questions to be answered are: What is the (minimum) dose of phenylpropanolamine that stimulates the CNS? And, what is the relationship between therapeutic dose and toxic dose?

Compared to the extensive clinical studies of cardiovascular toxicity of phenylpropanolamine, fewer studies have tested the potential for CNS toxicity. Several large-scale clinical safety studies have been conducted to evaluate whether phenylpropanolamine changes affective state or mood, to determine the subjective rating of drug effects, and to assess phenylpropanolamine's abuse liability. In these studies phenylpropanolamine has uniformly produced minimal CNS effects and very low abuse liability. Studies in experimental animals likewise demonstrate that phenylpropanolamine has very low abuse liability. Furthermore, the incidence of CNS side effects has been consistently low in extensive clinical efficacy studies.

Of the 108 adverse drug reactions and overdose cases, 64 cases involved CNS effects. Most of the cases involved acute phenylpropanolamine ingestion at doses ranging from 25 to approximately 2500 mg. Most of the CNS reactions occurred at lower doses of phenylpropanolamine (usually 100 mg or less); the CNS toxicity appears to be unrelated to the dose ingested.

The most frequently reported CNS effects were nervousness, hallucinations, psychotic episodes, and seizures. As with the cardiovascular toxicity, these effects usually were relatively brief. In most patients, the symptoms abated in a few hours without medical treatment. It should be noted that several of the patients had histories of psychiatric disturbance or drug abuse, suggesting that people with preexisting psychiatric or neurologic conditions may be predisposed to phenylpropanolamine-induced CNS reactions.

Many of the adverse reactions and overdose cases involved combination products that contained other CNS-active drugs: caffeine, ephedrine, antihistamines, or belladonna alkaloids. These components undoubtedly contribute to the reported CNS toxicity.

Thus, clinical efficacy studies demonstrate that most individuals taking recommended doses of phenylpropanolamine experience no significant CNS stimulation; however, some individuals do have idiosyncratic responses. Furthermore, clinical safety studies demonstrate that phenylpropanolamine produces minimal CNS stimulation and has very low abuse potential. Analysis of the adverse drug reaction and overdose case reports reveals that phenylpropanolamine is associated with a low incidence of CNS stimulation. People with preexisting neurologic or psychiatric conditions may be at higher risk for phenylpropanolamine-related CNS toxicity.

REFERENCES

Achor, M. B., & Extein, I. (1981). Diet aids, mania, and affective illness (Letter). *Am J Psychiatry, 138,* 392.

Altschuler, S., Conte, A., Sebok, M., Marlin, R. L., & Winick, C. (1982). Three controlled trials of weight loss with phenylpropanolamine. *Internatl J Obes, 6,* 549-556.

Aselton, P., Jick, H., & Hunter, J. R. (1985a). Phenylpropanolamine exposure and subsequent hospitalization. *JAMA, 253,* 977.

Aselton, P., Jick, H., Milunsky, A., Hunter, J. R., & Stergachis, A. (1985b). First-trimester drug use and congenital disorders. *Obstet Gynecol, 65,* 451-455.

Bale, J. F., Fountain, M. T., & Shaddy, R. (1984). Phenylpropanolamine-associated CNS complications in children and adolescents. *Am J Dis Child, 138,* 683-685.

Barrett, W. E., Hanigan, J. J., & Snyder, D. L. (1981). The bioavailability of sustained-release tablets which contain phenylpropanolamine and chlorpheniramine. *So Curr Ther Res, 30,* 640-654.

Bennett, W. M. (1979). Hazards of the appetite suppressant phenylpropanolamine (Letter). *Lancet, 2,* 42-43.

Bernstein, E., & Diskant, B. M. (1982). Phenylpropanolamine: A potentially hazardous drug. *Ann Emerg Med, 11,* 311-315.

Biaggioni, I., Onron, J., Parrish, C. K., & Robertson, D. (1986). Marked hypertensive effect of low dose phenylpropanolamine, an over-the-counter appetite suppressant, in subjects with autonomic impairment. Presented at the American Heart Association Meeting, Nov. 17–20, 1986, Dallas, Texas.

Bigelow, G. E. (1985). Quantitative assessment of mood and behavioral reinforcing effect of phenylpropanolamine. In J. P. Morgan, D. V. Kagan, and J. S. Brody (Eds.). *Phenylpropanolamine: Risks, Benefits, and Controversies,* Clinical Pharmacology and Therapeutics Series, Vol. 5. Praeger Scientific, New York (pp. 328-342).

Bigelow, G. E., Brady, J. B., Griffiths, R. R., Stitzer, M. L., Ator, N. A., Higgins, S. T., Liebson, I. A., & Lucas, S. E. (1985). Progress report from the Division of Behavioral Biology, John Hopkins University School of Medicine. In L. S. Harris (Ed.). *Problems of Drug Dependence: 1984.* NIDA Research Monograph Series. U.S. Government Printing Office, Washington (pp. 66-75).

Bigelow, G. E., Liebson, I. A., Griffiths, R., Trieber, R., & Nowowieski, P. (1984). Assessment of phenylpropanolamine (PPA) abuse risk in weight control patients [Abstract]. *Proceedings of the Federation of Am Soc Exp Biol, 43,* 571.

Black, N. J. (1937). The control of allergic manifestations by phenylpropanolamine (Propadrine) hydrochloride. *Lancet, 57,* 101-102.

Boyer, W. E. (1938). The clinical use of phenylpropanolamine hydrochloride (Propadrine) in the treatment of allergic conditions. *J. Allergy, 9,* 509-513.

Bradley, M. H., & Raines, J. (1987). Single-blind pilot and double-blind follow-up evaluations of the safety and efficacy of phenylpropanolamine HCl in obese patients with controlled hypertension. *New Engl J Med* (in press).

Broms, P., & Malm, L. (1982). Oral vasoconstrictors in perennial non-allergic rhinitis. *Allergy, 37,* 67-74.

Burton, B. T., Rice, M., & Schmertzler, L. E. (1985). Atrioventricular block following overdose of decongestant cold medication. *J Emerg Med, 2,* 415-419.

Caperton, E. (1983). Raynaud's phenomenon. Role of diet pills and cold remedies. *Postgrad Med, 73,* 291-292.

Castellani, S. (1985). Catatonia associated with phenylpropanolamine overdose and fluphenazine treatment: Case report. *J Clin Psychiatr, 46,* 288-289.

Chait, L. D., Uhlenhuth, E. H., & Johanson, C. E. (1984). Drug preference and mood in humans: Mazindol and phenylpropanolamine. In L. S. Harris (Ed.). *Problems of Drug Dependence: 1984.* NIDA Research Monograph Series. U.S. Government Printing Office, Washington (pp. 327-328).

Chait, L. D., Uhlenhuth, E. H., & Johanson, C. E. (1986). The discriminative stimulus and subjective effects of phenylpropanolamine, mazindol and *d*-amphetamine in humans. *Pharmacol Biochem Behav, 24,* 1665-1672.

Chouinard, G., Ghadirian, A. M., & Jones, B. D. (1978). Death attributed to ventricular arrhythmia induced by thioridazine in combination with a single Contac C capsule. *Can Med Assoc, 119,* 729-730.

Clark, J. E., & Simon, W. A. (1983). Cardiac arrhythmias after phenylpropanolamine ingestion. *Drug Intell Clin Pharm, 17,* 737-738.

Cornelius, J. R., Soloff, P. H., & Reynolds, C. F., 3rd. (1984). Paranoia, homicidal behavior, and seizures associated with phenylpropanolamine. *Am J Psychiatry, 141,* 120-121.

Cuthbert, M. F., Greenberg, M. P., & Morley, S. W. (1969). Cough and cold remedies: A potential danger to patients on monoamine oxidase inhibitors. *Br Med J, 1,* 404-406.

Cuthbert, M. F., & Vere, D. W. (1971). Potentiation of the cardiovascular effects of some catecholamines by a monoamine oxidase inhibitor. *Br J Pharmacol, 43,* 471p-472p.

Cutting, W. C. (1943). The treatment of obesity. *J Clin Endocrinol, 3,* 85-88.

Davis, W. M., & Pinkerton, J. T., 3rd. (1972). Synergism by atropine of central stimulant properties of phenylpropanolamine. *Toxicol Appl Pharmacol, 22,* 130-145.

Deocampo, P. (1979). Convulsive seizures due to phenylpropanolamine. *J Med Soc NJ, 76,* 591-592.

Dietz, A. J., Jr. (1981). Amphetamine-like reactions to phenylpropanolamine. *JAMA, 245,* 601-602.

Dreisbach, R. H. (Ed.) (1983). *Handbook of Poisoning: Diagnosis and Treatment,* 11th ed. Lange Medical Publications, Los Altos, CA.

Duffy, W. B., Senekjian, H. O., Knight, T. F., Gyorkey, F., & Weinman, E. J. (1981). Acute renal failure due to phenylpropanolamine. *South Med J, 74,* 1548-1549.

Dungal, H., & Griffiths, D. E. (1984). Visual hallucinations induced by a sympathomimetic drug. *Can Med Assoc J, 131,* 1186.

Duvernoy, W. F. (1969). Positive phentolamine test in hypertension induced by a nasal decongestant. *New Engl J Med, 280,* 877.

Ekins, B. R., & Spoerke, B. G., Jr. (1983). An estimation of the toxicity of non-prescription diet aids from seventy exposure cases. *Vet Hum Toxicol, 25,* 81-85.

Elliott, C. F., & Whyte, J. C. (1981). Phenylpropanolamine and hypertension. *Med J Aust, 1,* 715.

Fairchild, M. D., & Alles, G. A. (1967). The central locomotor stimulatory activity and acute toxicity of the ephedrine and norephedrine isomers in mice. *J Pharmacol Exp Ther, 158,* 135-139.

Fallis, R. J., & Fisher, M. (1985). Cerebral vasculitis and hemorrhage associated with phenylpropanolamine. *Neurology, 35,* 405-407.

Federal Register (1976). Establishment of a monograph for OTC cold, cough, allergy, broncho-dilator and antiasthmatic drug products. Docket No. 76N-0052. (Reference 10. Pugliese, P.T., "Sine-Aid II. Human Safety Study," Draft of unpublished data is included in OTC Volume 040298).

Federal Register (1983). Enforcement action under the new drug provisions of the Federal, Food, Drug and Cosmetic act; Certain OTC drug products; Advisory opinion. Docket No. 83A-0339.

Frewin, D. B., Leonello, P. P., & Frewin, M. E. (1978). Hypertension after ingestion of Trimo-lets. *Med J Aust, 2,* 497-498.

Gibson, G. J., & Warrell, D. A. (1972). Hypertensive crises and phenylpropanolamine. *Lancet, 2,* 492-493.

Gilmer, G., Swartz, M., Teske, M., & Crandall, A. S. (1986). Over-the-counter phenylpropa-nolamine: A possible cause of central retinal vein occlusion. *Arch Ophthalmol, 104,* 642.

Goodman, R. P., Wright, J. T., Jr., Barlascini, C. O., McKenney, J. M., & Lambert, C. M. (1986). The effect of phenylpropanolamine on ambulatory blood pressure. *Clin Pharmacol Ther, 40,* 144-147.

Gosselin, R. E., Smith, R. P., & Hodge, H. C. (1984). *Clinical Toxicology of Commercial Prod-ucts: Acute Poisoning,* 5th ed., Williams & Wilkins, Baltimore.

Griboff, S. I., Berman, R., & Silverman, H. I. (1975). A double blind clinical evaluation of a phenylpropanolamine-caffeine-vitamin combination and a placebo in the treatment of exoge-nous obesity. *Curr Ther Res, 17,* 535-543.

Grigg, J. R., & Goyer, P. R. (1986). Phenylpropanolamine anorexiants and affective disorders. *Mil Med, 151,* 387-388.

Groves, W. G., Macko, E., & Saunders, L. Z. (1970). Pharmacological and toxicological study of a pharmaceutical combination of phenylpropanolamine-isopropamide and chlor-pheniramine. *Boll Chim Farm, 109,* 132-154.

Hampel, G., Horstkotte, H., & Rumpf, K. W. (1983). Myoglobinuric renal failure due to drug induced rhabdomyolysis. *Hum Toxicol, 2,* 197-203.

Hartung, W. H. (1945). Sympathomimetic agents; beta-phenthylamine derivatives. *Ind Eng Chem, 37,* 126-137.

Hartung, W. H., & Munch, J. C. (1929). Amino alcohols. I. Phenylpropanolamine and *para-*tolylpropanolamine. *J Am Chem Soc, 51,* 2262-2266.

Heinonen, O. P., Slone, D., & Shapiro, S. (1977). *Birth Defects and Drugs in Pregnancy.* Bos-ton: Publishing Sciences Group.

Higgins, J. T., Oppenheimer, E. Y., & Gershman, M. (1985). Phenylpropanolamine-associated headache. *Am J Dis Child, 139,* 331.

Hill, R. M., & Tennyson, L. M. (1985). The effect of maternal allergy medications on the fetus. *Immunol Allergy Pract, 7,* 80-91.

Hoebel, B. G., Cooper, J., Kamin, M.-C., & Willard, D. (1975). Appetite suppression by phen-ylpropanolamine in humans. *Obesity/Bariatric Med, 4,* 192-197.

Horowitz, J. D., Lang, W. J., Howes, L. G., Fennessy, M. R., Christophidis, N., Rand, M. J., & Louis, W. J. (1980). Hypertensive responses induced by phenylpropanolamine in anorectic and decongestant preparations. *Lancet, 1,* 60-61.

Horowitz, J. D., McNeil, J. J., Sweet, B., Mendelsohn, F. A., & Louis, W. J. (1979). Hyperten-sion and postural hypotension induced by phenylpropanolamine (Trimolets). *Med J Austr, 1,* 175-176.

Howrie, D. L., & Wolfson, J. H. (1983). Phenylpropanolamine-induced hypertensive seizures. *J Pediatr, 102,* 143-145.

Huestis, R. D., & Arnold, L. E. (1974). Possible antagonism of amphetamine by decongestant-antihistamine compounds. *J Pediatr, 85,* 579-580.

Hyams, J. S., Leichtner, A. M., Breiner, R. G., Hill, D. W., McComb, R. B., & Manger, W. M. (1985). Pseudopheochromocytoma and cardiac arrest associated with phenylpropanolamine. *JAMA, 253,* 1609-1610.

Jackson, C., Hart, A., & Robinson, M. D. (1985). Fatal intracranial hemorrhage associated with phenylpropanolamine, pentazocine, and tripelennamine overdose. *J Emerg Med, 3,* 127-132.

James, C. R. H., & Price, N. C. (1984). Bilateral acute angle closure glaucoma after phenylpropanolamine. *Br Med J, 288,* 1346.

Jick, H., Aselton, P., & Hunter, J. R. (1984). Phenylpropanolamine and cerebral hemorrhage. *Lancet, 2,* 1017.

Jick, H., Holmes, L. B., Hunter, J. R., Madsen, S., & Stergachis, A. (1981). First-trimester drug use and congenital disorders. *JAMA, 246,* 343-346.

Johnson, D. A, Etter, H. S., & Reeves, D. M. (1983). Stroke and phenylpropanolamine use (Letter). *Lancet, 2,* 970.

Johnson, D. A., Stafford, P. W., & Volpe, R. J. (1985). Ischemic bowel infarction and phenylpropanolamine use. *West J Med, 142,* 399-400.

Kane, F. J., Jr., & Green, B. Q. (1966). Psychotic episodes associated with the use of common proprietary decongestants. *Am J Psychiatry, 123,* 484-487.

Katz, N. L., Hare, M., Davis, J. M., & Schlemmer, R. F., Jr. (1985a). Comparison of racemic phenylpropanolamine (PPA) with its (+)-isomer on spontaneous locomotor activity in rats [Abstract]. *Proceedings of the Federation of Am Soc Exp Biol, 45,* 429.

Katz, N. L., King, M., Jazwiec, N., Williams, E. A., Davis, J. M., & Schlemmer, R. F., Jr. (1985b). Adrenergic blockade antagonizes the lethality in rats by phenylpropanolamine (PPA) alone and in combination with caffeine (C) [Abstract]. *Proceedings of the Federation of Am Soc Exp Biol, 44,* 1637.

Kikta, D. G., Devereaux, M. W., & Chandar, K. (1985). Intracranial hemorrhages due to phenylpropanolamine. *Stroke, 16,* 510-512.

King, J. (1979). Hypertension and cerebral hemorrhage after Trimolets ingestion (Letter). *Med J Aust, 2,* 258.

Kizer, K. W. (1984). Intracranial hemorrhage associated with overdose of decongestant containing phenylpropanolamine. *Am J Emerg Med, 2,* 180-181.

Knochel, J. P., & Carter, N. W. (1976). The role of muscle cell injury in the pathogenesis of acute renal failure after exercise. *Kidney Internatl, 10,* (suppl), 58-64.

Knochel, J. P., Dotin, L. N., & Hamburger, R. J. (1974). Heat stress, exercise, and muscle injury: Effects on urate metabolism and renal function. *Ann Int Med, 81,* 321-328.

Koffler, A., Friedler, R. M., & Massry, S. G. (1976). Acute renal failure due to nontraumatic rhabdomyolysis. *Ann Int Med, 85,* 23-28.

Krakoff, L. R. (1985). Review of recent studies on the effect of phenylpropanolamine on systemic arterial blood pressure in human subjects. In J. P. Morgan, D. V. Kagan, and J. S. Brody (Eds.). *Phenylpropanolamine: Risks, Benefits, and Controversies,* Clinical Pharmacology and Therapeutics Series, Vol. 5. Praeger Scientific, New York (pp. 210-222).

Krosnick, A., Eppel, N., & Hoebel, B. G. (1982). Negative results with phenylpropanolamine in hyperglycemic patients. Presented at the Third Annual Regional Meeting of the Philadelphia, Delaware, and New Jersey Chapters of the Society for Neuroscience, Philadelphia, Pa.

Krupka, L. R., & Vener, A. M. (1983). Over-the-counter appetite suppressants containing phenylpropanolamine hydrochloride (PPA) and the young adult: Usage and perceived effectiveness. *J Drug Educ, 13*, 141-152.

Lai, K-N., & Lai, D-L-S., (1982). Intracerebral hemorrhage associated with anorectic (phenylpropanolamine) abuse. *Bull Hong Kong Med Assoc, 34*, 133-135.

Lake, C. R., Tenglin, R., Chernow, B., & Holloway, H. C. (1983). Psychomotor stimulant-induced mania in a genetically predisposed patient: A review of the literature and report of a case. *J Clin Psychopharmacol, 3*, 97-100.

Larson, W. L., & Rogers, A. (1986). Overdosage from phenylpropanolamine: Experience of the hennepin regional poison center. *Vet Hum Toxicol, 28*, 546-548.

Lee, K. Y., Beilin, L. J., & Vandongen, R. (1980). Severe hypertension following ingestion of an appetite suppressant (phenylpropanolamine) with indomethacin. *Aust NZ J Med, 10*, 122.

Lewith, G. T., & Davidson, F. (1981). Dystonic reactions to Dimotapp elixir. *J Royal Coll Gen Pract, 31*, 241.

Logie, A. W., & Scott, C. M. (1984). Fatal overdosage of phenylpropanolamine. *Br Med J, 289*, 591.

Loman, J., Rinkel, M., & Myerson, A. (1939). Comparative effects of amphetamine sulfate (benzedrine sulfate), paredrine and propadrine on the blood pressure. *Am Heart J, 18*, 89-93.

Lorhan, P. H., & Mosser, D. (1947). Phenylpropanolamine hydrochloride: Vasopressor drug, for maintaining blood pressure during spinal anesthesia. *Ann Surg, 125*, 171-176.

McDowell, J. R., & LeBlanc, H. J. (1985). Phenylpropanolamine and cerebral hemorrhage. *West J Med, 142*, 688-690.

McEwen, J. (1983). Phenylpropanolamine-associated hypertension after the use of 'over-the-counter' appetite-suppressant products. *South Med J, 2*, 71-73.

McLaren, E. H. (1976). Severe hypertension produced by interaction of phenylpropanolamine with methylidopa and oxprenolol. *Br Med J, 2*, 283-284.

McLaurin, J. W., Shipman, W. F., & Rosedale, R. (1961). Oral decongestants. *Laryngoscope, 71*, 54-67.

Mesnard, B., & Ginn, D. R. (1984). Excessive phenylpropanolamine ingestion followed by subarachnoid hemorrhage. *South Med J, 77*, 939.

Mitchell, C. A. (1968). Possible cardiovascular effect of phenylpropanolamine and belladonna alkaloids. *Curr Ther Res Clin Exp, 10*, 47-53.

Morgan, J. P. (1984). Problems of mass urine screening for misused drugs. *J Psychoact Drugs, 16*, 305-317.

Morgan, J. P. (1985a). Over-the-counter medication: Availability and issues. In J. P. Morgan, D. V. Kagan, and J. S. Brody (Eds.). *Phenylpropanolamine: Risks, Benefits, and Controversies*, Clinical Pharmacology and Therapeutics Series, Vol. 5. Praeger Scientific, New York (pp. 3-10).

Morgan, J. P. (1985b). Discussion. In J. P. Morgan, D. V. Kagan, and J. S. Brody (Eds.). *Phenylpropanolamine: Risks, Benefits, and Controversies*, Clinical Pharmacology and Therapeutics Series, Vol. 5. Praeger Scientific, New York (pp. 402-409).

Morgan, J. P. (1986). *Phenylpropanolamine: A Critical Analysis of Reported Adverse Reactions and Overdosage*. Jack K. Burgess, Inc., New Jersey.

Mueller, S. M. (1983). Neurologic complications of phenylpropranolamine use. *Neurology, 33*, 650-652.

Mueller, S. M., Graham, J. D. 2d., & Duggan, D. (1985). Neurologic signs and symptoms related to over-the-counter diet pills. *Indiana Med, 78*, 388-390.

Mueller, S. M., Muller, J., & Asdell, S. M. (1984). Cerebral hemorrhage associated with phenyl-propanolamine in combination with caffeine. *Stroke, 15,* 119-123.

Mueller, S. M., & Solow, E. B. (1982). Seizures associated with a new combination 'pick-me-up' pill (Letter). *Ann Neurol, 11,* 322.

Noble, R. E. (1982). Phenylpropanolamine and blood pressure (Letter). *Lancet, 1,* 1419.

Norvenius, G., Wilderlov, E., & Lonnerholm, G. (1979). Phenylpropanolamine and mental disturbances (Letter). *Lancet, 2,* 1367-1368.

Nuotto, E., & Seppala, T. (1984). Phenylpropanolamine counteracts diazepam effects in psychophysiological tests. *Curr Ther Res, 36,* 604-616.

Ostern, S., & Dodson, W. H. (1965). Hypertension following Ornade ingestion (Letter). *J Am Med Soc, 194,* 240.

Patterson, F. K. (1980). Delayed fatal outcome after possible Ru-Tuss overdose. *J Forens Sci, 25,* 349-352.

Paulman, P. M., Commers, J., & Goode, D. L. (1986). Leukocytosis following intravenous phenylpropanolamine use—possible association. *Nebr Med J, 71,* 40-41.

Penn, A. S., Rowland, L. P., & Fraser, D. W. (1972). Drugs, coma and myoglobinuria. *Arch Neurol, 26,* 336-343.

Pentel, P., Jentzen, J., Apple, F., & Sievert, J. (1984). Phenylpropanolamine (PPA)-induced myocardial necrosis in rats. *Vet Hum Toxicol, 26,* 402.

Pentel, P., & Mikell, F. (1982). Reaction to phenylpropalamine/chlorpheniramine/belladonna compound in a woman with unrecognised autonomic dysfunction (Letter). *Lancet, 2,* 274.

Pentel, P. R., Aaron, C., & Paya, C. (1985a). Therapeutic doses of phenylpropanolamine increase supine systolic blood pressure. *Int J Obes, 9,* 115-119.

Pentel, P. R., Asinger, R. W., & Benowitz, N. L. (1985b). Propranolol antagonism of phenylpropanolamine-induced hypertension. *Clin Pharmacol Ther, 37,* 488-494.

Pentel, P. R., Mikell, F. L., & Zavoral, J. H. (1982). Myocardial injury after phenylpropanolamine ingestion. *Br Heart J, 47,* 51-54.

Perkoff, G. T., Dioso, M. M., Bleisch, V., & Klinkerfuss, G. (1967). A spectrum of myopathy associated with alcoholism. I. Clinical and labortory features. *Ann Int Med, 67,* 481-492.

Peterson, R. B., & Vasquez, L. A. (1973). Phenylpropanolamine induced arrhythmias. *JAMA, 223,* 324-325.

Proctor, K. G., & Howards, S. S. (1983). The effect of sympathomimetic drugs on post-lymphadenectomy aspermia. *J Urol, 129,* 837-838.

Puar, H. S. (1984). Acute memory loss and nominal aphasia caused by phenylpropanolamine. *South Med J, 77,* 1604-1605.

Ratnasooriya, W. D., Gilmore, D. P., & Wadsworth, R. M. (1979). Antifertility effect of sympathomimetic drugs on male rats when applied locally to the vas deferens. *J Reprod Fertil, 56,* 643-651.

Ratnasooriya, W. D., Gilmore, D. P., & Wadsworth, R. M. (1980). Effect of local application of sympathomimetic drugs to the epididymis on fertility in rats. *J Reprod Fertil, 58,* 19-25.

Ratnasooriya, W. D., Gilmore, D. P., & Wadsworth, R. M. (1981). Effect of norephedrine locally applied to the vas deferens on semen quality of rabbits. *Indian J Exp Biol, 19,* 20-25.

Renvall, U., & Lindqvist, N. (1979). A double-blind clinical study with Monydrin tablets in patients with non-allergic rhinitis. *J Int Med Res, 7,* 235-239.

Richter, R. W., Challenor, Y. B., & Pearson, J. (1971). Acute myoglobinuria associated with heroin addiction. *JAMA, 216,* 1172-1176.

Rives, J. J., Olives, J. P., & Ghisolfi, J. (1985). Oesophagite aiguë médica menteuse. *Arch Fr Pediatr, 42,* 33-34.

Rosenblum, I., Wohl, A., & Stein, A. A. (1965). Studies in cardiac necrosis. I. production of cardiac lesions with sympathomimetic amines. *Toxicol App Pharmacol, 7,* 1-8.

Rumack, B. H., Anderson, R. J., Wolfe, R., Fletcher, E. C., & Vestal, B. K. (1974). Ornade and anticholinergic toxicity: hypertension, hallucinations and arrhythmias. *Clin Toxicol, 7,* 573-581.

Rumpf, K. W., Kaiser, H. F., Horstkotte, H., & Bahlmann, J. (1983). Rhabdomyolysis after ingestion of an appetite suppressant (Letter). *JAMA, 250,* 2112.

Ryan, J., Vargas, R., McMahon, F. G., & Gotzkowsky, S. (1987). Cardiovascular effects of phenylpropanolamine (PPA) [Abstract]. *Clin Pharm Ther, 41,* 179.

Salmon, P. R. (1965). Crisis with Eskornade (Letter). *Br Med J, 1,* 193.

Saltzman, M. B., Dolan, M. M., & Doyne, N. (1983). Comparison of effects of two dosage regimens of phenylpropanolamine on blood pressure and plasma levels in normal subjects under steady-state conditions. *Drug Intell Clin Pharm, 17,* 746-750.

Sandahl, B. (1985). A prospective study of drug use, smoking and contraceptives during early pregnancy. *Acta Obstet Gynecol Scand, 64,* 381-386.

Schaffer, C. B., & Pauli, M. W. (1980). Psychotic reaction caused by proprietary oral diet agents. *Am J Psychiatry, 137,* 1256-1257.

Schlemmer, R. F., Heinze, W. J., Asta, C. L., Katz, N. L., & Davis, J. M. (1984). Caffeine potentiates phenylpropanolamine (PPA) lethality but not motor behavior [Abstract]. *Proceedings of the Federation of Am Soc Exp Biol, 43,* 572.

Schrier, R. W., Henderson, H. S., Tischer, C. C., & Tannen, R. L. (1967). Neuropathy associated with heat stress and exercise. *Ann Int Med, 67,* 356-376.

Schuster, C. R., & Johanson, C. E. (1984). Anorectic drugs: Efficacy, reinforcing and discriminating aspects [Abstract]. *Proceedings of the Federation of Am Soc Exp Biol, 43,* 89.

Schuster, C. R., & Johanson, C. E. (1985). Efficacy, dependence potential and neurotoxicity of anorectic drugs. In L. S. Seiden and R. L. Balster (Eds.). *Behavioral Pharmacology: The Current Status,* Alan R. Liss, Inc., New York (pp. 263-279).

Sebok, M. (1985). A double-blinded, placebo-controlled, clinical study of the efficacy of a phenylpropanolamine/caffeine combination product as an aid to weight loss in adults. *Curr Ther Res, 37,* 701-708.

Seppala, T., Nuotto, E., & Korttila, K. (1981). Single and repeated dose comparison of three antihistamines and phenylpropanolamine: Psychomotor performance and subjective appraisals of sleep. *Br J Chem Pharmac, 12,* 179-188.

Shinn, A. F., Hogan, M. J., & Hebel, S. K. (1985). *Evaluations of Drug Interactions.* St. Louis, Mosby.

Silverman, H. I., Kreger, B. E., Lewis, G. P., Karabelas, A., Paone, R., & Foley, M. (1980). Lack of side effects from orally administered phenylpropanolamine and phenylpropanolamine with caffeine: A controlled three-phase study. *Curr Ther Res Clin Exp, 28,* 185-194.

Smookler, S., & Bermudez, A. J. (1982). Hypertensive crisis resulting from an MAO inhibitor and an over-the-counter appetite suppressant. *Ann Emerg Med, 11,* 482-484.

Speer, F., Carrasco, L. C., & Kimura, C. C. (1978). Allergy to phenylpropanolamine. *Ann Allergy, 40,* 32-34.

Stoessl, A. J., Young, G. B., & Feasby, T. E. (1985). Intracerebral hemorrhage and angiographic beading following ingestion of catecholaminergics. *Stroke, 16,* 734-736.

Sunshine, I. (Ed.) (1969). *Handbook of Analytical Toxicology*. Cleveland Chemical Rubber Company, Cleveland, OH.

Swenson, R. D., Golper, T. A., & Bennett, W. M. (1982). Acute renal failure and rhabdomyolysis after ingestion of phenylpropanolamine-containing diet pills. *JAMA, 248*, 1216.

Szefler, S. J., Rogers, R. J., & Strunk, R. C. (1984). Drug abuse and the asthmatic patient: a case report. *J Allergy Clin Immunol, 74*, 201-204.

Teh, A. Y. F. (1979). Phenylpropanolamine and hypertension. *Med J Aust, 2*, 425-426.

Terry, R., Kaye, A. H., & McDonald, M. (1975). Sinutab (Letter). *Med J Aust, 1*, 763.

Tornatore, F. L., & Gilderman, A. M. (1982). Substance induced organic mental disorders. *Am Pharmacy, NS22*, 43-46.

Traynelis, V. C., & Brick, J. F. (1986). Phenylpropanolamine and vasospasm. *Neurology, 36*, 593-594.

Unger, D. L., Unger, L., & Temple, D. E. (1967). Effect of an anti-asthmatic compound on blood pressure of hypertensive asthmatic patients. *Ann Allerg, 25*, 260-261.

Warren, M. R., & Werner, H. W. (1946a). Acute toxicity of vasopressor amines I. Effect of temperature. *J Pharmacol Exp Ther, 86*, 280-282.

Warren, M. R., & Werner, H. W. (1946b). Acute toxicity of vasopressor amines II. Comparative data. *J Pharm Exp Ther, 86*, 284-286.

Weesner, K. M., Denison, M., & Roberts, R. J. (1982). Cardiac arrhythmias in an adolescent following ingestion of an over-the-counter stimulant. *Clin Pediatr* (Philadelphia), *21*, 700-701.

Weintraub, M., Ginsberg, G., Stein, E. C., Sundaresan, P. R, Schuster, B., O'Connor, P., & Byrne, L. M. (1986). Phenylpropanolamine OROS (Acutrim) vs. placebo in combination with caloric restriction and physician-managed behavior modification. *Clin Pharmacol Ther, 39*, 501-509.

Weiss, L. R., & Vick, J. A. (1985). Heart rate monitoring as an indicator of acute toxicity of antiappetite drugs in rats [Abstract]. *Toxicologist, 5*, 112.

Wendkos, M. H. (1979). Death attributed to ventricular arrhythmia (Letter). *Can Med Assoc J, 190*, 1058-1060.

Wenger, A. P., & Lapsa, P. (1970). Three-way measurement of an oral nasal decongestant. *Clin Med, 77*, 15-18.

Wesson, D. R., & Morgan, J. P. (1982). Stimulant look-alikes. *NEWS, California Soc Treat Alcohol Other Drug Depend, 9*, 1-3.

Wharton, B. K. (1970). Nasal decongestants and paranoid psychosis. *Br J Psychiatry, 117*, 439-440.

Woo, O. F., Benowitz, N. L., Bialy, F. W., & Wengert, J. W. (1985). Atrioventricular conduction block caused by phenylpropanolamine. *JAMA, 253*, 2646-2647.

Woolverton, W. L., Johanson, C. E., de la Garza, R., Ellis, S., Seiden, L. S., & Schuster, C. R. (1986). Behavioral and neurochemical evaluation of phenylpropanolamine. *J Pharmacol Exp Ther, 237*, 926-930.

5

CLINICAL EFFICACY STUDIES

The studies of the clinical efficacy of phenylpropanolamine and phenylpropanolamine-containing products are reviewed in this chapter. The use of phenylpropanolamine in clinical medicine began shortly after the initial chemical synthesis of phenylpropanolamine during the second decade of this century (Chen et al., 1929) (see also Chapter 1, this volume) and the demonstration that this drug had marked effects on the nasal mucosa (Stockton et al., 1931) and various smooth muscles. Late in the 1930s the use of phenylpropanolamine as a nasal decongestant (Black, 1937; Boyer, 1938) and appetite suppressant in the treatment of obesity (Hirsh, 1939) was reported. Since that time a large number of case reports, clinical management studies, controlled clinical trials, laboratory studies in humans, and drug safety studies have been reported. Most of these studies have investigated the efficacy of phenylpropanolamine-containing preparations as decongestant drugs. To date, more than 36 clinical studies investigating some 20 drug formulations as decongestants have been published, as well as eight controlled clinical trials of phenylpropanolamine-containing anorectic drugs and several case report studies; the results of an additional eight unpublished clinical trials were reviewed (Weintraub, 1985). The efficacy of phenylpropanolamine-containing products in the management of urinary incontinence has been investigated in 12 clinical trials. Several of these trials in treatment of urinary incontinence have utilized objective laboratory techniques as well as clinical assessment to investigate the effects of the drugs on urinary tract function. Finally, several case reports and one clinical trial have been published that tested the efficacy of phenylpropanolamine in the therapeutic management of retrograde ejaculation.

Phenylpropanolamine is approved in the United States for only two clinical indications: as a decongestant and as an appetite suppressant. In other countries, notably in Europe, phenylpropanolamine and norephedrine are also used for treatment of urinary incontinence and retrograde ejaculation.

EFFICACY OF PHENYLPROPANOLAMINE AS A DECONGESTANT IN COUGH-COLD PREPARATIONS

Phenylpropanolamine was first used in human medicine as a nasal decongestant. Since local application of sympathomimetic amines to the nasal mucosa caused local vasoconstriction and decreased swelling of the mucosa (Chen et al., 1929; Stockton et al., 1931), phenylpropanolamine was investigated and shown to be effective as a decongestant in patients with asthma (Black, 1937; Boyer, 1938). Subsequent investigations have demonstrated that phenylpropanolamine, either alone or (usually) combined with other drugs, is effective in the symptomatic relief of respiratory and bponchial conditions. However, as discussed in the following sections, phenylpropanolamine selectively suppresses certain respiratory symptoms and is ineffective in suppressing others. Also, while phenylpropanolamine is at least partially effective in the symptomatic treatment of many cough-cold syndromes, it is ineffective in treatment of other related conditions, especially otitis media in children.

PATHOPHYSIOLOGY OF RHINITIS

Undoubtedly, the rationale for including phenylpropanolamine in cough-cold remedies is that phenylpropanolamine causes vasoconstriction of the vascular beds in the nasal mucosa, thereby decreasing the swelling of the erectile tissue and decreasing congestion. Nasal congestion, however, is only one of the signs and symptoms of rhinitis. A comprehensive review of the pathophysiology of rhinitis is beyond the scope of this chapter; several reviews have been recently published that detail the pathophysiology of rhinitis (Berman & Ross, 1983; Bristow, 1978; Fagin et al., 1981; Mullarkey, 1981; Wright, 1981). A brief review of rhinitis is presented here.

In general, there are two major categories of rhinitis: allergic and nonallergic. Allergic rhinitis is further classified as seasonal allergic rhinitis ("hay fever," which is not necessarily associated with hay, and does not involve fever) and perennial allergic rhinitis. Allergic rhinitis is a widespread condition, affecting 10-15% of the population (Berman & Ross, 1983; Bristow, 1978; Fagin et al., 1981; Mullarkey, 1981). The primary difference between seasonal and perennial allergic rhinitis is, as the names indicate, that seasonal rhinitis occurrs only during certain periods of the year whereas perennial rhinitis occurs throughout the year. The signs and symptoms of allergic rhinitis include (in order of increasing severity): frequent sneezing, nasal pruritus, rhinorrhea, and nasal obstruction. The etiology of allergic rhinitis includes atopic familial predisposition and exposure to allergens. Commonly the allergens include pollens, mold spores, animal dander, and dust. Therapeutic management of allergic rhinitis involves identification and avoidance of the allergen, pharmacotherapy, and immunologic desensitization. Pharmacological therapy may include antihistamines, α-adrenergic decongestants, corticosteroids, and cromolyn sodium.

The second major category of rhinitis is nonallergic rhinitis. The subcategories of nonallergic rhinitis are as follows: acute or vasomotor rhinitis (the "common cold"), perennial rhinitis, eosinophilic rhinitis, and sinusitis. The signs and symptoms of nonallergic rhinitis are similar to the signs and symptoms of allergic rhinitis. The primary difference between allergic and nonallergic rhinitis is that in nonallergic rhinitis no specific causative allergen can be identified, and the etiology is commonly assumed to be viral or bacteriologic. Treatment of nonallergic rhinitis consists primarily in the symptomatic use of decongestants and analgesics (Brummett, 1983), although antibiotics are indicated in some cases of sinusitis (Wright, 1981).

The nasal airway is a specialized portion of the nasobronchial system [see the review by Bristow (1978)]. The airway is susceptible to various factors that can decrease its patency and produce congestion. The airway is lined with mucous membranes, which are supplied with blood vessels and contain erectile tissue. The venous return from the mucous membranes is via sinusoids, which contain smooth muscle specialized into sphincterlike arrangements. In addition, the nasal mucosa is supplied by glands that secrete either watery or viscous mucous secretions and keep the nasal membranes moist. The volume of nasal secretions in normal humans is approximately 2 qt/day, but in allergic rhinitis the secretions greatly exceed this volume.

The symptomatic treatment of rhinitis is based partly on an understanding of the pathophysiology of the nose and partly on empirical evidence. Several important mechanisms that regulate the nasal airways have been identified (Berman & Ross, 1983). The cardiovascular system plays a major role in the normal function of the nasal airways. The small arteries in the nasal mucosa serve to warm the incoming air, whereas the fenestrated capillaries regulate the flow of interstitial fluid and the capacitance venules function to humidify the air. The seromucous glands in the nasal mucosa are stimulated by cholinergic mechanisms. The adrenergic system exerts multiple influences on the nasal airways. α-Adrenergic receptors are involved in presynaptic inhibition of norepinephrine release and contraction of smooth muscles in the erectile tissues of the nasal mucosa and in the vasculature. β-Adrenergics, on the other hand, cause relaxation of smooth muscles at various sites in the nasopharyngeobronchial pathway. Histamine can cause dilation of capillaries and increased capillary permeability in the nasal mucosa, as well as bronchoconstriction. Finally, gamma globulins, IgA, and lysozymes are involved in both mucociliary transport and immunologic protection of the airways. Obviously, rhinitis may result from disturbances in any or several of these regulatory mechanisms. Furthermore, symptomatic treatment of rhinitis can be mediated by various anticholinergic, adrenergic, and antihistaminic drugs.

METHODS USED TO INVESTIGATE CLINICAL PHARMACOLOGY OF DECONGESTANTS

In general, two types of investigative methods have been used to study the clinical pharmacology of phenylpropanolamine as a decongestant: subjective and objective. Subjective methods include evaluation by either the patient or the physician (or other health care practitioner) of the effectiveness of drug treatment in symptomatic relief. Controls for eliminating biases in such studies include the use of the double-blind technique and placebos. In many of the studies, patients were issued daily symptom card diaries and instructed to record the severity of such symptoms as nasal congestion, rhinorrhea, nasal obstruction, and sneezing (hence the term "sneeze cards"). These symptoms are commonly rated on an ordinal scale (e.g., a 4-point scale from 0 indicating absence of the symptom to 3 indicating severe). Ordinal data theoretically should not be analyzed by parametric statistics, but rather by nonparametric statistics. (In fact, ordinal data are commonly analyzed by parametric techniques; fortunately, the conclusions are seldom invalidated by this breach of statistical dogma.) Sneezing can be quantitated in terms of number of sneezes per unit of time and can be analyzed by conventional parametric statistics. Clinical assessment of effectiveness of treatment, even by an experienced physician in a double-blind study, is generally based on subjective evaluation of the severity of signs such as nasal congestion, edema, obstruction, and moistness. Such signs are usually evaluated by ordinal rating scales.

On the other hand, several studies have utilized more objective measures of nasal airway function in order to assess the efficacy of treatment with phenylpropanolamine. The most common objective measure of nasal airway function is measurement of nasal airway resistance (NAR) using rhinomanometric techniques. Although several variations in technique have been utilized, the basic principle involved in measurement of NAR is to determine the air pressure required to move air through the nose at a given airflow rate (see Aschan,

1974; Broms et al., 1982; Hamilton, 1978; McLaurin et al., 1961). Nasal airway resistance then is measured by the ratio of the transnasal pressure difference to the nasal airflow difference. Since rhinomanometric measurement of NAR is rarely used, a brief description of the technique is presented here. The subject is fitted with a face mask that covers the nose and mouth (see Figure 5.1). The face mask is equipped with a mouthpiece which is held in the subject's mouth. The subject is instructed to breathe through the nose while keeping the mouthpiece firmly in place. Intranasal pressure is measured from the pressure difference between the nasal portion of the mask and the mouthpiece. Airflow through the nose is measured by a pneumotachometer transducer attached to the face mask. The subject is instructed to breathe at various rates and depths in order to produce a range of intranasal pressure and airflow values (see Figure 5.2). From these values, the NAR-transnasal pressure relationship is plotted and the nasal airway resistance at a predetermined airflow rate calculated (see Figure 5.3). Nasal congestion is thus indicated by an increase in the NAR above the normal value, and the decongestant effect of drug treatment can be assessed by a decrease in the NAR from the predrug value. Experimental studies have demonstrated that a 20% decrease in airway resistance is the minimum response that can be detected by patients as an improvement in congestion (Cohen, 1978). One advantage of this technique, in addition to the quantitative nature of the measurement, is that the NAR can be measured serially in a subject before and after drug administration. Thus the technique is readily adaptable to a repeated measures experimental

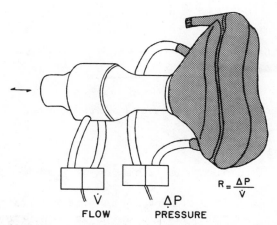

$$R = \frac{\Delta P}{\dot{V}}$$

$\dot{V}$ **FLOW** ΔP **PRESSURE**

Figure 5.1. Diagram of apparatus for measuring nasal airway resistance by rhinomanometric technique. From *Hamilton (1978)*.

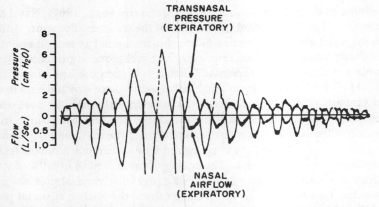

Figure 5.2. Recordings of nasal airflow and pressure from rhinomanometric study. From *Hamilton (1978)*.

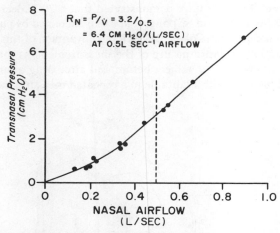

Figure 5.3. Graph of nasal airflow versus transnasal pressure for determining nasal airway resistance. From *Hamilton (1978)*.

design and can be used to determine both the intensity and the time course of drug action.

In these studies, ideally both subjective and objective measures of drug response should be analyzed. In fact, in several studies both subjective and rhinomanometric measures of drug response were evaluated. In most cases, the results of the subjective and objective measures correlated quite well. In cases when the objective and subjective measures did not correlate, it was necessary to determine which measure of drug response was more valid. In evaluation of decongestants for symptomatic relief of rhinitis, the response is essentially subjective, and the objective technique may not measure a parameter that is tightly related to the symptomatic response. Also, the rhinomanometric technique measures only one parameter of drug response, nasal congestion, whereas the subjective techniques measure multiple parameters, including congestion, rhinorrhea, obstruction, and sneezing.

EVALUATION OF PHENYLPROPANOLAMINE ALONE OR IN COMBINATION PRODUCTS

Many of the commercially available cough-cold products that contain phenylpropanolamine are combination products. In these products phenylpropanolamine is frequently combined with one or more of the following: antihistamines, anticholinergics, analgesics, expectorants, or antitussives. Ideally, in order to assess the efficacy of these combination products it would be desirable to investigate each of the components alone as well as in the combination formulation. However, very few clinical studies have investigated the efficacy of phenylpropanolamine both alone and in combination with other components of the combination product. Consequently, the following discussion is divided into three sections: (1) evaluation of studies in which the efficacy of phenylpropanolamine alone was investigated, (2) evaluation of studies in which the contribution of phenylpropanolamine as a component of combination products was specifically investigated, and (3) evaluation of studies in which combination products containing phenylpropanolamine were investigated but the contributions of individual components were not investigated.

Most of the cough-cold remedies that contain phenylpropanolamine are formulated for oral dosing, in either tablet, capsule, or syrup form. Although there are products available that contain sympathomimetic amines formulated for topical nasal decongestion ("nose drops"), no such products currently available in the United States contain phenylpropanolamine. Nonetheless, several of the published reports have evaluated the decongestant effects of phenylpropanolamine when applied topically to the nasal mucosa.

STUDIES INVESTIGATING THE EFFICACY OF PHENYLPROPANOLAMINE ALONE AS A DECONGESTANT

LABORATORY STUDIES

Only one preclinical study using experimental animals to test for decongestant effects of phenylpropanolamine has been reported. In this study, the effects of a series of sympathomimetic amines on carotid blood pressure and intranasal pressure were measured in anesthetized dogs (Aviado et al., 1959). Phenylpropanolamine (100 μg, intraarterially into the carotid artery) decreased carotid blood flow and decreased intranasal pressure. A secondary rise in nasal pressure, indicating a rebound congestion, was not observed following administration of phenylpropanolamine but was consistently observed following administration of epinephrine.

On the other hand, many laboratory studies using human subjects have demonstrated that phenylpropanolamine produces a decongestant effect in patients with rhinitis. These studies have used the rhinomanometric technique for measuring NAR. Phenylpropanolamine was shown to be an effective decongestant in patients with allergic rhinitis (Aschan, 1974; Cohen, 1975), acute or vasomotor rhinitis (Broms & Malm, 1982; Cohen, 1975; Lea, 1984; Pipkorn & Rundcrantz, 1982), or nasal obstruction from various causes (Bende et al., 1984, 1985; Bende & Laurin, 1986; Loth & Bende, 1985; McLaurin et al., 1961).

One of the earliest laboratory investigations of the decongestant effect of phenylpropanolamine in humans was that by McLaurin et al. (1961). A total of 88 patients with nasal obstruction, congestion, and edema were studied. The diagnoses in these patients included coryza, sinusitis, rhinitis, and hypothyroidism. Four drugs were compared (25 mg of phenylpropanolamine, 25 mg of ephedrine, 60 mg of pseudoephedrine, 10 mg of phenylephrine) in a double-blind, crossover, placebo-controlled design. Each patient received one dose of one drug for 5 consecutive days; thus a total of 440 office visits were included in the study. The following parameters were measured both before and 60 min after drug administration in a paired comparison experimental design: blood pressure, heart rate, and NAR as measured by a rhinomanometric method. In addition, the patients were interviewed 60 min after the drug dose and asked about their subjective rating of the change in the nasal airway and the occurrence of any nervousness or other side effects. The patients also took a second dose of the drug 60 min before bedtime. The following morning they were interviewed regarding the effects of the bedtime dose on the nasal airway and whether the drug caused insomnia. None of the drug treatments was rated by the patients as better than the placebo in the subjective rating of the effect on the nasal airway. Analysis of the rhinomanometric measurement of NAR was difficult because of the very high level of unexplained variance. Regression analysis of pre- versus posttreatment NAR scores in ungrouped data showed that, on the average, there was no significant improvement in NAR in any treatment group, including phenylpropanolamine. However, when the data were grouped by pretreatment values into groups that had low pretreatment NAR (slight congestion) and high pretreatment NAR (significant congestion), the following results were obtained. There was a significantly higher proportion of patients with a positive response to treatment in patients receiving placebo, phenylpropanolamine, or ephedrine (χ^2 test, $p < 0.05$). Analysis of the scattergrams of pre- versus post-treatment NAR indicated the following results. Placebo was effective in reducing the NAR only in patients with low pretreatment NAR values. Phenylpropanolamine decreased NAR in patients with high pretreatment values but actually increased the NAR in patients with low pretreatment values. Finally, ephedrine significantly reduced the NAR regardless of the pretreatment NAR. The overall analysis of the effects of the drug treatment on NAR is summarized in Table 5.1. Finally, there was no statistically significant effect of any drug treatment on heart rate or blood pressure. The incidence of nervousness was actually less with phenylpropanolamine than placebo.

However, more recent investigations have revealed a dose-related effect of phenylpropanolamine in decreasing NAR (Table 5.2). A dose of 37.5 mg of phenylpropanolamine produced a modest decrease in NAR (Cohen, 1978), whereas doses ranging up to 100 mg produced significant decreases in NAR (Broms & Malm, 1982; Pipkorn & Rundcrantz, 1982). When given in equivalent 50-mg doses, phenylpropanolamine was more effective in the sustained-release formulation than in the immediate-release formulation [5 out of 5 vs. 2 out of 5 patients, respectively (Aschan, 1974)].

Effects of phenylpropanolamine on NAR are illustrated in Figure 5.4. Nasal airway resistance was measured by rhinomanometric technique in 10 patients with chronic nonallergic rhinitis (Broms & Malm, 1982). Measurements, made in both the sitting and recumbent positions, were taken at 10-min intervals for a total of 200 min. Placebo or phenylpropanolamine (100 mg; Monydrin) was given 75 min after the first NAR measurement. As shown in the figure, the placebo produced no significant effect on the NAR, whereas phenylpropanolamine produced a prompt decrease in the NAR. The effect of phenylpropanolamine was sustained for the duration of the study.

TABLE 5.1. Effects of Four Sympathomimetic Amines on NAR in Patients with Nasal Obstruction[a]

Drug	Dose (mg)	NAR (mm H_2O) Predrug	Postdrug	p
Placebo	0	20.40	19.84	NS
Phenylpropanolamine	25	19.03	19.88	NS
Ephedrine	25	20.25	12.53	<.05
Pseudoephedrine	60	18.53	17.18	NS
Phenylephrine	10	24.38	21.45	NS

Source: Data from McLaurin et al (1961).
[a]Data are means; n = 88 per dose group; NS—not significant.

TABLE 5.2. Dose–Response Relationship for Effects of Acute Administration of Phenylpropanolamine on NAR[a]

Phenylpropanolamine		Patients				Results		Reference
Dose (mg)	Dosing formulation	n	Sex	Age (years)	Diagnosis	Design	Effects on NAR	
25	Generic	88	NS	NS	Nasal obstruction	DB PC Crossover	No significant effect on NAR (slight, nonsignificant increase in NAR)	McLaurin et al. (1961)
37.5	Syrup	80	M, F	NS	Acute rhinitis	DB Parallel groups	Decrease NAR 18.3%	Cohen (1978)
50	NS	15	11F, 4M	NS	Allergic rhinitis	PC	Significant decrease in NAR	Cohen (1975)
50 50	IR SR	85	NS	NS	Acute rhinitis	PC	Decrease in NAR in 2/5 patients Decrease in NAR in 5/5 patients	Aschan (1974)
100	Rinexin	6	3M 3F	25–29	Healthy	Single blind Placebo controlled	Decrease in OAR and NAR	Melen et al. (1986a)
100	Monydrin	10	5M, 5F	16–64	Chronic nonallergic rhinitis	Paired comparison	Approximately 40% decrease in NAR	Broms & Malm (1982)
100	Rinexin	34	31M, 3F	18–34	Acute infectious rhinitis	Single-blind	Approximately 50% decrease in NAR	Pipkorn & Rundcrantz (1982)
100	Rinexin	12	7M 5F	21–60	Chronic maxillary sinusitis	Open clinical trial	Decrease in OAR and NAR	Melen et al. (1986b)

[a]NAR—nasal airways resistance.
[b]NS—not specified.
[c]DB—double-blind.
[d]PC—placebo-controlled.
[e]IR—immediate-release.
[f]SR—sustained release.

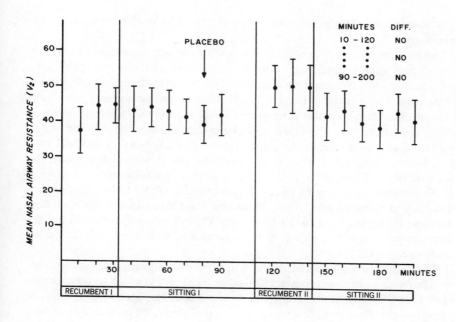

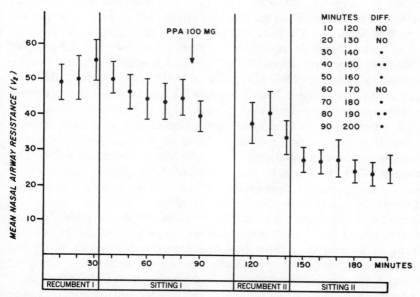

Figure 5.4. Effects of placebo (top panel) and 100 mg phenylpropanolamine (bottom panel) on nasal airway resistance in ten patients. Mean ± s.e.m. From *Broms and Malm (1982)*.

The body position did not significantly interact with the effects of phenylpro-panolamine.

Another technique that utilized the rhinomanometric method to evaluate the efficacy of phenylpropanolamine was reported by Brooks et al. (1981). In this study, pollen extracts were aerosolized and sprayed directly into the nares of patients with seasonal allergic rhinitis. Nasal airway resistance, sneezing, itching, and nasal secretions were measured at intervals after the allergen challenge. By varying the dilution of the pollen extract, the dilution which produced an unequivocal response was determined for each individual subject. In a randomized, double-blind, crossover, placebo-controlled study, the increase in NAR due to the pollen extract challenge was decreased following administration of 20 mg of phenylpropanolamine (PO). However, this is a relatively low dose of phenylpropanolamine, and it produced only a modest decrease in the response to the challenge. Phenylpropanolamine did not re-duce the sneeze count, itching, or nasal secretions associated with the pollen challenge.

The decongestant effect of topically applied phenylpropanolamine was in-vestigated using rhinomanometry and other techniques in four studies. Bende et al. (1984) investigated the decongestant effect of various concentrations of phenylpropanolamine nose drops. In this open study, 40 patients (16 males, 24 females, 15–65 years old), without common colds or nasal polyps who were attending an ear, nose, and throat (ENT) clinic with complaints of nasal ob-struction, were randomly divided into four groups and given nose drops con-taining 0, 0.5, 2.5, or 5% phenylpropanolamine. Bilateral NAR was mea-sured in a sitting position at rest several times until a steady baseline value was reached; three drops (about 0.1 ml) of solution were then instilled in the most congested nostril; 10 min later bilateral NAR was determined. Bilateral NAR was again determined 2 min after vigorous exercise on a bicycle ergome-ter (strenuous exercise induces maximum nasal decongestion and an exercise test can differentiate between nasal obstruction caused by skeletal stenosis and that caused by mucosal swelling). The three phenylpropanolamine con-centrations produced a significant dose-dependent decongestant action. The maximum effect, produced by three drops of 2.5% phenylpropanolamine (about 2.5 mg) per nostril, lowered NAR by about 42%. This was comparable to the reduction induced by exercise (about 50%).

In the second study, Bende et al. (1985) investigated the duration of decon-gestion produced by 2.5% phenylpropanolamine nose drops and the effect of the drug on mucosal blood flow. Eleven healthy subjects (5 males, 6 females, 16–35 years old) whose only complaint was nasal obstruction were included. Bilateral NAR was measured as described previously until baseline values were determined. Three drops (about 0.1 ml) of 2.5% phenylpropanolamine were instilled into each nostril, after which NAR was determined at intervals for up to 320 min. Bilateral NAR was again determined 2 min after vigorous exercise on a bicycle ergometer. Blood flow in nasal mucosa was determined in five subjects (2 males, 3 females) 30 min after dosing using the ^{133}Xe-washout method (0.1 ml ^{133}Xe in saline solution containing 1–10 MBq was injected into inferior turbinate mucosa; isotope elimination was followed using a scintillation detector; blood flow was calculated from initial slope of the first 5 min of the washout curve). A significant decongestant effect lasting up to 3 hr was noted (this is comparable to the duration of effect noted for other phenylamine nasal decongestants but less than that of the imidazoline derivatives). Because the first postdose NAR was not determined until 20 min after phenylpropanolamine application, the exact onset of action could not be determined. There was no significant effect of phenylpropanolamine on mucosal blood flow. Additionally, no secondary engorgement was noted; this observation suggests that phenylpropanolamine produced no "rebound congestion."

In the third study, Loth & Bende (1985) evaluated the effect of 2.5% phenylpropanolamine nose drops on nasal secretion after histamine challenge. Nasal secretion and congestion are principal symptoms of the common cold and other nasal disorders. Histamine challenge can produce these symptoms and is therefore a useful experimental model for studying drugs used to treat them. This double-blind, placebo-controlled, randomized, crossover study included 10 healthy subjects (4 males, 6 females, 20–43 years old) with no history of chronic recurrent airway disease or acute rhinitis symptoms. Baseline NAR values were determined by rhinomanometry as described previously, after which 0.1 ml of 2.5% phenylpropanolamine (about 2.5 mg) or saline solution was instilled into each nostril. NAR was measured for 15 min after dosing, histamine challenge (nasal spray containing about 260 μg of histamine chloride) was performed, and NAR was measured for an additional 50 min. Sneezes were counted. Nasal secretion was determined on the provoked side by weighing paper handkerchiefs used during the test period. Nasal blockage and secretion were also estimated by the subjects according to the following scale: 0 = no symptoms, 1 = mild symptoms, 2 = moderate symptoms, and 3 = severe symptoms. Compared to placebo, phenylpropanolamine significantly reduced the amount of nasal secretion collected after histamine challenge. Nasal secretion and blockage as estimated by the subjects and sneezing were noted only during the first 15 min after histamine challenge. Compared to placebo, phenylpropanolamine significantly reduced the former symptoms, while there was no difference in regard to sneezing score between the two treatments. Also, compared to placebo, phenylpropanolamine significantly reduced NAR both before and after histamine challenge.

In the fourth study, Bende & Laurin (1986) investigated the effect of 2.5% phenylpropanolamine nose drops on nasal secretion and NAR after nasal allergen challenge. This double-blind, placebo-controlled, randomized, crossover study included 10 subjects (7 males, 3 females, 21–38 years old) with seasonal allergic rhinitis who were asymptomatic during the test period. Baseline NAR values were determined as described previously after which nasal allergen challenge was performed (an 8-mm^2 paper disc soaked in pollen-allergen solution was applied for 5 min to the anterior part of the lower turbinate) in one nostril only; 15 min after challenge 0.1 ml of phenylpropanolamine (about 2.5 mg) or saline was dropped on the challenged turbinate. NAR was measured for an additional 45 min. Sneezes were counted and nasal secretion and blockage were estimated by the subjects as described previously. Allergen challenge significantly increased NAR, nasal obstruction, secretion, and sneezing in both treatment series. After phenylpropanolamine administration, NAR and nasal blockage were significantly reduced compared to placebo. However, no significant differences were noted between phenylpropanolamine and placebo treatments with regard to nasal secretion or sneezing.

Additionally, effects of phenylpropanolamine on the size of the maxillary ostium in humans were investigated (Aust et al., 1979; Melen et al., 1986a, 1986b). The maxillary ostium is a tubular canal connecting the maxillary sinus and the middle meatus of the nasal cavity. This ostium is involved in drainage of the paranasal sinuses and may be involved in the pathophysiology of rhinitis. One study investigated the possibility that either acute or repeated administration of phenylpropanolamine to patients with rhinitis may decrease the functional size of the maxillary ostium, thus contributing to the symptomatic relief of rhinitis (Aust et al., 1979). The experimental setup for measuring the size of the maxillary ostium is shown in Figure 5.5. Two cannulas were inserted into the ostium. Airflow was introduced into the sinus via one of the cannulas, and pressure changes in the sinus were measured from the second cannula. The size of the functional maxillary ostium was determined from a nomogram of airflow versus antral pressure change versus ostial size. These laboratory results were confirmed by clinical examination and x-rays of the maxillary sinuses. The patient population in this study was 20 adults (8 females and 12 males, ages 16–56 years) with acute rhinosinusitis. Phenylpropanolamine was administered both acutely and by repeated dosing schedule. Phenylpropanolamine (100 mg) or placebo (PO) was administered acutely in a double-blind experimental design. The size of the maxillary ostium was measured before and at intervals 30–120 min after the dose. In the repeated administration schedule, the patients took 100 mg of phenylpropanolamine b.i.d. for 7 days in a double-blind experimental design. The patients also were given antibiotics. The results showed that after neither acute nor repeated administration of phenylpropanolamine were there any effects on the size of the maxillary ostium that could be attributed to phenylpropanolamine. However, the interpretation of these negative results is limited,

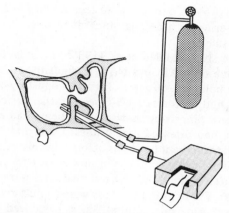

Figure 5.5. Experimental set-up for measuring the size of the maxillary ostium in humans. From *Aust et al. (1979)*.

since analysis of the subjective rating by the patients of the effects of drug treatment indicated that phenylpropanolamine did not provide symptomatic relief from nasal symptoms. In contrast, this dose of phenylpropanolamine significantly reduced the nasal airway resistance and relieved the nasal symptoms in patients with acute infectious rhinitis (Pipkorn & Rundcrantz, 1982) or with chronic nonallergic rhinitis (Broms & Malm, 1982).

Melen et al. (1986a) studied the effects of phenylpropanolamine on ostial and nasal airway resistance (OAR and NAR) in healthy subjects. OAR was measured using a pressure-flow technique similar to Aust et al. (1979), and NAR was measured as described previously. In this single-blind study, the participants were six healthy subjects (3 males, 3 females, 25–29 years old) with no history of sinusitis. OAR and NAR were determined in sitting and recumbent positions before administration of phenylpropanolamine (two 50-mg Rinexin tablets in slow-release form) or placebo, and again after dosing every 30 min for 2 hr. The experiments concluded with NAR measurement after physical exercise in the sitting position; postexercise OAR was also tested in the placebo but not the phenylpropanolamine group. First the right maxillary sinus and entire nasal cavity were tested; 48 hr later the left maxillary sinus was tested and the entire nasal cavity retested; 4 weeks later the same series was repeated. Compared with placebo, phenylpropanolamine significantly reduced OAR and NAR. The exercise test significantly reduced OAR at the end of the placebo series (phenylpropanolamine not tested); exercise significantly reduced NAR further for both the placebo and phenylpropanolamine series. In the phenylpropanolamine experiments, the greatest reductions in OAR and NAR were noted in recumbency 1–2 hr after dosing, suggesting that the drug has a decongestant effect when the ostial and nasal mucosae are blood-filled.

In a second open study, Melen et al. (1986b) investigated the effects of phenylpropanolamine on OAR and NAR in sinusitis patients. Twelve patients (7 males, 5 females, 21–60 years old) with no history of nasal polyposis or allergy, but who had been treated 1–5 years earlier for chronic maxillary sinusitis, participated. Sinoscopy showed six patients had normal or healed membranes and six had diseased membranes. OAR and NAR were determined in sitting and recumbent positions before administration of phenylpropanolamine (two 50-mg Rinexin tablets in slow-release form), 60 and 90 min after dosing, and after a final exercise test. All tests were performed twice about a month apart. Findings in this study were similar to those in the study of healthy volunteers: A decongestant effect, as evidenced by reduced OAR and NAR values, was noted in sitting and recumbent positions, with the effect more pronounced in recumbency; again, exercise further reduced OAR and NAR in both the "healed" and "diseased" groups. The authors suggested that the decongestant effect of phenylpropanolamine is probably more conspicuous on inflamed than on normal mucosa.

CLINICAL STUDIES OF THE EFFICACY OF PHENYLPROPANOLAMINE ALONE IN RHINITIS

The earliest clinical studies of the decongestant effects of sympathomimetic amines were those by Chen et al. (1929) and Stockton et al. (1931). Chen et al. (1929) demonstrated that topical application of a 1% solution of various sympathomimetic amines to the congested nasal mucous membranes in humans decreased the congestion. Phenylpropanolamine was not investigated in that study, however. Stockton et al. (1931) demonstrated that topical application of a 3% solution of phenylpropanolamine in humans with either acute or chronic sinusitis produced effective decongestion with no evidence of local irritation.

The efficacy of orally administered phenylpropanolamine for symptomatic relief in a bronchial-respiratory disorder was reported by Boyer (1938). This was a clinical case study of 44 patients with asthma. Each patient had used at least one other drug for symptomatic relief of the asthmatic symptoms. The patients were allowed to take Propadrine ($3/8$ grain = 24.375 mg) as required for symptomatic relief. The patients were interviewed for their self-report of the effectiveness of Propadrine and any side effects. The results showed that the daily dose of Propadrine ranged from one tablet t.i.d. to two tablets every 2 hr. The effectiveness of Propadrine relative to other drugs that the patients had used previously was as follows: 80% of patients rated Propadrine as better than other drugs, 11% rated it as equal to other drugs, and 9% rated it as less effective than other drugs. Clearly, Propadrine was preferred to other available drugs for relief of asthmatic symptoms. The subjective effects of Propadrine were relief of bronchospasm, rhinitis, and sneezing. The reported incidence of side effects was low. Few patients reported nervousness or insomnia. No patients experienced urinary retention, even though two patients were known to have prostatic hypertrophy. Finally, no patient reported palpitations or tachycardia while taking Propadrine. The lack of reported side effects is especially remarkable since the doses of Propadrine were as high as two tablets every 2 hr (equivalent to 48.75 mg of phenylpropanolamine q. 2 h.).

Few clinical studies have investigated the effects of phenylpropanolamine alone as a decongestant, although numerous studies have investigated the efficacy of phenylpropanolamine-containing combination products. Several factors contribute to this paucity of data regarding efficacy of phenylpropanolamine alone. Early studies indicated that phenylpropanolamine alone was only mildly to moderately effective alone but was very effective in combination with other drugs, especially antihistamines (Aschan, 1974; Cohen, 1975). Also, all the commercially available cough-cold products currently available in the United States are combination products. In Scandinavia, two cough-cold products that contain phenylpropanolamine alone are available: Monydrin and Rinexin.

Five clinical studies have been published that investigated phenylpropanolamine alone as a decongestant. In one study, generic phenylpropanolamine was used (McLaurin et al., 1961). In another study, phenylpropanolamine alone was investigated as a part of a study to determine the contribution of various components to the efficacy of a combination product (Cohen, 1975). In the other three studies, the Scandinavian products that contain phenylpropanolamine alone were investigated (Broms & Malm, 1982; Forsberg et al., 1983; Renvall & Lindqvist, 1979). In three of these five studies, the clinical results were correlated with the results of rhinomanometric testing of the NAR. In addition, one study investigated the efficacy of phenylpropanolamine in treatment of acute maxillary sinusitus (Axelsson et al., 1981).

The relatively low dose of 25 mg of phenylpropanolamine was shown to be ineffective in symptomatic relief of decongestion in patients with nasal obstruction, congestion, and edema (McLaurin et al., 1961). The overall study design of this investigation was described in detail in the previous section (see also Table 5.2). Briefly, this was a double-blind, crossover, placebo-controlled study of 88 patients with nasal obstruction due to various conditions. One dose of phenylpropanolamine was taken during a laboratory investigation during the day and a second dose, 1 hr before bedtime. The patients were interviewed regarding their subjective rating of changes in the nasal airway and the occurrence of nervousness and other side effects. This dose of phenylpropanolamine was rated as not better than placebo in reducing nasal airway obstruction. However, there was a pronounced placebo effect on nasal congestion. Nervousness was listed as a side effect of treatment more often when the drug was taken at bedtime than when taken in the laboratory study. However, phenylpropanolamine actually caused less nervousness than did the placebo. The results of the rhinomanometric measurements correlated well with the subjective report of symptomatic effects: phenylpropanolamine produced no significant effect on NAR.

A higher dose of phenylpropanolamine (50 mg) was effective in symptomatic relief of nasal congestion in patients with chronic allergic rhinitis (Cohen, 1975). The experimental design of this study is described in detail in the subsequent section (see also Table 5.2). Briefly, the design was as follows. In a placebo-controlled, crossover study, 15 patients with chronic allergic rhinitis were given phenylpropanolamine or placebo (as well as other components of the combination product Contac). The subjective ratings of efficacy and adverse effects were determined, and the NAR was measured. The percentages of patients reporting that phenylpropanolamine caused an improvement, no change, or worsening of their symptoms were 80.0, 13.3, and 6.6%, respectively. Thus phenylpropanolamine was significantly better than placebo in symptomatic relief, and these results were confirmed by rhinomanometric measurements (Table 5.2). In this study, 40% of the patients reported mild adverse effects while taking phenylpropanolamine. Of the 15 patients, three reported feeling "jittery"; two "gassy"; and one each, drowsy, sleepy, or nervous or experiencing dryness of the mouth.

The efficacy of 50 mg of phenylpropanolamine as a decongestant was confirmed by Forsberg et al. (1983). In a randomized, double-blind, placebo-controlled study, 116 patients (25 females, 91 males) with acute rhinitis received either Rinexin (50 mg of phenylpropanolamine in sustained-release formulation) or placebo twice daily for 3 days. The patients kept a daily record of nasal blockage, nasal secretion, feeling of deafness, and other side effects. Rinexin was significantly better than placebo in decreasing nasal symptoms, and there was no difference between the groups in the incidence of side effects. These authors suggested that the maximum dose of phenylpropanolamine for decongestant effects should be 50 mg (b.i.d.).

In a randomized, double-blind, placebo-controlled study, Renvall and Lindqvist (1979) used 70 patients (32 males, 38 females, 15–78 years old) with chronic nonallergic rhinitis to evaluate the nasal decongestant effect of phenylpropanolamine (Monydrin, 50 mg slow-release tablet). There were three dose groups: placebo, 50 mg, and 100 mg. Dosing was twice daily (8 A.M., 8 P.M.) for 3 days. Patients subjectively assessed their symptoms and side effects on a questionnaire; physicians evaluated nasal obstruction, nasal secretion, and blood pressure. The high dose of phenylpropanolamine (100 mg b.i.d.) significantly reduced nasal obstruction; the low dose

(50 mg b.i.d.) did not show any significant relief of nasal symptoms. No side effects such as CNS stimulation or blood pressure changes were noted at either dose level.

The decongestant effects of 100 mg of phenylpropanolamine (Monydrin, sustained release) twice daily for 10 days were investigated (Broms & Malm, 1982). Nineteen patients with chronic nonallergic rhinitis were included in this randomized, crossover, placebo-controlled study. Daily ratings of symptoms (nasal obstruction and secretion), number of sneezes, and side effects were recorded on a diary card. Phenylpropanolamine significantly reduced the nasal obstruction, secretion, and sneezing. Furthermore, phenylpropanolamine produced a low incidence of side effects. The incidence of headaches in the placebo and phenylpropanolamine groups was 7/19 and 2/19 (i.e., 7 out of 19 and 2 out of 19), respectively. Phenylpropanolamine produced urinary retention in only 2/19 patients, and these were older males (ages 60 and 64 years). Phenylpropanolamine had no effect on the subjective rating of sleep.

In summary, the efficacy of phenylpropanolamine alone as a decongestant was investigated in five studies using three different doses from 25 to 100 mg. The low dose of phenylpropanolamine (25 mg) was ineffective in producing decongestant effect. The two higher doses (50 and 100 mg) were effective in relief of nasal symptoms, with a low incidence of mild side effects.

STUDIES INVESTIGATING THE EFFICACY OF PHENYLPROPANOLAMINE AS A COMPONENT OF COMBINATION PRODUCTS

Most of the commercially available cough-cold preparations that contain phenylpropanolamine are combination products; that is, they contain phenylpropanolamine in combination with other active drugs. By far the most common combination is phenylpropanolamine and an antihistamine. Other components of combination products include anticholinergic drugs that decrease the nasal secretions, expectorants, and analgesics. Some combination products contain other sympathomimetic amines in addition to phenylpropanolamine. Finally, some antiasthmatic combination products contain bronchodilator drugs such as theophylline combined with phenylpropanolamine.

To fully investigate the efficacy of such combination products, it is necessary to compare the efficacy of each component separately with the efficacy of the combination of the components. Additionally, if the combination product contains more than two active drugs, each possible combination of the individual drugs should be tested for efficacy. Finally, the results must be analyzed to determine whether the combination of two active drugs produces additive, synergistic, or antagonistic effects. If the effects are additive, the effect of the combination is equal to the sum of the effects of the two components. If the effects are synergistic, the effect of the combination is greater than the sum of the effects of the components; if the drugs are antagonistic, the effects of the combination are less than the sum of the components. In the case of combination cough-cold preparations there is an additional confounding factor: the range and number of symptoms involved in the various rhinitis syndromes. In fact, the rationale for using combination products for cough-cold remedies is that each component of the product provides symptomatic relief of a different subset of rhinitis symptoms. Thus, ideally, to investigate the efficacy of the combination product, each component and all combinations should be tested for effects on a variety of rhinitis symptoms.

The efficacy of phenylpropanolamine-containing combination products as decongestants has been investigated in 26 published reports. However, the contribution of phenylpropanolamine to the efficacy of the combination was specifically investigated in only six of these studies. The results of these studies are reviewed in this section ("Studies Investigating the Efficacy of Phenylpropanolamine as a Component of Combination Products"). The results of studies which investigated the efficacy of the combination products without investigating the components will be reviewed in the following section ("Studies Investigating the Efficacy of Phenylpropanolamine-Containing Combination Products: Decongestant Efficacy").

COMBINATION OF PHENYLPROPANOLAMINE WITH AN ANTIHISTAMINE

In one of the most extensive investigations of the combination of phenylpropanolamine with an antihistamine clemastine was used as the antihistamine (Aschan, 1974). Clemastine was investigated because it is an antihistamine with low sedative potency. Two patient populations were investigated. One population consisted of 85 patients with acute rhinitis. The tests were conducted within 2–3 days of onset of symptoms, to minimize the influence of the time course of the rhinitis. The tests were also conducted at a time of year when the pollen count was negligible, to minimize the possible influence of allergic rhinitis. The second population consisted of 50 healthy volunteers who participated in histamine challenge tests. For the histamine challenge test, 1.5–2.0 ml of a 1:1000 solution of histamine was sprayed into each nostril. The time course and intensity of the effect of the histamine challenge on NAR were measured. Nasal airway resistance was measured in both the rhinitis patients and in the histamine challenge tests by rhinomanometric technique. The experimental design in both phases was double-blind and placebo-controlled. Rhinomanometric recordings were taken before drug administration, and repeatedly every 30–50 min after drug administration, for a total of 9 hr. The pretreatment airflow in these patients with acute rhinitis was considerably less than normal, and the intensity of the response was related to the pretreatment NAR level. Since the data were converted to quantal (all-or-nothing) responses, in the following discussion the results are expressed as the number of patients responding as a proportion of the total population.

Six separate studies were conducted. In each of the six studies, the placebo treatment produced no response in any subject. The combination of phenylpropanolamine and clemastine was investigated in the acute rhinitis patients in three separate studies. In the first study, neither placebo (0/5 patients) nor clemastine (0/5) alone produced a positive response in the rhinomanometric test. The combination of the two active drugs, however, produced a significant effect (4/5 patients). Since the effects of phenylpropanolamine alone were not investigated in this preliminary study it is not possible to evaluate the contribution of phenylpropanolamine to the combination. Thus the effects of phenylpropanolamine alone and in combination with clemastine were investigated in the second part of the study. Furthermore, the effects of immediate- and sustained-release phenylpropanolamine preparations were compared. As in the preliminary study, placebo alone had no effect (0/5) and clemastine alone had no (0/5) or limited effect (2/5) on airway resistance. Immediate-release phenylpropanolamine produced a moderate effect (2/5), whereas the sustained-release preparation was very effective (5/5). The author claimed that the immediate-release phenylpropanolamine and clemastine had synergistic effects on NAR, but because of the small number of subjects per group, this conclusion is questionable. However, the effects appeared additive.

The results from the histamine challenge studies support the results of the studies in patients with acute rhinitis. Thus clemastine alone was poorly effective (1/5), whereas phenylpropanolamine alone was very effective (5/5 for immediate-release preparation, 4/5 for sustained-release) in reducing the histamine-stimulated decrease in airway resistance. In this study, clemastine plus the sustained-release phenylpropanolamine formulation was more effective (5/5) than clemastine plus the immediate-release preparation (3/5). Although the author suggested that the results with the combination "supported the hypothesis of synergism between antihistamine and adrenergic substance...," critical examination of the results does not support this conclusion. In fact, clemastine and the sustained-release phenylpropanolamine were simply additive, whereas clemastine and the immediate-release phenylpropanolamine were actually antagonistic. Nonetheless, this report is often cited as evidence that phenylpropanolamine and antihistamines are synergistic. It is not clear why phenylpropanolamine, a sympathomimetic amine, effectively reversed the effects of histamine, whereas clemastine, an antihistamine, was ineffective against histamine.

The efficacy of the phenylpropanolamine-clemastine combination (HSP

525A) was confirmed by Aschan and Tham (1974). In this study, patients with allergic rhinitis and confirmed allergy to Timothy grass pollen were studied. The HSP 525A compound was effective (6/11 patients) or partially effective (3/11) in reducing the elevation of NAR after acute challenge with Timothy grass pollen. It was ineffective in only 2 of 11 patients, and placebo was effective in 2 of 11 patients. The effects of the individual components of this mixture were not investigated.

The effects of phenylpropanolamine and an antihistamine, alone and in combination, on several symptoms of rhinitis were investigated by means of the challenged allergic nose paradigm (Brooks et al., 1981). In this study the antihistamine was hydroxyzine, which is an H_1 histamine receptor antagonist with antianxiety effects. The experimental population was 20 patients with seasonal allergic rhinitis and a nasal sensitivity to pollen. The challenged allergic nose test is accomplished by spraying a dilute pollen extract directly into the nostrils and measuring the nasal response. A range of dilutions of the pollen extract was studied to determine the dilution that produced an unequivocal response in each patient. The following responses were measured: sneeze count, nasal secretions, the patient's subjective rating of itching and congestion, and increase in NAR. The nasal secretion was quantitated by patients blowing their noses into preweighed tissues. Nasal airway resistance was measured by standard rhinomanometric technique. The experimental design was randomized, double-blind, crossover, and placebo-controlled. Each patient received each of the following treatments: placebo, phenylpropanolamine (20 mg), hydroxyzine (25 mg), and phenylpropanolamine combined with hydroxyzine. Each drug treatment involved four doses of the treatment, one on the evening of the pretest day and three on the test day, with the last dose 45 min prior to the test. A 1-week washout period was allowed between drug groups for each patient. Phenylpropanolamine decreased the nasal congestion associated with the pollen challenge but had no effect on the sneezing, nasal secretion, or itching. However, the dose of phenylpropanolamine used was lower than those required to produce adequate decongestion in naturally occurring rhinitis. It may be that the efficacy of phenylpropanolamine in naturally occurring rhinitis is different from that in this artificially induced rhinitis paradigm. Hydroxyzine, in contrast, decreased sneezing, nasal secretions, and itching but had no effect on nasal congestion. Thus the combination of phenylpropanolamine and hydroxyzine was effective in decreasing all four of the major symptoms, presumably as a result of the additive effects of the two active compounds.

The additive effects of phenylpropanolamine and the antihistamine brompheniramine were demonstrated in a study that used both rhinomanometric measurements of airway resistance and clinical evaluation of patient responses (Broms & Malm, 1982). Two commercially available phenylpropanolamine-containing products were compared in this study: Monydrin (100 mg of phenylpropanolamine, sustained-release) and Lunerin (50 mg of phenylpropanolamine and 12 mg of brompheniramine, sustained-release). Changes in NAR were measured by rhinomanometric methods following acute administration of placebo, Monydrin, or Lunerin. In this portion of the study, 10 patients with chronic nonallergic rhinitis were investigated. The clinical evaluation of drug efficacy was conducted using a randomized, cross-over, placebo-controlled design. The drugs were administered b.i.d. for 10 days, and symptoms were rated on a daily diary card.

Monydrin significantly reduced the NAR whereas Lunerin had no significant effect. Both Monydrin and Lunerin decreased the symptom scores for sneezing, nasal obstruction, and nasal secretion. Lunerin produced a greater decrease in the symptom score than Monydrin for each of these three symptoms, but the difference between the two drugs was statistically significant only for sneezing. Since the two preparations contain different doses of phenylpropanolamine, and since the effects of brompheniramine alone were not tested, it is not possible to state whether the effects of phenylpropanolamine and brompheniramine were additive or synergistic. Nonetheless, the combination products (which also had a lower dose of phenylpropanolamine) produced greater symptomatic relief than did phenylpropanolamine alone. In this study, the results of the clinical evaluation and the rhinomanometric study were inconsistent, since the phenylpropanolamine alone significantly reduced the NAR whereas the combination product did not. Thus the results of the clinical evaluation indicate that Lunerin was a more effective product, whereas the results of the rhinomanometric study indicate that Monydrin was the more effective.

COMBINATION OF PHENYLPROPANOLAMINE WITH AN ANTIHISTAMINE AND BELLADONNA ALKALOIDS

Contac is a triple combination product containing 50 mg of phenylpropanolamine, 4 mg of chlorpheniramine, and 0.2 mg of belladonna alkaloids (0.0375 mg of atropine and 0.1906 mg of hyoscyamine) in a sustained-release formulation. The efficacy of phenylpropanolamine, alone and in combination with each of the other components of Contac, and of the triple combination mixture have been investigated (Cohen, 1975). Fifteen patients with chronic allergic rhinitis were enrolled in this randomized, double-blind, placebo-controlled clinical trial. Nasal airway resistance was measured by electronic posterior rhinometry before and at intervals after drug treatment. The total observation period was 12 hr. In addition, the patients rated the efficacy of treatment by a subjective rating scale and were asked to report any side effects. Each patient was given each of the five drug treatments, with at least 3 days between successive drug treatments for any given patient.

Each of the four treatment groups that contained active drugs was significantly better than placebo in producing subjective relief from rhinitis. However, there were no significant differences between the active treatment groups, indicating that there were no interactions between phenylpropanolamine and any of the other components of the combination product. All the treatments produced a very high proportion of positive responses, and under such conditions it is very difficult to detect any additive or synergistic interactions between the treatments. These results were confirmed by the results from the rhinomanometric study. The mean NAR in the pretreatment condition was 4.91–5.21 mm $H_2O \cdot liter^{-1} \cdot sec^{-1}$ in this patient population, compared to 2.58 mm $H_2O \cdot liter^{-1} \cdot sec^{-1}$ in normal healthy adults. Thus these patients with chronic allergic rhinitis had considerably elevated baseline levels of NAR, indicating chronic nasal congestion. Phenylpropanolamine produced a prompt decrease in this elevated airway resistance with the onset to effect in 1 hr. The decrease in airway resistance with phenylpropanolamine alone was statistically significant 2–8 hr after drug administration. The effects of the drug combinations were not significantly different from the effects of phenylpropanolamine alone, except that the duration of action was longer for the triple combination. The triple combination (i.e., Contac per se) was significantly more effective than phenylpropanolamine alone at 10–12 hr after the dose.

MISCELLANEOUS COMBINATIONS

The efficacy of combination products used topically as decongestants was investigated in humans with nasal congestion (Hamilton, 1978). Twenty-one males with elevated baseline nasal airway resistance were studied. Elevated nasal airway resistance was defined as a resting value of greater than 2.0 cm $H_2O \cdot liter^{-1} \cdot sec^{-1}$. Airway resistance was measured by rhinomanometric techniques. The diagnoses in these patients included allergic rhinitis and acute coryza. The effects of acute topical application of drug mixtures into the nostrils were measured. The drug mixtures were applied to the nostrils from a spray dispenser, with the spray applied twice to each nostril. This was a repeated-measures, crossover design, with at least a 1-day interval between drugs for any given individual. A pretreatment measurement of NAR was taken, and the measurements were repeated at intervals after drug application for a total of 180 min. The drug combinations were as follows: drug A—saline; drug B—phenylpropanolamine, phenylephrine, thonzylamine; drug C—phenylephrine, thonzylamine; drug D—phenylpropanolamine, phenylephrine, thonzylamine, volatile oil. Phenylpropanolamine and phenylephrine are adrenergic agonists, and thonzylamine is an antihistamine. Preliminary analysis of the data revealed that the data were skewed, and consequently the data were subjected to a logarithmic transformation in order to allow statistical analysis by conventional parametric tests. All treatments produced a significant change in NAR. In the placebo group there was a very brief increase in airway resistance, lasting approximately 5 min. The combination of 0.25% phenylephrine and 1.0% thonzylamine (drug C) produced a transient, moderate decrease in NAR. Addition of 0.25% phenylpropanolamine to this mixture (i.e., drugs B and D) produced a marked and prolonged decrease in airway resistance. This enhancement of the decongestant effects was particularly marked for the triple combination, drug B. Airway resistance was significantly reduced during the time period of 10–150 min following topical application of drug B, with the peak effect occurring 60 min after drug application. Unfortunately, the effects of topical application of phenylpropanolamine alone were not investigated in this study, and the full nature of the drug interaction cannot be evaluated. Topical application of a 3% solution of phenylpropanolamine alone was shown to produce effective decongestion in humans with sinusitis (Stockton et al., 1931). Further studies would be required to determine whether the interactions between phenylpropanolamine, phenylephrine, and thonzylamine are additive or synergistic.

Finally, the efficacy of phenylpropanolamine and aromatic oils, alone and in combination, was investigated (Cohen, 1978). The drugs were given in hydroalcoholic syrup to 80 patients with common colds of less than 48-hr duration. Nasal airway flow-resistance was measured by electronic posterior rhinometry before and at intervals after drug administration. This was a double-blind, randomized, parallel-groups study. The four treatments were as follows: 37.5 mg of phenylpropanolamine, aromatic oils, 37.5 mg of phenylpropanolamine plus aromatic oils, and placebo. Either placebo or aromatic oils alone produced a mild but statistically significant decrease in airway resistance, specifically, 10.3 and 7.3%, respectively. The effect of aromatic oils alone was not significantly different from placebo. Phenylpropanolamine alone produced a significant decrease in airway resistance for up to 180 min, with a maximum decrease of 18.3%. The greatest decrease in airway resistance occurred in the group given phenylpropanolamine plus aromatic oils. In this group the maximum decrease was 22.4%. Airway resistance was significantly decreased for up to 180 min, and the total duration of drug effect was approximately 4 hr. Subjective rating of drug effect by the patients confirmed the results of the rhinomanometric test. Furthermore, it was noted that a 20% decrease in NAR was the minimum response that the patients were able to report as a subjective improvement of the congestion.

STUDIES INVESTIGATING THE EFFICACY OF PHENYLPROPANOLAMINE-CONTAINING COMBINATION PRODUCTS: DECONGESTANT EFFICACY

Clinical trials investigating the decongestant efficacy of commercial products that contain phenylpropanolamine are reviewed in this section. This review includes studies of combination products that contain phenylpropanolamine as one of the active components but in which the contribution of each of the various components was not specifically evaluated. The combination products and their active components and doses, and manufacturers are listed in Table 5.3.* These products are subdivided as follows: products containing phenylpropanolamine and antihistamine(s); triple combination products containing phenylpropanolamine, an antihistamine, and an anticholinergic (antimuscarinic) drug; and multicomponent combinations. The multicomponent combinations contain phenylpropanolamine and two or more of the following: another sympathomimetic amine, an antihistamine, an anticholinergic, an analgesic, an antitussive, an expectorant, or a bronchodilator. In addition, Table 5.3 lists commercial products that do not contain phenylpropanolamine but were compared to phenylpropanolamine-containing products in the clinical trials.

COMBINATIONS OF PHENYLPROPANOLAMINE AND ANTIHISTAMINES

Clinical trials have been conducted to test the efficacy of drug combinations containing phenylpropanolamine and antihistamines (summarized in Table 5.4). The antihistamines were brompheniramine (Lunerin and Lunerin-mite), cinnarizine (Rinomar and Rinomar syrup), and pheniramine and pyrilamine (Triaminic). As can be seen in Table 5.4, the recommended daily doses of phenylpropanolamine-containing products produced symptomatic relief of all four of the major symptoms of rhinitis: sneezing, nasal itching, rhinorrhea, and nasal congestion. In some patients, twice the daily recommended dose was required for adequate response (Axelsson, 1972). The phenylpropanolamine-antihistamine combinations were effective in both adult (Aaronson et al., 1968; Axelsson, 1972; Lofkvist & Svensson, 1978; Mercke & Wihl, 1973a,b; Wenger & Lapsa, 1970) and pediatric patients (Horak, 1982; Kjellman, 1975; Moller & Bjorksten, 1980). In addition, the phenylpropanolamine-antihistamine combinations were effective in both allergic and vasomotor rhinitis. The duration of action in most patients was 10–12 hr.

The efficacies of two combination products, Lunerin and Rinomar, were

---

*Table 5.3 lists only those commercial products tested in the clinical trials reviewed in this chapter. It is not a complete list of phenylpropanolamine-containing commercial products.

TABLE 5.3. Commercial Decongestant Products Containing Phenylpropanolamine

Trade Name	Composition (mg)[a]	Manufacturer	Reference
A. Products containing phenylpropanolamine alone			
Monydrin	Phenylpropanolamine 100 (SR)[b]	AB Draco, Sweden	Broms & Malm (1982)
Rinexin	Phenylpropanolamine 50 (SR) Phenylpropanolamine 100 (SR)	NR	Forsberg et al. (1983)
B. Phenylpropanolamine–antihistamine combinations			
Lunerin	Phenylpropanolamine 50 Brompheniramine 12 (SR)	AB Draco, AB Astra, Sweden	Broms & Malm (1982) Mercke & Wihl (1973a,b) Kjellman et al. (1978)
Lunerin-mite	Phenylpropanolamine 25 Brompheniramine 6 (SR; pediatric)	AB Draco, AB Astra, Sweden	Moller (1980) Sorri et al. (1982)
Rinomar	Phenylpropanolamine 25 Cinnarizine 10	NR	Mercke & Wihl (1973a) Moller & Bjorksten (1980)
Rinomar syrup	Phenylpropanolamine 12.5 Cinnarizine 5	Janssen, Tournhout	Horak (1982)
Triaminic	Phenylpropanolamine NR Pheniramine NR Pyrilamine NR	Dorsey Laboratories, Lincoln, NE	Forquer & Linthicum (1982)
C. Phenylpropanolamine–antihistamine–anticholinergic combinations			
Contac	Phenylpropanolamine 50 Chlorpheniramine 4 Belladonna alkaloids 0.2 (SR)	Menley and James, Philadelphia, PA	Cohen (1975)
Eskornade	Phenylpropanolamine 50 Diphenylpyraline 5 Isopropamide 2.5 (spansules)	NR	Heron (1972)
Ornade	Phenylpropanolamine 50 Chlorpheniramine 8 Isopropamide 2.5	Smith, Kline and French, Philadelphia, PA	Ashe (1968)

TABLE 5.3. Continued.

Trade Name	Composition (mg)[a]	Manufacturer	Reference
	D. Multicomponent combinations		
Asbron	Phenylpropanolamine 25 Theophylline sodium glycinate 300	Dorsey Laboratories, Lincoln, NE	Parrillo & Humoller (1966)
Benylin Day and Night	Glyceryl guaiacolate 100 "Day" tablet Phenylpropanolamine 25 Acetaminophen 500 "Night" tablet Diphenhydramine 25 Acetaminophen 500	Warner-Lambert (UK)	Middleton (1981)
Day Nurse	Phenylpropanolamine 25 Acetaminophen 500 Vitamin C 60 Dextromethorphan 15 Alcohol 3.08 ml	Beecham Proprietaries (UK)	Lea (1984)
Dimetapp L.A.	Phenylpropanolamine 15 Phenylephrine 15 Brompheniramine 12 (SR)	Robins	Forquer & Linthicum (1982)
Naldecon syrup	Phenylpropanolamine NR Phenylephrine NR Chlorpheniramine NR Phenyltoloxamine NR	Bristol Laboratories	Moran et al (1983)
Pholcolix syrup	Phenylpropanolamine 12.5 Paracetamol 150 Pholcodine 5	Warner Lambert	Jaffe & Grimshaw (1983)
Ru-Tuss	Phenylpropanolamine 50 Phenylephrine 25 Chlorpheniramine 8	Rucker Pharmacal, Shreveport, LA	Jackson et al. (1975) Pou et al. (1970)

Product	Ingredients (mg)[a]	Manufacturer	Reference
Rymed	Hyoscyamine 0.1936 Atropine 0.0362 Scopolamine 0.0121 (SR) Phenylpropanolamine 45 Phenylephrine 5 Guaifenesin 200	NR	Erffmeyer et al. (1982)
Sinulin	Phenylpropanolamine 37.5 Chlorpheniramine 2 Acetaminophen 325 Salicylamide 250 Homatropine methylbromide 0.75	Carnrick Laboratories, Cedar Knolls, NJ	Rhea (1971)
Sinutab Pediatric Suspension	Phenylpropanolamine 12.5 Acetaminophen 300 Phenyltoloxamine 10	Warner-Chilcott Laboratories, Morris Plains, NJ	Carter (1965)

E. Products not containing phenylpropanolamine; used as comparisons to phenylpropanolamine-containing products

Product	Ingredients (mg)[a]	Manufacturer	Reference
Actifed	Pseudoephedrine 60 Triprolidine 2.5	Burroughs Wellcome, Tuckahoe, NY	Ashe (1968)
Actifed Compound Syrup	Pseudoephedrine 30 Triprolidine 1.25 Codeine 10	Burroughs Wellcome, Tuckahoe, NY	Jaffe & Grimshaw (1983)
Demazin	d-Isoephedrine 120 Dexchlorpheniramine 6 (chronsules)	NR	Heron (1972)
Disophrol Syrup	Pseudoephedrine 30 Dexbrompheniramine 1.5	Schering Corp., U.S.A.	Horak (1982)
Drixoral	d-Isoephedrine 120 Dexbrompheniramine 6	Schering Corp., U.S.A.	Ashe (1968)

[a]Milligrams per tablet or per 5 ml (for syrups or suspensions).
[b]SR—sustained release; NR—not reported.

TABLE 5.4. Efficacy of Combination Products Containing Phenylpropanolamine and Antihistamines[a]

	Drug			Patients			
Tradename	Total Daily Dose of PPA (mg)	Dosing Schedule	Duration of Drug Intake[b] (days)	n	Sex	Age (years)	Diagnosis
Lunerin	100	b.i.d.	5	23	NS	A	Vasomotor rhinitis
Lunerin	100	b.i.d.	5	27	9M, 18F	20–53	Perennial allergic rhinitis
Lunerin	100	b.i.d.	14	31	17M, 14F	20–60	Vasomotor rhinitis
Lunerin vs. Rinomar	100 75	b.i.d. t.i.d.	5	32	NS	>15	Allergic rhinitis
Rinomar	50–400[c]	b.i.d.	31	40	26M, 14F	5–18	Seasonal allergic rhinitis
Rinomar syrup	55	3–4/day	14	78	M, F	5–12	Seasonal allergic rhinitis
Lunerin-mite	50	b.i.d.	7	17	14M, 3F	4–14	Chronic rhinitis
Triaminic	150	t.i.d.	10	104	38M, 66F	NS	Rhinitis
Triaminic	NS	Acute	NS	80[d] 45[e]	NS	A	Rhinitis

[a]Symbols: + —symptom relieved by drug treatment; 0—no effect; A—adult; NR—not reported; NS—not specified.
[b]Duration of drug treatment for a single drug.
[c]Dose adjusted to the age of the patient.
[d]Double-blind study.
[e]Uncontrolled study.

TABLE 5.4. Continued

Results					
Symptoms Relieved					
Sneez-ing	Itch-ing	Rhinor-rhea	Conges-tion	Comments	Reference
+	0	+	+	Additional uncontrolled study showed that Lunerin was effective at higher doses	Axelsson (1972)
+	+	+	+	Duration of action >10 hr in 17/19 patients	Mercke & Wihl (1973a)
NR	NR	+	+	Rhinoscopic examination showed no effect on edema or secretions; Lunerin and Disofrol were equally effective	Lofkvist & Svensson (1978)
+	+	+	+	Lunerin was more effective than Rinomar for all symptoms except secretions	Mercke & Wihl (1973b)
+	+	+	+		
NR	NR	NR	NR	Reduced symptoms when pollen count was low; no effect when pollen count was high	Moller & Bjorksten (1980)
NR	NR	+	+	Favorable response in 86% of patients; Rinomar and Disophrol syrups equally effective	Horak (1982)
+	+	+	+	Lunerin-mite reduced symptoms and improved clinical status; duration of action 0–12 hr (mean 9.4 hr)	Kjellman (1975)
NR	NR	NR	NR	Triaminic produced fair to excellent response; time to onset was 50 min and duration of effect was 6 hr; Drixoral was more effective than Triaminic	Aaronson et al. (1968)
NR	NR	NR	NR	Triaminic more effective than placebo when evaluated by patient rating, physician examination or by rhinomanometric test	Wenger & Lapsa (1970)

tested and compared by Mercke and Wihl (1973a,b). There were two randomized, double-blind, crossover clinical trials in patients with allergic rhinitis. The duration of drug administration in each phase was 5 days, with 2 drug-free days between treatments. Lunerin was taken b.i.d., whereas Rinomar was taken t.i.d. Thus the total daily doses of phenylpropanolamine in the two groups were 100 and 75 mg, respectively. In the comparison study (Mercke & Wihl, 1973b), all patients took one tablet t.i.d. during both the Lunerin and Rinomar treatment periods. During the Lunerin treatment, the morning and evening doses were active drug and the midday dose was placebo, whereas during the Rinomar treatment all three doses were active drug. These precautions were followed in order to maintain the double-blind conditions of the study. The drug efficacy was evaluated from the patients' subjective ratings of nasal symptoms (irritation, obstruction, secretion), by number of sneezing attacks recorded on "sneeze cards," and by clinical evaluation by a physician. Both Lunerin and Rinomar were effective in reducing all four major symptoms of allergic rhinitis. Furthermore, Lunerin was more effective than Rinomar, and the differences between the drug treatments were statistically significant for all the symptoms except nasal secretions. The differences between the drug treatments are difficult to evaluate, however, since Lunerin contains more phenylpropanolamine than Rinomar (50 and 25 mg, respectively) and the two products contain different antihistamines (brompheniramine and cinnarizine, respectively). Thus Lunerin may be more effective because it contains more phenylpropanolamine or because brompheniramine is more effective than cinnarizine. Also Lunerin is a sustained-release product, whereas Rinomar is not.

COMBINATIONS OF PHENYLPROPANOLAMINE, ANTIHISTAMINES AND ANTICHOLINERGICS

Contac, Eskornade, and Ornade are triple-combination products containing phenylpropanolamine, an antihistamine, and anticholinergic drugs. The clinical trials with Contac, Eskornade, and Ornade are summarized in Table 5.5. These products were shown to be moderately effective in symptomatic treatment of rhinitis or upper respiratory tract infections. Ornade was rated poorly effective in treatment of sinusitis in the double-blind clinical trial.

The therapeutic efficacy of Ornade spansules was systematically compared in three groups of patients with different diagnoses (Ashe, 1968). The patients all had nasal congestion, and the diagnoses were allergic rhinitis, upper respiratory infection, and sinusitis. Ornade was equally effective in symptomatic treatment of patients with allergic rhinitis and upper respiratory infections, but much less effective in patients with sinusitis.

Presumably, the rationale for including the anticholinergic drugs in these triple-combination products is to decrease the nasal secretions, since the seromucous glands of the nasal mucosa are stimulated by cholinergic influences. Unfortunately, the effects of these drugs on the nasal secretions was not specifically tested in any of the three studies, and it is not possible to determine whether this was indeed the contribution of the anticholinergic drugs to the therapeutic efficacy.

MULTIPLE COMPONENT COMBINATIONS

Clinical trials testing the decongestant efficacy of multicomponent combinations that contain phenylpropanolamine are summarized in Table 5.6.

Ru-Tuss contains the triple combination (phenylpropanolamine-antihistamine-anticholinergic) plus another sympathomimetic amine, phenylephrine (see Table 5.3). Ru-Tuss was shown to be an effective decongestant in a controlled clinical trial in patients with allergic rhinitis (Jackson et al., 1975) and an uncontrolled clinical case study in patients with maxillary sinusitis (Pou et al., 1970). Dimetapp L.A., a triple-combination product containing phenylpropanolamine, another sympathomimetic amine, and an antihistamine, was also shown to be an effective decongestant in patients with rhinitis or postnasal discharge (Edwards et al., 1973). Rymed, a triple-combination product that contains no antihistamine (Table 5.3), was an effective decongestant in patients with allergic or nonallergic perennial rhinitis (Erffmeyer et al., 1982), suggesting that the antihistamine is not absolutely required for effective decongestion. Finally, Sinulin, which contains two analgesics in addition to the phenylpropanolamine-antihistamine-anticholinergic combination (Table 5.3), was effective in therapy of pansinusitis caused by environmental pollution (Rhea, 1971).

In a randomized, double-blind, between-groups clinical study, Middleton (1981) evaluated the nasal decongestant effect of a combination phenylpropanolamine-containing product in male and female patients (18–75 years old) who had a common cold or related upper respiratory tract infection. Ninety-one patients received Benylin Day and Night: the "Day" formulation contained 500 mg of acetaminophen and 25 mg of phenylpropanolamine; in the "Night" formulation phenylpropanolamine is replaced with 25 mg of the antihistamine diphenhydramine. Three Day tablets and one Night tablet were given daily for 5 days. Ninety patients received 500 mg of acetaminophen q.i.d. for 5 days. Subjects kept daily diaries to record symptoms and side effects. There was a significant reduction in severity of symptoms during the 5-day trial for both treatment groups, and in both groups more patients thought their tablets helped more at night than by day. However, a significantly greater number of patients felt that Benylin Day and Night helped their cold symptoms more than did acetaminophen, irrespective of day or night use. Benylin Day and Night seemed to reduce headache severity more than acetaminophen did throughout the trial (the difference was significant on day

TABLE 5.5. Efficacy of Combination Products Containing Phenylpropanolamine, Antihistamines, and Anticholinergicas[a]

	Drug			Patients			
Tradename	Total Daily Dose of PPA (mg)	Dosing Schedule	Duration of Drug Intake[b] (days)	n	Sex	Age (years)	Diagnosis
Contac	50	acute	—	15	11F, 4M	NS	Allergic rhinitis
Eskornade	100	b.i.d.	7	45	22M, 23F	15–>50	Rhinitis
Ornade	100	b.i.d.	10	126	M, F	NS	Allergic rhinitis; URI; sinusitis

[a]Abbreviations and symbols: NR—not reported; NS—not specified; URI—upper respiratory tract infection; + —symptom reduced.
[b]Duration of drug treatment per each drug (or placebo).

3). The number of patients given Benylin Day and Night who reported "treatment-related upset" was similar to the acetaminophen group on day 1 but fell to zero on days 3–5; from day 3 this difference was significant.

Lea (1984) used rhinomanometry to measure nasal patency and thus evaluate the nasal decongestant effect of a single oral dose of a combination product containing a low (25 mg) dose of phenylpropanolamine. The study was double-blind, placebo-controlled, randomized, and noncrossover. Subjects were 18 volunteers (sex not specified, 18–70 years old) with complaints of nasal congestion due solely to a common cold (i.e., nonallergic rhinitis). Onset

TABLE 5.5 Continued

| | | | | Results | |
| Symptoms Relieved | | | | | |
Sneez- ing	Itch- ing	Rhinor- rhea	Conges- tion	Comments	Reference
NR	NR	NR	+	93.3% of the patients reported subjective improvement of symptoms following Contac	Cohen (1975)
NR	NR	NR	NR	Clinical response rated fair to excellent; Demazin and Eskornade were equally effective	Heron (1972)
NR	NR	NR	NR	Ornade was rated good in the majority of patients with rhinitis or URI, but poor in patients with sinusitis; overall, Ornade and Actifed were equally effective, but Drixoral was rated better than either drug	Ashe (1968)

of symptoms (coryza, lacrimation, irritated nasopharynx, chilliness, malaise) was 24–72 hr prior to study and no nasal decongestant medication had been used for at least 12 hr prior to study. Eight subjects received a single 20 ml dose of Day Nurse (25 mg of phenylpropanolamine, 500 mg of acetaminophen, 60 mg of vitamin C, 15 mg of dextromethorphan, 3.08 ml of alcohol); 10 subjects received placebo. For the Day Nurse group a significant reduction in nasal congestion was obtained at the 1-, 2-, 3-, and 4-hr postdosing measurement times from initial values compared to placebo values. The maximum decongestant effect was achieved during the first hour after dosing and remained approximately constant over the next 3 hr.

TABLE 5.6. Efficacy of Multicomponent Combinations[a]

	Drug			Patients			
Tradename	Total Daily Dose of PPA (mg)	Dosing Schedule	Duration of Drug Intake[b] (days)	n	Sex	Age (years)	Diagnosis
Day Nurse	25	o.d.	1	18	NS	18–70	Common cold
Benylin Day & Night	75	b.i.d.	5	91	M,F	18–75	Common cold or related infection
Ru-Tuss	100	b.i.d.	7	24	NS	NS	Allergic rhinitis
Ru-Tuss	100	b.i.d.	(≤ 4 months)	10	8F, 2M	4–58	Maxillary sinus disease
Dimetapp L.A.	30	b.i.d.	28	48	19M, 29F	10–70	Vasomotor rhinitis, post-nasal discharge
Rymed	180	q.i.d.	14	22	8M, 14F	22–60	Perennial rhinitis
Sinulin	300	2 tablets q.i.d.	$3\frac{1}{2}$–4	35	NS	18–73	Pansinusitis

[a]Symbols: NS—not specified; NR—not required; NA—not applicable; + —symptom relieved; 0—no effect.
[b]Duration of drug treatment per each drug (or placebo).

SPECIAL STUDIES

STUDIES IN PEDIATRIC PATIENTS
The decongestant efficacy of phenylpropanolamine-containing products in pediatric patients was investigated in several studies. Rinomar and Rinomar syrup were shown to be effective decongestants in children with allergic rhinitis (Horak, 1982; Moller & Bjorksten, 1980), and Lunerin-mite was

TABLE 5.6 Continued

Results					
Symptoms Relieved					
Sneez-ing	Itch-ing	Rhinor-rhea	Conges-tion	Comments	Reference
NR	NR	NR	+	Day Nurse caused significant decongestion 1–4 hr after a single dose	Lea (1984)
NR	NR	+	+	Benylin Day & Night was more effective than acetaminophen	Middleton (1981)
+	0	+	0	Ru-Tuss significantly reduced 7/11 symptoms of rhinitis	Jackson et al. (1975)
NA	NA	NA	NA	Clinical case studies, confirmed by x-rays; subjective and objective evidence of relief from sinusitis	Pou et al. (1970)
NR	NR	+	+	81.5% of patients rated Dimetapp L.A. better than placebo	Edwards et al. (1973)
+	+	+	+	Good decongestion without antihistamines	Erffmeyer et al. (1982)
NR	NR	NR	NR	Sinusitis believed to be due to atmospheric pollution; uncontrolled study; Sinulin rated "very effective" in symptomatic treatment in 35/35 patients	Rhea (1971)

shown to be effective in children with chronic rhinitis (Kjellman, 1975). The study designs and results of these three studies are summarized in Table 5.4. Phenylpropanolamine-containing products were also effective in symptomatic treatment of children with upper respiratory disorders (Carter, 1965) and acute cough (Jaffe & Grimshaw, 1983). However, most studies have concluded that phenylpropanolamine-containing products are ineffective in treatment of children with otitis media (see the paragraphs that follow).

Phenylpropanolamine-containing products were ineffective either in therapy of acute cases of otitis media or in prevention of otitis media when given prophylactically.

It is well recognized in pediatric clinical pharmacology that drug dosages in children need to be adjusted to both the age and body weight of the child. In some of the pediatric studies, products specifically formulated for pediatric use were investigated, including Lunerin-mite and Sinutab pediatric suspension. In other studies, general-formulation products were investigated, with the dosages adjusted for pediatric patients. The age-adjusted dosages for selected phenylpropanolamine-containing products are summarized in Table 5.7. The differences in the dose-response relationships for phenylpropanolamine between children and adults have not been investigated. Furthermore, none of the studies systematically investigated the dose-response relationship as a function of the age of the child. Kjellman (1975) claimed that a fixed dose of Lunerin-mite was less effective in children over the age of 10 than in children less than 10 years old. However, the data do not demonstrate a clear difference in the response as a function of age, and no statistical analysis of this effect was presented.

The efficacy of Sinutab pediatric suspension in symptomatic treatment of upper respiratory disorders was investigated in 100 permanently hospitalized, mentally retarded patients (Carter, 1965). Epidemics of upper respiratory disorders are a particular problem in institutionalized patients, and especially among nonambulatory or semiambulatory patients. In this study, 100 patients (48 female, 52 male; ages 2–15 years) with an average mental age of 2 years were studied. The upper respiratory disorders (and incidences) were as follows: allergy (59), upper respiratory infection (33), pharyngitis (7), and

TABLE 5.7. Dosages of Phenylpropanolamine-Containing Products in Pediatric Patients

Product	Formulation	Age (years)	Dose of PPA (mg)	Dosing Schedule	Reference
Generic	Tablets (SR)[a]	4–9	50	b.i.d.	Meistrup-Larsen et al.
		≥ 10	100	b.i.d.	(1978); Thomsen
	Syrup	0.5–2	16.5	t.i.d.	et al. (1979)
		3–5	25	t.i.d.	
		6–9	33	t.i.d.	
Generic	Combination	0.5–1.5	8.33	q. 4–6 hr	Randall & Hendley
	syrup[b]	1.5–3	12.5	q. 4–6 hr	(1979)
		3–5	18.75	q. 4–6 hr	
Lunerin-mite	Tablets	<7	25	b.i.d.	Moller (1980)
		>7	50	b.i.d.	

[a]SR—sustained release.
[b]Ingredients: 25 mg of phenylpropanolamine and 2 mg of brompheniramine per teaspoon.

chronic rhinitis (1). The dose of Sinutab was adjusted to the age of the patient and ranged from 1/2 to 2 teaspoons (phenylpropanolamine dose 6.25–25 mg), q.i.d. The following signs were rated on an ordinal scale after 24 hr on the medication: mucosal congestion, airway obstruction, nasal secretion, malaise, and pain. The results were analyzed separately for each diagnostic category. Sinutab was most effective in patients with allergies. In patients with allergy, 100% had excellent or good response to Sinutab. Therapeutic response in patients with upper respiratory infection, pharyngitis, or rhinitis was also favorable, with the response rated excellent in at least 30% of the patients in each group. The greatest symptomatic response was decrease in nasal secretions, although all symptoms responded well to therapy with Sinutab. The time to onset of the effects of Sinutab was 15–30 min.

Otitis media is a common problem in pediatric medicine. It is estimated that 20% of 5-year-old children have medical problems related to the middle ear and that 60% of surgery in children under 10 years old is for correction of otitis media (Fraser et al., 1977). Otitis media is a serious problem that may cause recurrent otalgia or conductive deafness. The diagnostic criteria for otitis media are reddening, bulging, edema, and immobility of the tympanic membrane (Thomsen et al., 1979). The etiology of otitis media includes swelling of the mucosa in the eustachian tube (Kjellman et al., 1978), allergy, and complications secondary to the common cold (Randall & Hendley, 1979). Children with cleft palate are particularly susceptible to otitis media (Moller, 1980). Treatment includes antibiotics, nasal decongestants, and surgery to relieve the excess pressure in the middle ear. It has been suggested that α-adrenergic decongestants are ineffective in therapy of otitis media because the mucosa of the eustachian tube is devoid of erectile tissue (Meistrup-Larsen et al., 1978).

The results of clinical trials testing the efficacy of phenylpropanolamine-containing products in treatment of otitis media are summarized in Table 5.8. Phenylpropanolamine-containing products were ineffective in acute therapy of otitis media, and prophylactic administration did not prevent or reduce the occurrence of otitis media (Kjellman et al., 1978; Randall & Hendley, 1979; Renvall & Nilsson, 1982). Phenylpropanolamine, either alone or combined with an antihistamine, was ineffective against otitis media (Haugeto et al., 1981). Nonhospitalized children with secretory otitis media who were awaiting operation for adenoid removal and were given a phenylpropanolamine-antihistamine product showed significant increase in adenoid histamine content of mass cells, but no change in histamine content of middle-ear fluid or nasopharyngeal secretions (Collins & Church, 1983). The only report in the literature citing beneficial effects of a phenylpropanolamine-antihistamine combination in treating secretory otitis media is by Saunte and Johansson (1978). In their study of 21 children, healing time and

TABLE 5.8. Clinical Studies of Phenylpropanolamine-Containing Products in Treatment of Otitis Media

| Drug | | | | Patients | | | |
Trade-name	PPA Formulation	Dosing Schedule	Duration	n	Sex	Age (years)	Diagnosis
—[b]	50-mg tablet; syrup[c]	Adjusted for age	1–2 wk	100	53M, 47F	0.5–>10	Acute OM
—	50-mg SR, syrup[c]	Adjusted for age	1–2 wk	93	50M, 43F	0.5–10	Acute OM
—	Combination syrup[d]	Adjusted for age	32 wk	104	NS	0.5–5	Common cold
—	100 mg	b.i.d.	Acute vs. 1 wk	17	NS	8–56	SOM
Monydrin vs. Lunerin	100-mg tablet 50-mg tablet	NS NS	4 wk	77	NS	1–14	SOM
Lunerine-mite	25-mg tablet	NS	10–21 days	44	M, F	<13	OM; SOM
Lunerine-mite	25-mg tablet	Adjusted for age	6 wk	26	10F, 16F	5–19	Cleft palate or cleft lip and palate SOM or negative middle ear pressure

340

TABLE 5.8 Continued

Design	Measurements	Results	Reference
Randomized DB parallel groups	Otoscopy; tympanometry; symptom score cards	No improvement attributed to PPA	Meistrup-Larsen et al. (1978)
Randomized PC parallel groups	Otoscopy; tympanometry; symptom score cards	No therapeutic effect attributed to PPA	Thomsen et al. (1979)
PC crossover	Symptom score cards; clinical evaluation	No prophylactic effect of PPA on development of OM secondary to common colds	Randall & Mendley (1979)
DB crossover	Eustachian tube function (aspiration and deflation technique)	No effect attributed to PPA; no effect of either acute or repeated dosing	Renvall & Nilsson (1982)
DB PC parallel groups	Clinical examination; otoscopy; audiometry	No effect of either drug on otoscopic findings, conduction threshold or tympanometry results; PPA ineffective either alone or with antihistamine	Haugeto et al. (1981)
DB parallel groups PC	ENT examination; audiometry; symptom score cards	No prophylactic effect on number of episodes of OM or SOM; no effect on symptoms	Kjellman et al. (1978)
ENT examination	ENT examination	No effect of Lunerin on hearing improvement; no effect of Lunerin on middle-ear infusions; no effect of Lunerin on middle-ear pressure	Moller (1980)

341

TABLE 5.8. Continued.

Drug				Patients			
Trade-name	PPA Formulation	Dosing Schedule	Duration	n	Sex	Age (years)	Diagnosis
Lunerine-mite or Lunerin-mixt	NS	NS	≤8 wk	73	48M, 25F	0.5–13	Recent episode of OM
Dimetapp	5 mg/5 ml	t.i.d.	6 wk	85 (10–11 per group)	47M, 38F	3–12	SOM
Dimetapp vs. Triaminic	NS	NS	NS	30	NS	<9	Chronic SOM
				31	NS	<9	
BPP	NS	Adjusted for age	1–28 days	58	39M, 21F	5–14	Bilateral SOM
Naldecon + anti-biotic[e]	syrup	q.i.d.; adjusted to body weight	14 days	53	25M, 28F	7 mo–15 yr	Acute OM with effusion
Dimetapp	5 mg/5 ml	t.i.d.	7 days	8	NS	NS	SOM

342

TABLE 5.8 Continued

Design	Measurements	Results	Reference
Parallel groups	Clinical assessment	No effect on development of SOM	Sorri et al. (1982)
8 combinations of 3 treatments	Clinical examination; audiometry; tympanometry	No therapeutic improvement attributed to Dimetapp; no improvement attributed to ephedrine nose drops	Fraser et al. (1977)
Retrospective	Clinical assessment	Either drug alone poorly effective; effectiveness increased when combined with antibiotics	Forquer & Linthicum (1982)
Randomized DB PC	Clinical examination, including otoscopy	No effect of BPP on hearing thresholds for either air or bone conduction	Khan et al. (1981)
DB parallel groups	Clinical evaluation; tympanometry; symptom diary	Naldecon + antibiotics reduced middle ear effusions more than antibiotics alone; no effect on tympanograms or physician's evaluation	Moran et al. (1982)
Randomized DB parallel groups Age- and sex-matched groups	Adenoid wt; histamine content of adenoids, middle-ear fluid, nasopharyngeal secretions	Significant increase in adenoid histamine content of mast cells; no effect on histamine content of middle-ear fluid or nasopharyngeal secretions	Collins & Church (1983)

TABLE 5.8. Continued.

Drug				Patients			
Trade-name	PPA Formulation	Dosing Schedule	Duration	*n*	Sex	Age (years)	Diagnosis
Dimetapp + Antibiotic[d]	5 mg/5 ml	Adjusted for age	10 days	33	M,F	< 15	Acute OM
Lunerin-mixt	1.7 mg/ml	t.i.d. adjusted for age	16–85 days	11	NS	3–10	SOM
Lunerin-mite	25 mg tablet	b.i.d.					

[a]Abbreviations: OM—otitis media; SOM—secretory otitis media; DB—double blind; PC—placebo controlled;
SR—sustained release; BPP—brompheniramine, phenylephrine, phenylpropanolamine;
ENT—ear, nose, throat; NS—not specified.
[b]Generic phenylpropanolamine.
[c]Syrup—333 mg phenylpropanolamine/100 ml.
[d]Combination syrup—25 mg phenylpropanolamine and 2 mg brompheniramine/teaspoon.
[e]Amoxicillin suspension.

otoscopy findings were significantly improved for the drug group compared to a placebo group.

The combined use of a phenylpropanolamine-containing product and antibiotics may be effective in therapy of otitis media (Forquer & Linthicum, 1982; Moran et al., 1982) although some studies suggest that no benefit can be expected from the use of phenylpropanolamine-antihistamine medication as an adjunct to antibiotic therapy in treating this common pediatric disorder (Schnore et al., 1986).

ANTITUSSIVE EFFICACY

The antitussive efficacy of phenylpropanolamine-containing products has been demonstrated in an experimental study in healthy human adults (Packman & London, 1977) and a clinical trial in pediatric patients (Jaffe & Grimshaw, 1983). The antitussive efficacy of phenylpropanolamine was also demonstrated in experimental animals (Winter & Flataker, 1954) (see also Chapter 3).

TABLE 5.8 Continued.

Design	Measurements	Results	Reference
Randomized DB, PC, parallel groups	Otoscopy, pneumatic otoscopy, symptom score card	No benefits seen in those children given phenylpropanolamine/antihistamine preparation	Schnore et al. (1986)
Randomized DB, PC	ENT examination Audiometry Otoscopy	Significant therapeutic improvement on every investigated parameter (hearing threshold, eardrum appearance and mobility, number of myringotomies, time to recovery)	Saunte & Johansson (1978)

The laboratory technique used in the experimental study in humans was the artificially induced cough technique (Packman & London, 1977). This is an objective technique for measuring antitussive effects in humans. The apparatus is shown in Figure 5.6. The subjects were fitted with a face mask. At intervals, aerosolized citric acid was delivered under positive pressure to the face mask. The citric acid spray was inhaled by the subject, and this irritation produced coughing. The coughs were measured polygraphically by a pneumotachometer and a microphone. Artificially induced coughs were measured before and at intervals after administration of the following drugs: (1) 25 mg of phenylpropanolamine and 20 mg of dextromethorphan; (2) 100 mg of glyceryl guaiacolate, an expectorant; (3) a combination of these three drugs; and (4) placebo. The results are summarized in Figure 5.7. Each drug treatment reduced coughing in the artificially induced cough test. The most effective drug treatment was the triple-drug combination. The time to onset of effect was approximately 30 min, and the duration of effect was 4–5 hr.

The efficacies of Pholcolix and Actifed cough linctus preparations were

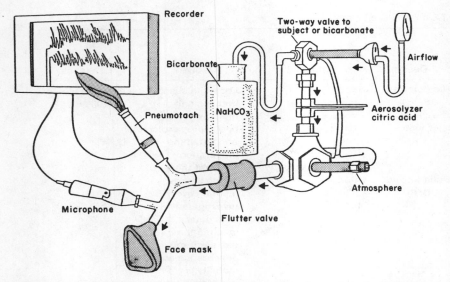

Figure 5.6. Apparatus for measuring artificially induced cough in humans. From *Packman and London (1977)*.

tested in a randomized, single-blind, between-group comparison clinical trial (Jaffe & Grimshaw, 1983). A total of 217 children aged 6–12 years with acute cough due to upper respiratory infection were studied. Pholcolix was given q.i.d. and Actifed t.i.d. for 72 hr. The overall effectiveness was rated by both a physician and the patient or a parent. Both Pholcolix and Actifed decreased coughing and the sore throat associated with the upper respiratory infections. Pholcolix was rated as more palatable, and produced fewer side effects, than Actifed.

EFFICACY OF A PHENYLPROPANOLAMINE-CONTAINING COMBINATION PRODUCT IN ASTHMA

Asbron is a combination product containing phenylpropanolamine, theophylline sodium glycinate, and glyceryl guaiacolate (see Table 5.3). Theophylline, a methylxanthine, is a bronchodilator often used in asthma therapy. Glyceryl guaiacolate is an expectorant. The efficacy of this combination product in symptomatic treatment of patients with bronchial asthma or asthmatic bronchitis was investigated by Parrillo and Humoller (1966). Nine patients took Asbron elixir (t.i.d.), and three patients took Asbron tablets (q.i.d.). Asbron produced good symptomatic treatment of bronchial asthma. The drug treatment decreased wheezing, coughing, and dyspnea and improved

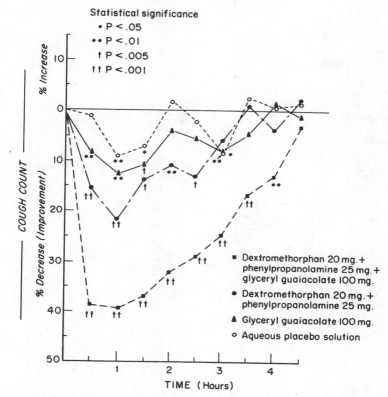

Figure 5.7. Effects of drugs on artificially induced cough in humans. From *Packman and London (1977)*.

expectoration. There was no difference in the efficacy of Asbron between elixir and tablet formulation.

SIDE EFFECTS OF PHENYLPROPANOLAMINE-CONTAINING DECONGESTANT PRODUCTS

Phenylpropanolamine, alone or in combination products, has been reported to produce a low incidence of side effects in published studies. The side effects described were mild, and rarely did any patient withdraw from a clinical trial due to the occurrence of side effects. The incidence of various side effects of phenylpropanolamine-containing products is summarized in Tables 5.9–5.13.

TABLE 5.9. Side Effects of Decongestants Containing Phenylpropanolamine Alone[a]

Tradename: PPA dose (mg): Reference:	Generic 25 McLaurin et al. (1961)		Generic[b] 50 (SR)[c] Cohen (1975)		Monydrin 100 Broms & Malm (1982)		Monydrin 50, 100 Renvall & Lindqvist (1979)		
	PPA	Placebo	PPA	Placebo	PPA	Placebo	50 mg PPA	100 mg PPA	Placebo
Blood pressure change ≥20 mm Hg	14/88	5/88	—	—	—	—	NS	NS	NS
Heart rate change ≥10 bpm	3/88	3/88	—	—	—	—	—	—	—
Headache	4/88	4/88	—	—	2/17	7/17	—	—	—
Dizziness	3/88	1/88	1/15	—	—	—	—	—	—
Nervousness	10/88	27/88	3/15	—	—	—	—	—	—
Jittery feeling	—	—	2/15	—	—	—	1/25	0/18	1/26
Drowsiness, sleepiness	1/88	0/88	—	—	0/17	0/17	—	—	—
Sleep disturbances	—	—	—	—	—	—	5/25[d]	2/18[d]	3/26[d]
Dry	0/88	1/88	1/15	1/15	—	—	—	—	—
Gassy feeling	—	—	2/15	—	—	—	—	—	—
Nausea	2/88	2/88	—	—	—	—	1/25	2/18	0/26
Micturition difficulty	—	—	—	—	2/17[e]	0/17	—	—	—
Urticaria, hives	1/88	0/88	—	—	—	—	—	—	—
Asthma	1/88	0/88	—	—	—	—	—	—	—

[a]Entries represent number of patients with side effects per total number of patients.
[b]Contac formulation containing phenylpropanolamine alone.
[c]SR—sustained release.
[d]Difficulty falling asleep on day 4.
[e]Two older males, ages 60 and 64 years.

TABLE 5.10. Effects of Phenylpropanolamine on Heart Rate and Blood Pressure in Patients with Chronic Nonallergic Rhinitis[a]

	Blood Pressure (mm Hg)		Heart Rate (bpm)
	Systolic	Diastolic	
Recumbent			
Predrug	121 ± 15	77 ± 6	68 ± 10
PPA[b]	122 ± 13	78 ± 5	66 ± 9
Sitting			
Predrug	122 ± 14	80 ± 6	69 ± 11
PPA[b]	126 ± 18	78 ± 4	66 ± 9

Source: Data from Broms & Malm (1982).
[a]n = 10 patients, ages 16–64 years.
[b]Monydrin, 100-mg phenylpropanolamine, sustained-release.

The side effects reported in patients taking phenylpropanolamine alone in doses of 25 to 100 mg are summarized in Table 5.9. In most cases the incidence of side effects was similar in patients taking phenylpropanolamine to that in patients on placebo. Phenylpropanolamine produced a low incidence of side effects indicating either CNS stimulation ("nervousness," "jittery" feelings) or sedation ("drowsy," "sleepy"). In fact, in one study the incidence of nervousness was lower in patients taking phenylpropanolamine than in those on placebo; whether the phenylpropanolamine was in immediate- or sustained-release formulation was not specified (McLaurin et al., 1961). Likewise, fewer patients complained of headache when taking phenylpropanolamine than when taking placebo (Broms & Malm, 1982). Two patients taking 100 mg of phenylpropanolamine in a sustained-release formulation had difficulty in micturition, but these were older male patients (Broms & Malm, 1982). Dry mouth was an infrequent side effect of phenylpropanolamine alone. There was no consistent dose-response relationship for side effects with phenylpropanolamine.

Cardiovascular side effects of phenylpropanolamine taken alone were not striking. In patients taking low doses of phenylpropanolamine, the incidence of patients with increased, decreased, or unchanged systolic blood pressure was 31/88, 18/88, and 39/88, respectively (McLaurin et al., 1961). Heart rate was not significantly changed by phenylpropanolamine. A more quantitative evaluation of cardiovascular side effects was conducted in patients taking the high dose of 100 mg of phenylpropanolamine (Broms & Malm, 1982). As shown in Table 5.10, this high dose produced virtually no effect on systolic or diastolic blood pressure or heart rate, measured in either the recumbent or sitting position.

Since both antihistamines and anticholinergic drugs produce side effects

TABLE 5.11. Side Effects of Combination Decongestant Products Containing Phenylpropanolamine and Antihistamines[a]

Tradename: PPA dose (mg):	Lunerin 50								Rinomar 25		Triaminic 50			
Reference:	Axelsson (1972)		Lofkvist & Svensson (1978)		Mercke & Wihl (1973a)		Mercke & Wihl (1973b)		Mercke & Wihl (1973b)		Aaronson et al. (1968)		Wenger & Lapsa (1970)	
	A	P	A	P	A	P	A	P	A	P	A	P	A	P
Sleepiness, drowsiness	4/23	1/23	3/31	3/31	—	—	—	—	—	—	8/104	—	56%	38%
Fatigue	—	—	—	—	5/27	5/27	+[b]	—	+	—	—	—	+	+
Dry mouth–throat–nose	—	—	—	—	4/27	—	+[b]	—	+	—	4/104	—	+	+
Headache	—	—	3/31	3/31	—	1/27	—	—	—	—	—	—	+	+
Dizziness	—	—	1/31	0/31	—	—	—	—	—	—	—	—	+	+
Restlessness	—	—	1/31	0/31	1/27	—	—	—	—	—	—	—	—	—
Impaired sleep	—	—	—	—	—	1/27	—	—	—	—	—	—	—	—
Nausea	—	—	1/31	1/31	1/27	1/27	—	—	—	—	—	—	—	—
Anxiety	—	—	—	—	—	1/27	—	—	—	—	—	—	—	—
Eyes itching, smarting	1/23	—	—	—	—	—	—	—	—	—	—	—	—	—

						Pediatric preparations			
Visual blurring	—	—	—	—	—	—	—	—	—
Palpitation, tachycardia	—	1/31	0/31	1/27	1/27	1/27	—	—	—
Urticaria	—	—	—	—	—	1/104	—	—	—
Thirst	1/23	—	—	—	+	—	+	—	—
Constipation	1/23	—	—	—	—	—	—	—	—
Tremor	(1/27)c	—	—	—	—	—	—	—	—
Total	—	—	—	9/32	—	6/32	—	—	—

	Lunerin-mite 25			Rinomar 25		Rinomar syrup 12.5	
Tradename: PPA dose (mg):							
Reference:	Max Kjellman (1975)			Moller & Bjorksten (1980)		Horak (1982)	
	A	P		A	P	A	P
Fatigue	1/17	2/17		5/13	—	No serious adverse reactions were reported	
Hair loss, slight	—	—		1/13	—		

aEntries represent number of patients with side effects per total number of patients (+ —side effect reported but incidence not specified; A—active drug; P—placebo).

bOne patient discontinued medication because of side effects.

cUncontrolled study.

TABLE 5.12. Side Effects of Combination Decongestant Products Containing Phenylpropanolamine, Antihistamines, and Anticholinergics[a]

Tradename: PPA dose (mg):	Contac 50		Eskornade 50	Ornade 50	Ru-Tuss 50
Reference:	Cohen (1975)		Heron (1972)	Ashe (1968)	Pou et al. (1970)
	A	P	A[b]	A[b]	
Drowsiness, yawning	1/15	—	+	3/24	Not associated with side effects of any kind[c]
Dry mouth, lips	3/15	1/15	+		
Dizziness	—	—	3/50	—	
Headache	—	—	3/50	—	
Nocturnal restlessness	—	—	—	0/42	
Total	—	—	57%	—	0/10

[a]Entries represent number of patients with side effects per total number of patients (+ —side effect reported but incidence not specified; A—active drug; P—placebo).
[b]No placebo control; double-blind study.
[c]Uncontrolled clinical case study.

TABLE 5.13. Side Effects of Multicomponent Decongestant Combinations Containing Phenylpropanolamine[a]

Tradename: PPA dose (mg): Reference:	Phocolix 12.5 Jaffe & Grimshaw (1983)	Sinutab 12.5 Carter (1965)	Dimetapp L.A. 15 Edwards et al. (1973)		Asbron 25 Parrillo & Humoller (1966)	Sinulin 37.5 Rhea (1971)	Rymed 45 Erffmeyer et al. (1982)		Benylin Day and Night 25 Middleton (1981)
	A[b]	A[b]	A	P	A[b]	A[b]	A	P	A
Drowsiness	28/105	—	4/48	2/48	—	5/35	—	—	4/96
Nausea	8/105	—	—	—	(2/18)[c]	—	—	1/22	5/96
Headaches	—	—	2/48	—	—	—	—	1/22	1/96
Anorexia	8/105	—	—	—	—	—	—	—	1/96
GI disturbances	—	—	1/48	1/48	—	—	—	—	5/96
Nervousness	0/105	—	—	—	—	1/35	—	—	—
Tremor	0/105	—	—	—	—	—	—	—	—
Heartburn	0/105	—	—	—	—	—	1/22	—	—
Urinary effects	—	—	—	—	—	—	—	—	—
Malaise	—	—	—	—	—	—	—	1/22	—
Diarrhea	—	—	—	—	—	—	—	1/22	0/96
Total	31/105	—	7/48	3/48	—	6/35	1/22[d]	1/22[d]	9/96

[a]Entries represent number of patients with side effects per total number of patients (A—active drug; P—placebo).
[b]No placebo control.
[c]Nausea when taking Asbron elixir but not when taking tablets.
[d]One patient from each group withdrew from the study because of side effects.

of sedation and dry mouth, it is to be expected that combinations of phenyl-propanolamine with antihistamines and/or anticholinergics will produce these side effects (Tables 5.11 and 5.12). Other side effects occurred with a low incidence and were not consistently observed with the various preparations. The pediatric preparations produced a low incidence of mild side effects (Table 5.11).

The multicomponent combinations were also associated with a low incidence of mild side effects (Table 5.13).

Surprisingly, only one clinical trial reported anorexia as a side effect of phenylpropanolamine-containing cough-cold preparations (Jaffe & Grimshaw, 1983) (see also Table 5.13), and this preparation contained a low dose of phenylpropanolamine. It cannot be determined whether the lack of reported anorexia could be attributed to the investigators' failure to specifically question the patients regarding possible effects on appetite and food intake. On the other hand, since the patients in most of these studies were being treated for rhinitis and related conditions, perhaps the patient population in general had poor appetites secondary to their disease conditions. Nonetheless, loss of appetite has not been a prominent side effect of phenylpropanol-amine-containing decongestant products.

EFFICACY OF PHENYLPROPANOLAMINE AS AN ANORECTIC DRUG IN THE TREATMENT OF OBESITY

Obesity, one of the major health problems in our society today, has been defined in various ways. In general, obesity is the condition in which an individual's body weight significantly exceeds the norm or the ideal body weight, adjusted for age, sex, and body size. Although the quantitative definition of obesity is somewhat arbitrary, obesity has been considered to exist when an individual's body weight exceeds the ideal body weight by 20% (House, 1981) to 25% (Baptista & Beauchemin, 1981). The incidence of obesity has been estimated to be 25–45% of adults and 2–15% of children (Baptista & Beauchemin, 1981). The medical consequences of obesity are well recognized. The incidence of cardiovascular disorders is much higher among obese than normal-weight individuals. For example, the incidence of hypertension among the obese is twice that for the general population (House, 1981). The incidence of obesity among patients with adult-onset diabetes is 85% (House, 1981). In addition, obese individuals have higher incidences of menstrual, reproductive, and cardiac disorders, as well as arthritis and gout (Krupka & Vener, 1983).

However, correction of obesity is a difficult medical problem. Since maintenance of body weight is determined by food intake and energy expenditure, it would seem that decreasing body weight would be a simple matter of either decreasing food intake, increasing energy expenditure, or both. In practice, however, decreasing body weight is not an easy process. For example, to lose 1 lb of body weight, one must reduce one's food intake by 3500 cal (House, 1981). Thus, reducing the diet by 500 calories per day would result in a body weight loss of 1 lb/week. Exercise is another way to lose weight. However, to lose 1 lb of body weight, a 250-lb individual would have to walk approximately 26 mi (Williams et al., 1948). Obviously, for an individual who is even moderately overweight, a considerable amount of time and effort is involved in effectively losing weight. One of the medical practices used as a supplement to dietary restriction and exercise programs has been the use of appetite-suppressant drugs. Such use constitutes an area of considerable controversy. Nonetheless, the development of safe and effective appetite-suppressant drugs has been a major pharmaceutical endeavor in this country.

One problem in assessing the efficacy of anorectic drugs is quantitation of the response. Since body weight loss is the ultimate goal of weight-loss programs, measurement of changes in body weight is a relatively simple and reliable measure of drug effect. Measurement of anorectic efficacy, on the other hand, requires the accurate and reliable measurement of food intake and appetite. Food intake can be measured either indirectly or directly (Silverstone, 1982). Indirect measurements of food intake include observation of eating behavior, or analysis of a diet diary in which the individual records daily food intake. Direct measurements of food intake are in general both more quantitative and more difficult than indirect measurements. Measurement of intake of a liquid diet is a relatively simple procedure but does not necessarily reflect an individual's normal eating habits. Several methods have been developed to measure the intake of solid foods. These methods include bomb calorimetry of duplicate meals, measurement of intake of standardized foods (such as nuts, crackers, sausages, or sandwiches, which can easily be counted). Automated measurements of food intake include various types of automated food dispensers, and the Bite Indicating Telemetering Eatometer (BITE). The BITE system is a complex electronic apparatus that includes a detector attached to an eating utensil, typically a fork. The subject is presented with a meal and instructed to eat. The movements of the fork-detector are monitored by remote telemetry to measure the number, rate, and frequency of bites of food eaten. In a further development of the system, the entire meal can be placed on a balance. Thus the weight of the food in each bite can be measured and the rate of food intake estimated. Because the BITE system involves a considerable amount of electronic and computer support, it is not suitable for large-scale investigations of the effects of drugs on food intake.

Phenylpropanolamine and phenylpropanolamine-containing products have been available and used in weight-reducing programs for well over

40 years. The clinical studies that have tested the anorectic efficacy of these products are reviewed in this section. In some of the studies the efficacy of phenylpropanolamine alone was investigated, and in other studies the efficacy of combination products containing phenylpropanolamine and caffeine was investigated.

EARLY STUDIES

The first publication reporting the anorectic efficacy of phenylpropanolamine was published in 1939 (Hirsh, 1939). Hirsh noted that ephedrine and Benzedrine were popular and effective drugs for treatment of obesity but produced unacceptable side effects (viz., nervousness and insomnia) in susceptible individuals. As an alternative therapy, Hirsh suggested that phenylpropanolamine (Propadrine; one or two tablets 20 min prior to meals) was effective in control of appetite and produced no side effects. Although no quantitative data were presented, Hirsh reported that he had been prescribing Propadrine to obese patients for 1 year and that no patient had reported nervousness or insomnia as a side effect of the drug. Six case reports were presented and are summarized in Table 5.14. Propadrine taken before meals and combined with a low-calorie diet produced weight loss without side effects, even in patients who experienced nervousness and insomnia while taking Benzedrine or ephedrine. The rate of weight loss ranged from 25 lb in 1 month to 24 lb in 4 months.

In a placebo-controlled study, the effects of phenylpropanolamine, phenylpropanolamine combined with the barbiturate Sodium Delvinal (vinbarbital), and d-amphetamine on appetite in humans were compared (Kalb, 1942). In this study, a total of 1880 patients who were 10–192% overweight were investigated. The patients were placed on a high-protein diet that was individualized to approximately 600–1500 cal. The results are summarized in Table 5.15. The method of assessing appetite suppression was not specified in this report. However, the percent of patients with appetite suppression was approximately the same in the three drug treatment groups. Unfortunately, the amount of weight lost while taking the drugs was not reported. The rationale for combining phenylpropanolamine with a barbiturate as an anorectic was not specified. The incidence of side effects was less in patients who received the Propadrine-Delvinal combination than in those who received Propadrine alone, but this difference is difficult to interpret since the doses of Propadrine were higher in the patients who received Propadrine alone. Although this study did not use a double-blind procedure, phenylpropanolamine was said to decrease the appetite when administered for periods as long as 16 weeks. Whether tolerance to phenylpropanolamine developed during this prolonged drug administration schedule was not reported.

TABLE 5.14. Case Histories of Obese Patients Given Propadrine for Appetite Control

Patient				Therapy		
Sex	Age (years)	Initial weight (lb)	Diagnosis	Diet (cal)	Drugs	Results
F	NS[a]	227	Hypopituitary	1400	2 Propadrine before meals	Lost 25 lb in 1 month
M	22	235	Hypopituitary	1500	Thyroid extract	Lost 1 lb in 12 days; complained of nervousness
				1500	2 Propadrine before meals	Lost 24 lb in 4 months
F	21	198.5	Hypopituitary	900	Benzedrine	Complained of nervousness and insomnia
				900	2 Propadrine before meals	Lost 33.5 lb in 2 months; no side effects
F	NS	189	Postpregnancy	None	1 Propadrine before meals	Lost 20 lb in 10 weeks
F	NS	212	NS	None	Ephedrine before meals	Lost 7 lb in one month; side effects: nervousness
				1500	None	Lost 4 lb in 3 weeks
				1500	Propadrine before meals	Lost 29 lb (duration not specified)
F	NS	178	Hypothyroid	1600	Thyroid medication; Pituitrin; 2 Propadrine before meals	Total weight loss 17 lb in 25 days[b]

Source: Data from Hirsh (1939).
[a]NS—not specified.
[b]Propadrine was taken on the last 6 days only.

TABLE 5.15. Effects of Sympathomimetic Amines on Appetite in Obese Patients[a]

Drug	Dose	Duration (weeks)	n	Appetite Suppression (Percent of patients)
Propadrine	3/4 grain,[b] b.i.d.	4–16	464	45
Propadrine	3/8 grain, b.i.d.	4–16	216	44
Na Delvinal	1/4 grain, b.i.d.			
Amphetamine	10–20 mg, b.i.d.	4–36	1200	40
—[c]	—	NS	100	12

Source: Data from Kalb (1942).
[a]All patients received 600–1500-cal diet.
[b]$\frac{3}{4}$ grain = 48.75 mg.
[c]Control group, received low-calorie diet only.

The efficacy of phenylpropanolamine (Propadrine) in producing weight loss was reported in a clinical management study of obese patients who had failed to lose weight by dietary restrictions alone (Cutting, 1943). Fifteen trials were conducted in 13 patients. The patients were placed on a 960-cal, balanced diet. The dose of phenylpropanolamine was individually adjusted. The initial dose was 25 mg t.i.d., 1/2 hr before meals, and the dose was increased to a maximum of 50 mg "every hour while awake"; the latter was an extremely high daily dose of phenylpropanolamine. The average weight loss in those on the regimen of phenylpropanolamine combined with the low-calorie diet was 5 lb in 10 weeks, which the author considered "decidedly unsatisfactory." One of the 13 patients lost 21 lb in 27 weeks. In 12 of the 13 patients, phenylpropanolamine produced no nervousness, dry mouth, thirst, insomnia, visual disturbances, sweating, or increase in blood pressure. One patient reported tachycardia and abdominal discomfort while taking phenylpropanolamine. The lack of reported side effects is particularly striking since at least some of the patients were given quite high doses of phenylpropanolamine. Finally, with regard to the anorectic effects of phenylpropanolamine, the author reported that "on pointed questioning, a few admitted some loss of appetite."

These three studies (Cutting, 1943; Hirsh, 1939; Kalb, 1942) were the only reports in the medical literature prior to 1959 in which the efficacy of phenylpropanolamine as an anorectic drug in humans was investigated. Nonetheless, the use of phenylpropanolamine as an anorectic was recommended in several articles (Colton et al., 1943; Reilly, 1950; Williams et al., 1948), although none of these presented any additional data. In addition, the efficacy of phenylpropanolamine as an anorectic drug in laboratory animals was reported (Tainter, 1944).

CONTROLLED CLINICAL TRIALS

The efficacy of phenylpropanolamine as an anorectic drug was investigated in institutionalized, obese, mentally retarded individuals (Fazekas et al., 1959). These subjects were not placed on restricted, low-calorie diets. The following drugs were administered in a "blind" procedure 1 hr before each meal: 25 mg of phenylpropanolamine, 50 mg of phenylpropanolamine, 5 mg of d-amphetamine, and placebo. The results are summarized in Table 5.16. Although no statistical analysis of the results was presented, the authors noted that neither dose of phenylpropanolamine produced significant weight loss compared with placebo, whereas d-amphetamine did produce significant weight loss.

The Fazekas et al. (1959) study was severely criticized in a Federal Trade Commission hearing (Federal Trade Commission, 1967). One of the coauthors of the study, K.D. Campbell, testified that there were faults in the experimental design: No dietary restrictions were followed; several of the patients had epilepsy or brain damage; some patients went home on weekends and it was impossible to verify their compliance; and 28 of the 81 patients were taking other concurrent medications (tranquilizers, anticonvulsants, insulin). Other expert witnesses likewise criticized the study. The FTC concluded that the study results were unreliable; specifically, "The testimony of Dr. Campbell, . . . especially on cross examination, raises serious questions as to the reliability of the so-called study."

The experimental design of the Fazekas et al. (1959) study was also criticized by Silverman (1963). The rationale for investigation of weight loss in mentally retarded patients was questioned since most individuals who use phenylpropanolamine are not mentally retarded. Investigation of weight loss in the absence of dietary restriction was questioned, since most weight reduction programs involve low-calorie diets. The validity of the "blind" procedure for drug administration was questioned since the overt behavioral effects of d-amphetamine could have been observed. Finally, Silverman (1963) demonstrated that the IQ of the patients could have confounded the results, since in all four groups subjects with an IQ higher than 33 lost more weight than did those with lower IQs.

EFFECTS OF PHENYLPROPANOLAMINE ON FOOD INTAKE IN HUMANS

Only one report has been published in which the effects of phenylpropanolamine on food intake in humans was investigated (Hoebel et al., 1975a). Food intake was quantitated by measuring the amount of a liquid diet consumed during an experimental lunch session. The liquid diet was a Metrecal shake, either chocolate or Dutch chocolate flavor. The liquid lunch was offered ad

TABLE 5.16. Anorectic Efficacy of Phenylpropanolamine and d-Amphetamine in Institutionalized, Mentally Retarded, Obese Patients[a]

Drug	Dose (mg) (t.i.d.)	n	Sex	Age (years)	IQ	Initial Weight (lb)
PPA	25	19	13F, 6M	33 (11–67)	33 (idiot—59)	167.5 (86.0–220.0)
PPA	50	18	9F, 9M	32 (8–48)	34 (idiot—64)	170.9 (67.0–252.5)
d-Amphetamine	5	21	13F, 8M	36 (13–61)	42 (imbecile—76)	163.5 (111.0–229.5)
Placebo	—	21	13F, 8M	35 (16–61)	37 (10–70)	157.6 (85.0–201.0)

Source: Data from Fazekas et al. (1959).
[a]Data are mean (range).
[b]Negative values indicate weight gain.

libitum, and the amount consumed was measured. One of the possible confounding variables in measurement of the amount of diet consumed is that subjects may tend to judge their intake according to the size of the meal. In order to minimize the influence of visual cues as to the amount of liquid diet consumed, in this study the subjects drank the Metrecal shake from a straw attached to a graduated cylinder reservoir. The reservoir was hidden from the subject's view so that the subject could not see the amount consumed. In addition to the quantitative measurement of food intake, a questionnaire was used to record subjective responses to the meal. The following responses were rated: taste (from "very bad" to "excellent"), reason for terminating the meal (from "very full" to "very tired of the taste"), amount of diet consumed in relation to the previous day (from "much more" to "a lot less"), and taste of the diet in relation to the previous day (from "much worse" to "much better").

The experiment employed a double-blind, placebo-controlled, crossover design with repeated measures for each subject. Each subject was tested on 10 days—on 5 days phenylpropanolamine was administered and on 5 days placebo was administered. The order of administration of phenylpropanolamine and placebo was randomly assigned. The subjects were instructed to eat a normal breakfast on the study days and to fast for 2 hr before and after each session. Phenylpropanolamine or placebo was administered 30 min prior to the lunch. The phenylpropanolamine formulation was Hungrex (Alleghany Pharmacal Corp.), which contains 25 mg of phenylpropanolamine.

In the first study, the subjects were 16 paid volunteers. They were adults who wished to lose weight. Individuals with hypertension, heart disease, or diabetes were not accepted into the study. The results are summarized in Table 5.17. Phenylpropanolamine decreased the food intake by approximately 27% ($p < .01$). The subjective ratings of the taste of the lunch, and the reason for terminating the lunch (i.e., feeling full or tired of the taste) were not

TABLE 5.16 Continued

	Weight Loss/2 weeks[b] (lb)		Total Weight
2	4	6	Loss (lb)
0.9 ([−5.3]−7.0)	0.6 ([−7.7]−5.0)	−0.7 ([−5.5]−2.0)	0.9 ([−11.5]−10.0)
1.5 ([−6.2]−8.0)	−0.1 ([−4.5]−4.5)	−0.5 ([−3.0]−2.5)	0.8 ([−7.0]−6.0)
2.2 ([−4.3]−8.5)	1.2 ([−2.5]−7.2)	0.7 ([−1.5]−4.5)	4.6 ([−2.3]−10.0)
−0.1 ([−3.0]−6.0)	−0.2 ([6.0]−4.5)	0 ([−3.0]−2.7)	−0.3 ([−6.0]−9.5)

significantly different under the phenylpropanolamine and placebo conditions. However, the subjects were able to estimate correctly whether their food intake was greater or less than on the previous session ($p < .05$).

The experimental design of the second study was similar to that of the first study but tested a larger number of subjects. Also, the commercially available Hungrex tablets and the placebo tablets were coated in gelatin in order to mask the taste. The results of the second study confirmed the results of the first. Phenylpropanolamine decreased food intake, and although the percent decrease (5%) was less than in the first study (27%), the effect of phenylpropanolamine was statistically significant. Also, in the second study, the subjects rated the taste of the liquid diet as significantly worse when they took phenylpropanolamine than when they took placebo ($p < .05$). However, the subjects' ratings regarding the reason for terminating the meal and the estimate of meal size relative to the previous session were not significantly different in the phenylpropanolamine and placebo treatments.

The experimental design in the third study was similar to the designs in the first two studies, except that the recruitment of subjects and the instructions to them were somewhat different. This group of subjects was not recruited on the basis of their motivation to lose weight, but rather simply as paid volunteers. Also, they were instructed that the test drug was a nasal decongestant, without mentioning the possible effects on appetite. The results of this study were different from the results of the first two studies. Phenylpropanolamine did not significantly decrease food intake in these subjects, although the data were not presented in the article. The authors suggest four possible explanations for the lack of anorectic effect of phenylpropanolamine in this population: the subjects were given different instructions regarding the nature of the study (decongestant rather than anorectic study), were younger than subjects in the previous studies, had a lower mean body weight, and were not necessarily motivated to lose weight.

TABLE 5.17. Effects of Phenylpropanolamine on Intake of Liquid Nutrition

	Drug				Patients				
Tradename	Dose	Dosing Schedule	n	Sex	Age (years)	Diagnosis	Experimental Design	Results	
Hungrex	25	Acute	16	9M, 7F	$\bar{x} = 26, \bar{x} = 25$	Healthy volunteers	DB[a], crossover, repeated measures	Food intake PPA 535.0 ml Placebo 390.5 ml	$p < .01$
			32	13M, 19F	$\bar{x} = 29, \bar{x} = 34$	Healthy volunteers	Same	PPA 707 ml Placebo 669 ml	$p < .01$
			32	M, F	$\bar{x} = 18, \bar{x} = 19$	Healthy volunteers	Same, except the subjects were instructed the test drug was a decongestant	PPA — Placebo —	NS[b]

Source: From Hoebel et al. (1975a).
[a]DB—double blind.
[b]NS—not significant.

In summary, these studies demonstrated that phenylpropanolamine significantly decreased food intake, at least in a motivated, weight-conscious population. There was some indication that phenylpropanolamine may make food less palatable, but phenylpropanolamine had no effect on the perception of the amount of food consumed. Finally, the results of the subjective questionnaire indicated that phenylpropanolamine had no effect on the individual's energy level and was not a "psychic energizer."

EFFECTS OF PHENYLPROPANOLAMINE ON BODY WEIGHT

Six articles have been published since 1959 in which the effects of phenylpropanolamine or phenylpropanolamine-containing products on body weight were investigated. These reports include the results of eight independent clinical trials. In two studies, the efficacy of phenylpropanolamine alone was investigated (Hoebel et al., 1975b; Weintraub, 1986). In the other studies, the efficacy of combination products containing phenylpropanolamine and caffeine were investigated (Altschuler et al., 1982; Bess & Marlin, 1984; Griboff et al., 1975; Sebok, 1985). In addition, eight clinical trials in obese patients [reviewed by Weintraub (1985)] and two clinical trials (one single-blind study and one double-blind study) in obese, hypertensive patients (Bradley & Raines, 1987) have been conducted. The commercial products used in these studies are shown in Table 5.18, and the study designs and results are summarized in Table 5.19.

The efficacy of phenylpropanolamine alone as a weight-reducing drug was investigated (Hoebel et al., 1975b). The study population was 70 weight-conscious, paid volunteers, who were paid $20 and received a 1-month supply of the drug if they completed the study. There were no drop-outs in this study. Individuals who had a heart condition, hypertension, thyroid disturbance, diabetes, or other diseases were not included in the study. The subjects were not given any particular dietary instructions. The results are summarized in Table 5.19 and Figure 5.8. Each drug treatment lasted 2 weeks, and the results were analyzed separately according to whether the subject received phenylpropanolamine or placebo as the first drug treatment. During the first drug treatment period, subjects in both the phenylpropanolamine and placebo groups lost weight, and the weight loss was greater in the phenylpropanolamine treatment group. The mean body weight in both groups decreased approximately 1-2 lb between the time of the pretreatment examination and the first day of the study. However, in the second treatment period, only the subjects in the phenylpropanolamine treatment group lost weight. In the combined overall analysis, the subjects lost nearly three times as much weight while taking phenylpropanolamine than while taking placebo (Table 5.19). The weight loss as a percent of initial body weight was signifi-

TABLE 5.18. Appetite-Suppressant Products Containing Phenylpropanolamine[a]

Tradename	Composition (mg)	Manufacturer	Reference
A. Products containing phenylpropanolamine alone			
Hungrex	PPA, 25	Alleghany Pharmacal Corp.	Hoebel et al. (1975a,b)
Vita Slim	PPA, 50 Kelp, 37.5 Multivitamins, NS[b] Lecithin, 150 Vitamin B$_6$, 0.5	Thompson Medical Co., NY, NY	Weintraub (1985)
Acutrim	Phenylpropanol- amine PPA, 75	Burroughs Wellcome	Weintraub et al. (1986)
B. Products containing phenylpropanolamine and caffeine			
Anorexin	PPA, 25 Caffeine, 100 Multivitamins, NS	SDA Pharmaceutical Co., NY, NY	Griboff et al. (1975)
Appedrine	PPA, 25 Caffeine, 100	Thompson Medical Co., NY, NY	Altschuler et al. (1982)
Prolamine	PPA, 37.5 Caffeine (SR)[c], 140	Thompson Medical Co., NY, NY	Altschuler et al. (1982)
Dexatrim	PPA, 50 Caffeine (SR), 200	Thompson Medical Co., NY, NY	Altschuler et al. (1982)

[a]This table contains a listing of phenylpropanolamine-containing products reviewed in Chapter 5; it is not a complete listing of phenylpropanolamine-containing appetite suppressants.
[b]NS—not specified.
[c]SR—sustained release.

cantly greater in the phenylpropanolamine group ($p < .001$). Also the drug x group interaction was significant ($p < .01$), confirming the observation that the order of drug treatment was important. Thus the subjects lost more total weight when the phenylpropanolamine was given first than when the placebo was given first. There was no difference between males and females in regard to the weight lost during phenylpropanolamine treatment.

Also in this study (Hoebel et al., 1975b), the subjects' eating habits were analyzed from diary cards kept by the subjects. Subjects ate smaller meals than usual when taking phenylpropanolamine but ate more than usual when taking placebo. Finally, the subjects reported eating significantly fewer between-meal snacks while taking phenylpropanolamine than while taking placebo. (The number of snacks per 2 weeks were 14.9 and 16.3 for phenyl-propanolamine and placebo, respectively, $p < .05$.)

Weintraub et al. (1986) added phenylpropanolamine to a physician-

TABLE 5.19. Clinical Trials Investigating the Efficacy of Phenylpropanolamine-Containing Appetite Suppressants[a]

Tradename and Reference	Drug Total Daily Dose of PPA (mg)	Dosing Schedule	Duration of Drug Intake (weeks)	Patients n	Sex	Age (years)	Diagnosis	Experimental Design		Results Weight Loss[b] (lb) A	P	p	Comments
Phenylpropanolamine alone													
Hungrex; see Hoebel et al. (1975b)	75	t.i.d.	2	70/70[c]	50F, 20M	18–64	2 underweight, 8 normal weight, 60 overweight, paid volunteers	Randomized, DB, PC, crossover, no special diet		1.7	0.54	—	PPA suppressed appetite more than placebo (subjective rating scale)
Generic diet cube; see Weintraub (1985)	75	t.i.d.	6	43/62	57F, 5M	19–45	Obese (at least 15% overweight)	Randomized, DB, PC, 1250-cal diet	2 wk 4 wk 6 wk	3 5 6.5	3 4 4	NS NS NS	Diet cubes taken with coffee or tea; PPA produced clinically but not statistically significant weight loss compared to placebo
Generic drops; see Weintraub (1985)	75	t.i.d.	6	50/64	58F, 6M	19–69	Obese (at least 3% overweight)	Randomized, DB, PC	2 wk 4 wk 6 wk	−2.81 4.47 4.65	2.44 3.22 3.72	— — .04	PPA was more effective than placebo in producing weight loss and appetite suppression
Acutrim; see Weintraub et al. (1985)	75	o.d.	12	106	F	18–44	Obese	DB, PC, reduced calorie diet, exercise, behavioral modification		13.4	9.5	<0.05	Acutrim was a safe, effective adjunct to weight-loss program

365

TABLE 5.19. Continued.

Drug				Patients				Experimental Design		Results			Comments
Tradename and Reference	Total Daily Dose of PPA (mg)	Dosing Schedule	Duration of Drug Intake (weeks)	n	Sex	Age (years)	Diagnosis			Weight Loss[b] (lb)		p	
										A	P		
Vita Slim; see Weintraub (1985)	100	b.i.d.	6	54/72	63F, 9M	19–65	Obese (10–30% overweight)	Randomized, DB, PC	2 wk	3.2	1.8	—	Vita Slim contains PPA, kelp, and vitamins; produced safe and effective weight loss (no statistical analysis reported)
									4 wk	5.1	3.6	—	
									6 wk	6.1	3.5	—	

Phenylpropanolamine and caffeine

Tradename and Reference	Total Daily Dose of PPA (mg)	Dosing Schedule	Duration of Drug Intake (weeks)	n	Sex	Age (years)	Diagnosis	Experimental Design		Weight Loss (lb) A	Weight Loss (lb) P	p	Comments
Anorexin; see Griboff et al. (1975)	75	t.i.d.	4	66/77	M, F	16–75	Exogenous obesity ($\geq 11\%$ overweight)	Randomized, DB, PC, parallel groups, 1200-cal diet	Females	4 [$0-15\frac{1}{2}$]	$[(-4\frac{1}{2})-17\frac{1}{2}]$	<.05	Appetite suppression: placebo—10/38; PPA—17/36
									Males	8 [$(-\frac{1}{2})-16$]	$4\frac{1}{2}$ [$2-11\frac{1}{2}$]	NS	
Prolamine; see Altschuler et al. (1982)	75	b.i.d.	6	56/72	15M, 41F	Ad[d]	Obese[e]	DB, PC, parallel groups, no special diet	6 wk	4.64 ± 0.72	2.07 ± 0.69	<.01	
Prolamine; see Sebok (1985)	70	b.i.d.	6	49/70	60F, 10M	18–60	Obese (at least 10% overweight)	Randomized, DB, PC, 1250-cal diet	2 wk	2.0	2.0	—	Prolamine plus diet produced significantly greater weight loss than placebo
									4 wk	4.0	3.0	—	
									6 wk	5.5 [$(-2)-19$]	4.0 [$(-0.5)-13$]	—	
Dexatrim; see Altschuler et al. (1982)	50	m.i.d.	6	55/67	58F, 9M	Ad[d]	Obese[e]	DB, parallel groups, 1250-cal diet	6 wk	8.11 ± 1.02	—	—	Weight loss with mazindol (2 mg): 9.00 ± 0.79 (NS)

Drug; reference	Dose (mg)	Schedule	Duration (wk)	No.[c]	Gender	Age[d]	Population	Design		Weight loss[b]		Comments
Appedrine; see Altschuler et al. (1982)	75	t.i.d.	6	48/62	59F, 3M	Ad[d]	Obese[e]	DB, parallel groups, 1250-cal diet	6 wk 8 wk		5.67 ± 0.80 6.84 ± 0.85	Weight loss with diethylpropion (25 mg): 6 wk 6.61 ± 1.17 (NS) 8 wk 7.96 ± 1.44 (NS)
Generic; see Weintraub (1985)	75	m.i.d.	8	45/60	53F, 7M	18–66	Obese (at least 15% overweight)	Randomized, DB, 1250-cal diet	2 wk 4 wk 6 wk 8 wk		5 6 6 8	PPA + caffeine was safe and effective anorectic when given m.i.d.; comparable to diethylpropion

Phenylpropanolamine with and without caffeine

Drug; reference	Dose (mg)	Schedule	Duration (wk)	No.[c]	Gender	Age[d]	Population	Design		PPA alone	PPA + caffeine	Comments
Generic; see Weintraub (1985)	100	b.i.d.	8	43/62	55F, 7M	18–60	Obese (≥10% overweight)	Randomized, DB, PC	2 wk 4 wk 6 wk 8 wk	5.7 7.9 9.6 10.9	7.1 9.8 12.4 13.5	Substantial weight loss in both groups; greater weight loss and appetite suppression in PPA + caffeine group than in PPA alone group

[a] Abbreviations: A—active drug; P—placebo; NS—not significant ($p > .05$); DB—double-blind; PC—placebo-controlled; Ad—adult.
[b] Negative values indicate weight gain.
[c] Final number/total.
[d] Adults age 18–65 for the three studies.
[e] 12–45% overweight for the three studies.

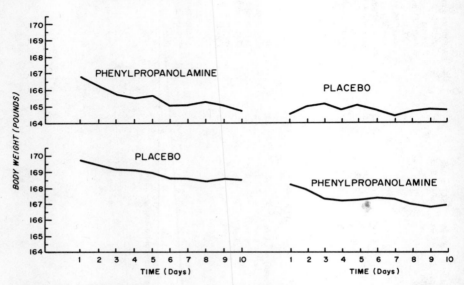

Figure 5.8. Body weight loss in human subjects taking placebo or phenylpropanol-amine. From *Hoebel et al. (1975b)*.

managed weight-control program that included behavior modification, mild caloric restriction, and exercise. The trial was a double-blind, parallel-group comparison of Acutrim and placebo. Each Acutrim tablet contained 75 mg of phenylpropanolamine in an osmotically controlled drug-delivery system (OROS). The external coating of the tablet contained 20 mg of phenylpro-panolamine that dissolved conventionally after ingestion; the remaining 55 mg was released slowly from the tablet over approximately 16 hr. This formulation, by releasing a fixed amount of drug per unit of time for absorp-tion, is designed to provide constant blood levels in the therapeutic range for long periods, thus avoiding concentration peaks, which may result in adverse side effects, and concentration valleys, which result in minimal drug effect. Subjects were 106 healthy, overweight (115–130% of ideal body weight) women, 18 to 44 years old. Before dosing, there was a 2-week period during which the women began dieting, behavior modification, and exercise. Diets were personalized, based on individual food preferences, eating habits, and ideal body weight; total caloric intake was 16–18 kcal/kg ideal body weight/ day. Behavior modification included instruction in charting food intake, eat-ing patterns, and stimuli; visual analog scales were used to rate diet difficulty, hunger, and drug effects. Under medical guidance, but based on personal preference, subjects gradually increased their exercise to expend 300 kcal three times weekly. Dosing was once daily (after the morning meal and not later than 10 A.M.) for 12 weeks. During biweekly clinic visits, physicians continued behavior modification, diet, and exercise counseling. The study period ran through Thanksgiving and Christmas.

Women who took Acutrim lost significantly more weight than those who took placebo. More than twice as many Acutrim subjects lost >3.0 kg. Data for weight loss and percent loss were statistically significant. Interestingly, during Thanksgiving and Christmas weeks, women who took Acutrim controlled their appetite, continued behavior modification, restricted caloric intake, and lost weight. The placebo group did not lose weight during Thanksgiving week and gained weight during Christmas week. Calculation of weight loss based on compliance (subjects took >90% of the drugs) showed a decrease in weight loss with a decrease in compliance in both the Acutrim and placebo groups. In both groups there were only slight changes in all measures of hunger at all times of day; although between-group differences were slight, women who took Acutrim had less difficulty adhering to their caloric restriction regimen at every time point throughout the trial. Subjects perceived much greater benefit in appetite control from Acutrim than from placebo. Adverse drug reactions caused 13/53 Acutrim subjects and 15/53 placebo subjects to withdraw. Dry mouth was the most frequent complaint from women given Acutrim. There were no serious cardiovascular effects. Both complaints and number of women reporting adverse reactions decreased with continued dosing. The authors concluded that sustained-release Acutrim was a safe, effective adjunct to a physician-managed, integrated weight-loss program.

Sebok (1985) investigated the efficacy of phenylpropanolamine (35 mg) combined with caffeine (140 mg) as an adjunct to a low-calorie (1250 cal/day) diet plan. The study was randomized, double-blind, and placebo-controlled. Patients were 70 obese (>10% overweight by Metropolitan Life Insurance Company tables) adults (10 males, 60 females) in general good health. Dosing was twice daily for 6 weeks. Efficacy of the phenylpropanolamine-caffeine combination was assessed in terms of weight loss. Patients were also asked to rate appetite suppression as none, mild, or moderate. Of 70 patients entering the study, 49 completed; 26 (3 males, 23 females) received phenylpropanolamine-caffeine and 23 (5 males, 18 females) received placebo. The 1250 cal/day diet plan produced significant mean weight loss in both groups. Patients given phenylpropanolamine-caffeine lost more weight than those given placebo: 50% lost 6 lb or more compared with 22% for the placebo group, and 19% lost 10 lb or more compared with 4% for the placebo group. In addition, 31% of the patients given the combination lost 5% or more of their initial body weight compared with only 4% of the placebo group. Patients in both groups reported minor side effects, but there were no significant differences between the groups in terms of nature or incidence of these reactions. Changes in blood pressure and heart rate were clinically insignificant in both groups.

Bess and Marlin (1984) evaluated the appetite-suppressant activity of phenylpropanolamine combined with supportive group therapy and behavior modification in 12 juvenile-onset obese physicians. The volunteers for this open study were seven men and five women, 27–62 years old, who were up to 62% overweight by Metropolitan Life Insurance Co. tables. All of the participants routinely advised their patients in private practice to lose weight and offered dietary and psychological programs for weight reduction. Yet despite their level of educational attainment and medical knowledge, none of the subjects in this study had previously been seriously motivated to lose weight. Additionally, all were opposed to the use of anorectants, ethical or OTC. The study medication was capsules containing 35 mg of phenylpropanolamine plus 140 mg of caffeine taken once or twice daily. Subjects also attended 90-min weekly group therapy sessions that focused on weight reduction, dietary compliance, physical appearance, and the psychodynamics of obesity. No particular diet regimen was prescribed, but subjects agreed to follow a high-protein, low-fat, and low-carbohydrate diet of about 1250 cal/day. Exercise or increased physical activity was encouraged, but not required.

Ten physicians completed the 6-week initial evaluation period with significant mean weight loss of 10 pounds, which averaged 1.1 lb/wk (one physician was lost due to professional relocation; one physician refused medication and was considered a nonmedicated control who participated for 2 weeks with no weight loss before withdrawing from the study). These 10 agreed to extend the study. By week 12, six were still in the study; mean cumulative weight loss was 23.3 lb, or about 2 lbs/wk/physician. Those who ceased medication but remained in the group gained an average of 2.7 lb. Five physicians were followed for an additional 10 weeks; the average weight loss for the 22-week study period was 32.2 lb, or about 1.5 lb/wk. This weight loss was maintained for up to 2 years. Their weight loss was significantly greater than that of the subjects who stayed in the group but stopped medication (these latter physicians actually gained weight during the medication-free period). There were no significant adverse effects related to the phenylpropanolamine. The study suggests that the group process alone was ineffective in weight loss and that OTC appetite-suppressant medication could be an important adjunct in assisting motivated patients to reduce weight and to maintain weight loss.

The efficacy of the commercial product Anorexin, which contains phenylpropanolamine and caffeine (Table 5.18), was investigated in individuals with exogenous obesity (Griboff et al., 1975). Obesity was defined in this study as body weight at least 11% greater than the ideal body weight as determined from the Metropolitan Life Insurance Tables. The subjects were placed on a 1200-cal diet and were given Anorexin or placebo for 4 weeks. The results are summarized in Table 5.19. Of the 77 subjects, 11 left the study before it was completed. Anorexin produced significantly more weight loss than did placebo in females ($p < .05$). Males lost even more weight than did females when taking phenylpropanolamine, but the weight loss in males taking Anorexin was not significantly different from that in the males taking placebo control ($p > .05$) probably due to the small number of males in the study. The amount of weight loss was approximately 1–2 lb/week, which is consistent with the rate of weight loss reported in other studies of patients taking phenylpropanolamine-containing products. Finally, weight loss during administration of phenylpropanolamine was correlated with the subjects' subjective ratings of appetite suppression.

The results of three independent, controlled clinical trials of the efficacy of phenylpropanolamine-caffeine combination products were reported by Altschuler et al. (1982). The subjects were obese adults who were 12–45% overweight. In one study, Prolamine (see Table 5.19) was compared to placebo in a parallel-groups design. The subjects were not given low-calorie diets. Eight patients in each group (Prolamine and placebo) dropped out of the study for various reasons. Phenylpropanolamine consistently produced greater weight loss than did placebo. The difference between the groups was not significantly different after 2 weeks of treatment, but was significantly different after 4 weeks ($p < .02$) and after 6 weeks ($p < .01$). The subjects taking Prolamine lost approximately twice as much weight as the subjects taking placebo. This 2:1 ratio of weight loss in phenylpropanolamine and placebo groups is consistent with the results of previous studies (Griboff et al., 1975; Hoebel et al., 1975b).

In another study, the weight-loss efficacy of Dexatrim (see Table 5.19) and mazindol (a prescription anorectic) were compared (Altschuler et al., 1982). This was a parallel-groups comparison study in obese adults placed on a 1250-cal diet. Seven patients treated with Dexatrim and five patients treated with mazindol dropped out of the study for various reasons. Both drug treatments produced significant weight loss, and there was no statistically significant difference between the drug treatments.

In the third study, the efficacies of Appedrine (see Table 5.19) and diethylpropion (a prescription anorectic) were compared (Altschuler et al., 1982). The study design was similar to the design just described for the comparison of Dexatrim and mazindol. Six patients treated with Appedrine and eight patients treated with diethylpropion dropped out of the study for various reasons. Both treatment groups lost weight, and there were no statistically significant differences between the groups. The amount of weight loss during

6 weeks of treatment with Appedrine was comparable to the amount of weight loss during 6 weeks of treatment with Prolamine but less than the weight loss with Dexatrim.

The results of eight unpublished clinical trials in obese patients [reviewed by Weintraub (1985)] confirm the efficacy and safety of phenylpropanolamine either alone or combined with caffeine (Tables 5.19 and 5.20). In one clinical trial, phenylpropanolamine was administered with or without caffeine; both weight loss and appetite suppression were greater in the group receiving phenylpropanolamine plus caffeine than in the group receiving phenylpropanolamine alone, but the difference was not statistically significant. In addition, one clinical trial tested the efficacy and safety of phenylpropanolamine in obese patients with controlled, stable hypertension (Bradley & Raines, 1987). Phenylpropanolamine produced significant weight loss and appetite suppression in these patients. (The design and results of this study are discussed more fully in Chapter 4.)

The results of these controlled clinical trials demonstrate a consistent effect of phenylpropanolamine-containing products in producing weight loss in obese individuals. Phenylpropanolamine, alone or combined with caffeine, produced approximately 1–2 lb of weight loss per week. In those studies that compared phenylpropanolamine treatment to placebo control, patients lost approximately twice as much weight while taking phenylpropanolamine-containing products. The total daily dose of phenylpropanolamine ranged from 50 to 100 mg, and the duration of drug administration ranged from 2 to 8 weeks. Unfortunately, the development of tolerance to the anorectic effects of phenylpropanolamine was not specifically assessed in any of these studies. In one study, however, the weight loss during treatment with Prolamine or placebo was compared after 2, 4, and 6 weeks of treatment. The results indicated that the difference between placebo and Prolamine treatment increased progressively during the 6 weeks. This suggests that tolerance to Prolamine did not develop.

Blumberg and Morgan (1985) described a statistical method for analyzing combined studies. Ten small, randomized, double-blind, matched-group, clinical studies of weight reduction were variously combined in order to extrapolate more definitive conclusions than were possible from separate examination of each individual study. Some of these studies have been summarized in this chapter (e.g., Altschuler et al., 1982; Griboff et al., 1975). In six of the 10 studies phenylpropanolamine was matched against placebo; in three studies phenylpropanolamine plus caffeine was matched against an active anorectic, diethylpropion or mazindol; and in one study phenylpropanolamine was matched against phenylpropanolamine plus caffeine. The efficacy of phenylpropanolamine as an appetite suppressant was statistically demonstrated. Significantly more weight (approximately 50% more) was lost per subject taking phenylpropanolamine (70–100 mg/day) than was lost by placebo subjects. Also, the rate of weight loss was significantly and consistently greater for phenylpropanolamine subjects than for placebo subjects throughout the 4- to 6-week study periods. More weight was lost by subjects on diethylpropion than those on phenylpropanolamine, but the difference was not statistically significant.

The authors also examined product safety by analyzing biweekly changes in radial pulse, systolic and diastolic blood pressures, and number of study dropouts. Statistical evaluation indicated that phenylpropanolamine produced no significant effect on pulse or blood pressure. The highest dropout rate occurred in the diethylpropion group, the second highest in the placebo group, and the third highest in the phenylpropanolamine group. The relatively high rate of placebo-group dropouts indicated there was no statistical evidence that dropout could be drug-related. The dropout pattern also suggested that a principal cause for leaving may have been failure to experience appetite suppression. Subjects who dropped out of a study because of adverse side effects often were from the placebo groups, which the authors suggested may have indicated that a weight-loss regimen was in itself stressful. The authors concluded that the combined sample size of over 500 completed cases generated confidence in their statistical demonstrations of phenylpropanolamine efficacy and safety.

SIDE EFFECTS OF PHENYLPROPANOLAMINE-CONTAINING ANORECTIC PRODUCTS

Side effects reported during these clinical trials of phenylpropanolamine-containing products for anorectic efficacy are summarized in Table 5.20. Consistent with the reports of side effects of phenylpropanolamine-containing decongestants (see Tables 5.9, 5.11, 5.12, 5.13), the incidence of side effects was low and the side effects were mild. Table 5.20 contains the results from those controlled clinical trials that systematically reported the incidence of side effects. In addition, the following observations were reported. Hirsh (1939) reported that Propadrine (one or two tablets before meals) produced no side effects, including no nervousness or insomnia, in obese patients. The number of patients was not specified. No side effects were observed in 12 out of 13 obese patients receiving Propadrine in doses ranging from 25 mg t.i.d to 50 mg each hour, whereas 1 out of 13 patients reported tachycardia and abdominal discomfort (Cutting, 1943). Fazekas et al. (1959) did not report the incidence of side effects in their mentally retarded, obese patients given 25 or 50 mg of phenylpropanolamine t.i.d. before meals.

The side effects reported during administration of phenylpropanolamine-containing anorectic drugs were qualitatively similar to the side effects re-

TABLE 5.20. Side Effects of Phenylpropanolamine-Containing Appetite Suppressants[a]

Tradename: PPA dose (mg): Caffeine dose (mg): Reference:	Hungrex 25 — Hoebel et al. (1975)		Generic 25 — Weintraub (1985)		Generic 25 — Weintraub (1985)		Vita Slim 50 — Weintraub (1985)		Acutrim 75 — Weintraub et al. (1986)	
	A	P	A	P	A	P	A	P	A	P
Nervousness	—	—	—	1/31	—	—	—	1/36	+[b]	+[b]
Blood pressure change	—	—	—	—	—	—	—	—	+	+
Heart rate change	—	—	—	—	—	—	—	1/36	+	+
Headache	—	—	—	—	—	—	—	—	+	+
Dry mouth	—	—	—	—	1/41	—	3/36	—	—	—
Nausea	—	—	—	—	—	—	2/36	—	+	+
Tiredness, sleepiness	—	—	—	—	—	—	1/36	—	+	+
Diarrhea	—	—	—	—	—	—	1/36	2/36	+	+
Constipation	—	—	1/31	—	—	—	—	1/36	+	+
Lightheadedness	—	—	—	—	—	—	—	1/36	—	—
Itching	—	—	—	1/31	—	—	—	—	—	—
Diuresis	—	—	—	—	—	—	—	—	—	—
Cramps	—	—	1/31	—	—	—	—	—	+	+
Insomnia	—	—	1/31	1/31	1/41	—	—	—	—	—
Increased energy	—	—	—	—	—	—	—	—	—	—
Total	—[c]	—	3/31[d]	3/31	2/41	0/23	10/36[e]	6/36[f]	—	—

Tradename:	Appedrine	Anorexin		Prolamine		Dexatrim	Generic		Generic
PPA dose (mg):	25	25		37.5		50	50	50	75
Caffeine dose (mg):	100	100		140		200	—	200	200
Reference:	Altschuler et al. (1982)	Griboff et al. (1975)		Altschuler et al. (1982)		Altschuler et al. (1982)	Weintraub (1985)	Weintraub (1985)	Weintraub (1985)
	A	A	P	A	P	A	PPA Alone	PPA + Caffeine	A
Nervousness	1/25	—	—	—	—	—	—	1/32	2/30
Blood pressure change	NE	—	—	NE	NE	NE	—	—	—
Heart rate change	NE	—	—	NE	NE	NE	—	—	—
Headache	1/25	—	—	—	—	—	—	—	3/30
Dry mouth	2/25	—	—	1/28	1/28	—	1/30	—	NE/30
Nausea	—	1/33[g]	—	—	—	—	—	—	NE/30
Tiredness, sleepiness	—	1/33[g]	2/33	1/28	—	—	—	—	1/30
Diarrhea	—	—	2/33	1/28	—	—	—	—	—
Constipation	—	—	2/33	—	—	—	—	—	—
Lightheadedness	—	—	1/33	—	—	—	—	—	1
Itching	—	—	—	—	1/28	—	1/30	—	—
Diuresis	—	2-6/33[h]	1-6/33[h]	1/28	1/28	—	1/30	—	1
Cramps	1/25	—	—	—	—	—	—	—	1
Insomnia	—	—	—	—	—	—	—	—	1/30
Increased energy	—	—	—	—	—	—	—	—	3/30
Total	5/25	—	—	4/28	2/28	0/28	5/30[i]	3/32[j]	6/30

[a] Data are number of patients with side effects per total number of patients (A—active drug; P—placebo; NE—no effect).
[b] Side effects tabulated biweekly.
[c] No effect on ability to fall asleep and no effect on energy level.
[d] One patient with pain on urination.
[e] One patient each with tingle or strange feeling in the head; two patients with urinary frequency.
[f] One patient with change in bowel movements; one patient with tingle in arms, stomach pain; one patient with visual disturbance.
[g] Transient.
[h] Incidence reported separately for each week.
[i] One patient thirsty; one patient with jittery stomach.
[j] One patient bloated; one patient with increased urination.

ported during administration of phenylpropanolamine-containing decongestants. Several of the anorectic products contained caffeine in addition to
phenylpropanolamine. Thus, some of the side effects could be attributed to
caffeine or to the caffeine-phenylpropanolamine mixture. Since caffeine produces CNS stimulation, cardiac stimulation, and diuresis, such side effects of
phenylpropanolamine-caffeine mixtures may be due to caffeine. Unfortunately, insufficient data are available for analysis of the contribution of each
component to the overall side effects.

EFFICACY OF PHENYLPROPANOLAMINE IN TREATMENT OF URINARY INCONTINENCE

PATHOPHYSIOLOGY OF URINARY INCONTINENCE

Urinary incontinence—the involuntary voiding of urine from the bladder—is
a complex medical problem. Micturition is controlled by a mixture of voluntary and involuntary reflexes and thus involves both the somatic and autonomic nervous systems as well as higher control centers in the brain. In addition, the activity of smooth muscles in the bladder and urethra as well as
smooth and striated muscles in the external urinary sphincter are involved in
the regulation of micturition. Consequently, urinary incontinence can origi-
nate from pathophysiological conditions at many sites within the nervous and
urinary systems.

The anatomy and physiology of the urinary system have been extensively
investigated in recent years [see reviews by Applebaum, (1980); Bradley &
Sundin, (1982); Finkbeiner & Bissada, (1980); Norlen & Sundin, (1982);
Robinson, (1982)]. Much of this research has focused on the influence of the
autonomic nervous system on the urinary tract. Anatomically and functionally the urinary bladder is divided into two parts: the detrusor and the trigone. Both the detrusor and the trigone receive innervation from the parasympathetic and sympathetic postganglionic nerves. The parasympathetic
innervation is involved primarily in the voiding of urine and causes contraction of both the detrusor and the trigone. The sympathetic innervation is involved in relaxation of the bladder during the period of bladder filling. The
adrenergic receptor distribution differs for the detrusor and the trigone. In
the detrusor, the primary sympathetic response is β-adrenergic relaxation,
whereas in the trigone the primary response is α-adrenergic contraction. In
the proximal urethra, the parasympathetic input produces contraction. The
sympathetic input produces both α-adrenergic contraction and β-adrenergic
relaxation of the urethra. Under normal physiological conditions the α-adre-
nergic response predominates in the urethra, and activation of the sympa-

thetic nervous system causes urethral contraction and increased tone. In addition, there is reciprocal cross-innervation between the sympathetic and parasympathetic systems, so that when the parasympathetic system is activated the sympathetic influences on the urinary system are inhibited, and vice versa. The external urinary sphincter receives innervation from both the somatic and sympathetic nervous systems. The somatic nervous system causes a cholinergically mediated contraction of the sphincter, and the sympathetic nervous system produces relaxation via release of norepinephrine. The balance between parasympathetic, sympathetic, and somatic influences on the urinary system is coordinated both within the spinal cord and by input from higher centers in the brain.

The effects of drugs in therapy of neurological disorders of the urinary system are summarized in Table 5.21. The effects are due to actions on the sympathetic, parasympathetic, or somatic nervous system. Thus drugs that cause bladder relaxation act via blockade of the parasympathetic nervous system, whereas drugs that cause bladder contraction stimulate the parasympathetic

TABLE 5.21. Effects of Drugs on Urinary Bladder, Urethra, and Sphincter

Effect	Mechanism	Drugs
Relaxation of bladder	Blockade of muscarinic receptors and ganglia	Propantheline, methantheline, oxybutynin (also smooth muscle relaxation), flavoxate (also smooth muscle relaxation), dicyclomine, imipramine
Contraction of bladder	Stimulation of cholinergic receptors	Bethanechol
	Inhibition of acetylcholinesterase	Neostigmine
Relaxation of bladder neck and urethra	α-Adrenergic blockade	Phentolamine, phenoxybenzamine
	Blockade of adrenergic neurons	Guanethidine, methyldopa
Contraction of bladder neck and proximal urethra	Stimulation of α-adrenergic receptors	Phenylpropanolamine, ephedrine, pseudoephedrine, phenylephrine
	Blockade of β-adrenergic receptors	Propranolol
Relaxation of external urethral sphincter	Relaxation of skeletal muscle	Dantrolene
	Inhibition of spinal cord reflexes	Baclofen

Source: Data from Applebaum (1980) and Robinson (1982).

nervous system. Drugs that cause relaxation of the trigone and proximal urethra act via blockade of α-adrenergic mechanisms, whereas drugs that cause contraction of the trigone and urethra act via α-adrenergic agonist or β-adrenergic antagonist activity. Drugs that relax the external urethral sphincter act via relaxation of skeletal muscle or inhibition of spinal cord reflexes.

Since phenylpropanolamine is a sympathomimetic amine with predominantly α-adrenergic activity, and since the trigone and proximal urethra have been shown to have α-adrenergic receptors (Ek et al., 1978a), it is reasonable to expect that phenylpropanolamine would produce α-adrenergic contraction of the bladder neck and the proximal urethra. Thus phenylpropanolamine may be useful in managing some forms of urinary incontinence.

Urinary incontinence has been categorized into many subtypes, including stress, urge, overflow, functional, iatrogenic, and total incontinence and incontinence due to detrusor instability (Diokno, 1983; Moen & Stein, 1982; Ouslander, 1981; Williams & Pannill, 1982). Each of these has a different set of signs and symptoms and results from different pathophysiological conditions. Consequently, the management of incontinence depends on the type of disorder involved. Phenylpropanolamine is useful in therapy of incontinence due to weakness of the bladder neck and proximal urethra, so-called urinary stress incontinence. Stress incontinence is defined as incontinence in which the pressure in the urethra involuntarily falls below the pressure in the bladder, thus causing leakage of urine (Williams & Pannill, 1982). This type of incontinence typically occurs when the intraabdominal pressure suddenly increases—for example, when the individual coughs or laughs, bends over, or lifts heavy objects (hence "stress" incontinence).

Urinary stress incontinence is most prevalent in the elderly, in women who have borne children by vaginal delivery, and in men who have undergone prostatectomy (Fossberg et al., 1982; Ouslander, 1981; Williams & Pannill, 1982). In the United States, approximately 3 million people have urinary stress incontinence. The incidence is related to age, gender, and state of health of the population. Among the elderly, the incidence of stress incontinence ranges from 5–42% among individuals living in the community, to 28–50% among individuals in nursing homes, and to 18–46% among hospitalized patients (Ouslander, 1981). Thus urinary stress incontinence is an important medical and social problem.

To evaluate the efficacy of treatment in urinary incontinence, it is necessary to develop a quantitative measure of continence-incontinence. Since micturition involves both voluntary and involuntary reflexes, and since incontinence is a process that occurs spontaneously and at irregular intervals, incontinence is difficult to quantify [see review by Robinson (1982)]. Two primary types of measurement have been used to quantify the number and frequency of episodes of incontinence: patient diaries and electronically telemetered underpads. Since diaries are subjective in nature, it is difficult to control the accuracy and reliability of the records and to quantify the volume of urine voided. The electronically telemetered underpad is a more objective measure. The underpad contains an electronic sensor that detects the presence of electrolytes in the urine voided during incontinence. The sensor can be monitored by telemetry to detect the time of occurrence of incontinence. The weight of the underpad can be used to estimate the volume of urine voided. Because of the nature of the equipment involved, this method is not suitable for routine monitoring of large numbers of patients.

More recently, urodynamic techniques have been developed to measure several parameters of urinary bladder and urethral function (Ek et al., 1978a,b; Robinson, 1982). Several variations of this technique have been utilized (Ek et al., 1978a,b). With the patient in a lithotomy position, a catheter is placed in the urethra, the residual urine volume is measured, and the residual urine is voided. The catheter is replaced by a recording catheter. The recording catheter consists of two microtransducers for recording bladder (intravesical) and urethra (intraurethral) pressures. The bladder is filled with a fixed volume of saline (100–300 ml), and the intravesical and intraurethral pressures are recorded. The recording catheter is then withdrawn at a slow, fixed rate in order to measure the pressure gradient along the urethra (see Figure 5.9). From these studies the following can be determined: maximal urethral pressure (MUP), urethral closure pressure profile (UCPP), functional length of the urethra, and bladder pressure (Figure 5.10). The urethral closure pressure is defined as the difference between the pressure in the urethra and in the urinary bladder. Furthermore, if the transducer catheter is positioned at the maximum urethral pressure zone, the urethral vascular pul-

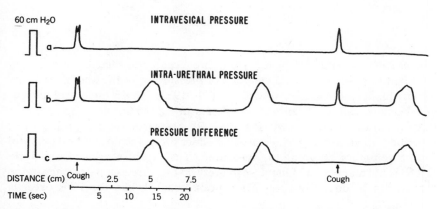

Figure 5.9. Measurement of urethral closure pressure profiles. From *Ek et al. (1978a)*.

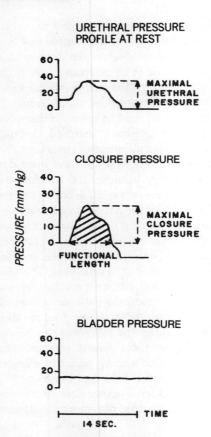

Figure 5.10. Measurement of the parameters from the urethral closure pressure profiles. From *Obrink and Bunne (1978)*.

sations can be recorded (Figure 5.11). More recently, this technique has been modified to measure the transmission of pressure from the abdomen to the urinary bladder and urethra (Fossberg et al., 1983). This is important to measure because adequate transmission of pressure to the urethra is required for micturition to occur. The MUP and UCPP pressures are measured as just described. In addition, the increase in bladder pressure and urethral pressure during voluntary coughing are measured. The pressure transmission ratio (PTR) is the magnitude of increase in urethral pressure as a percentage of the increase in bladder pressure. Micturition occurs when the PTR exceeds

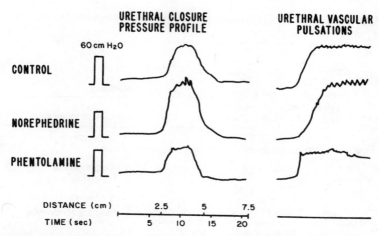

Figure 5.11. Urethral closure profile showing urethral vascular pulsations. From *Ek et al. (1978a)*.

100%. By measurement of these urodynamic parameters in both the empty bladder and the filled bladder in both the lithotomy and erect positions, quantitative assessment of bladder compliance, urethral function, and urethral sphincter tone can be made. These measures can be taken in a single individual before and after drug administration in a repeated-measures experimental design in order to assess drug effects on bladder and urethral function. Obviously, the technique is limited to a laboratory or inpatient setting and does not measure the actual occurrence of stress incontinence. Thus, in order to gain maximum clinical and scientific relevance, urodynamic measurements and clinical assessment of therapeutic efficacy need to be correlated.

EFFICACY OF PHENYLPROPANOLAMINE-CONTAINING PRODUCTS IN STRESS INCONTINENCE

The efficacy of phenylpropanolamine, either alone or in combination products, in symptomatic treatment of urinary stress incontinence has been investigated in several studies (summarized in Table 5.22). The results are summarized in this section. The efficacy of phenylpropanolamine-containing products in other types of urinary incontinence are reviewed in a subsequent section.

TABLE 5.22. Efficacy of Phenylpropanolamine-Containing Products in Urinary Stress Incontinence[a]

	Drug			Patients			
Tradename	Total Daily Dose of PPA (mg)	Dosing Schedule	Duration of Drug Intake	n	Sex	Age (years)	Diagnosis
Products containing phenylpropanolamine alone							
Generic	150	t.i.d.	4 wk	20	13F, 7M	NS	Modest stress incontinence
Generic	NS	NS	NS	36	26F, 10M	NS	Stress incontinence
Generic	100	b.i.d.	2 wk	23	F	36–77	Slight to severe stress incontinence
Combination products							
Ornade spansule	100	b.i.d.	3 months to 3 years	88	77F, 11M	NS	Mild to moderate stress incontinence
Ornade spansule	—	acute	—	12	F	NS	Moderate to marked stress incontinence

[a]Abbreviations: NS—not specified; PC—placebo controlled; MCP—maximum closure pressure; MUCP—maximum urethral closure profile; PTR—pressure transmission ratio; MUP—maximum urethral pressure.

EFFICACY OF PHENYLPROPANOLAMINE ALONE IN STRESS INCONTINENCE

The efficacy of phenylpropanolamine alone in therapy of urinary stress incontinence was investigated in two uncontrolled clinical studies (Awad et al., 1978, 1979) and one controlled clinical trial (Fossberg et al., 1983). The study designs and results are summarized in Table 5.22. Phenylpropanolamine was rated as a moderately effective therapy for stress incontinence as measured by both subjective rating and urodynamic studies. In one of the uncontrolled clinical studies of patients with a modest degree of urinary stress inconti-

TABLE 5.22 Continued

Experimental Design	Results		Reference
	Subjective Response	Urodynamic Responses	
Uncontrolled clinical study	Improvement	Significant increase in MCP in empty bladder but not in full bladder	Awad et al. (1978)
Uncontrolled clinical study	Improvement better in females than in males	—	Awad et al. (1979)
Randomized; PC; crossover	Improvement in 12/20 patients	MUCP increased; PTR slightly increased; bladder pressure not changed; functional length not changed	Fossberg et al. (1983)
Uncontrolled clinical study	Improvement in 67% of females and 36% of males	—	Stewart et al. (1976)
Repeated-measures experimental study	—	MUP increased >20% in 11/12 patients	Montague & Stewart (1979)

nence, the effectiveness of phenylpropanolamine was better in women than men (Awad et al., 1978). In women, the responses were rated good in 8/13 patients, improved in 3/13, and failed in 2/13. In men, the ratings were good in 2/7 patients, improved in 4/7, and failed in 1/7. In six of the seven men the stress incontinence was secondary to prostatectomy. Also in this study, it was noted that in one patient the dosage of phenylpropanolamine was increased from 50 to 75 mg t.i.d. in order to achieve adequate therapeutic response.

In a randomized, placebo-controlled, crossover clinical investigation, phenylpropanolamine was effective in reducing incontinence and improved the urodynamic status of the patients (Fossberg et al., 1983). The population included 20 women with slight, moderate, or severe stress incontinence (grades I, II, or III on the Ingleman-Sundberg Scale, respectively). The clinical response was rated subjectively as good (no incontinence), improved, unchanged, or worse. Phenylpropanolamine produced an improvement in stress incontinence in 12/20 patients, although none became completely continent. No patient experienced a worsening of incontinence while taking phenylpropanolamine. Furthermore, the efficacy of phenylpropanolamine was not related to the severity of the stress incontinence.

Urodynamic studies also demonstrated that phenylpropanolamine produced a significant improvement in the function of the urethra (Fossberg et al., 1983). The maximum urethral closure pressure was significantly increased in both the empty and filled bladder when the patients were in the lithotomy position (Table 5.23). The maximum closure pressure in the filled bladder in the erect position was also increased, but the effect was not statistically significant ($p = .056$). Also, the pressure transmission ratio showed a tendency to increase following administration of phenylpropanolamine. Phenylpropanolamine had no effect on the functional length of the urethra or on bladder pressure. In six patients, the relationship between serum levels of phenylpropanolamine and effects on urodynamic status was investigated. Serum levels of phenylpropanolamine were determined by mass fragmentographic technique with gas chromatography. Peak serum concentrations of approximately 175 ng/ml were achieved 1.5 hr after administration of 50 mg of phenylpropanolamine (PO). The serum concentration required to produce a subjective improvement in incontinence was at least 150 ng/ml. There was

TABLE 5.23. Effects of Phenylpropanolamine on Maximum Urethral Closure Pressure in Patients with Stress Incontinence[a]

Bladder Volume	Position	Drug	Maximum Urethral Closure Pressure (cm H_2O)	p
Empty	Lithotomy	Predrug	42.0 ± 3.5	—
		Placebo	44.6 ± 4.9	0.33
		PPA	55.8 ± 5.0	0.015
300 ml	Lithotomy	Predrug	36.9 ± 3.7	—
		Placebo	41.7 ± 5.6	0.23
		PPA	50.3 ± 5.3	0.024
300 ml	Erect	Predrug	41.9 ± 3.7	—
		Placebo	43.8 ± 5.6	0.39
		PPA	51.7 ± 4.6	0.056

Source: From Fossberg et al. (1983).
[a]Data are mean ± SEM.

no correlation between serum levels of phenylpropanolamine and the increase in maximum urethral closure pressure, but the increase in pressure transmission ratio was greater in patients with serum levels of phenylpropanolamine higher than 150 ng/ml than it was in patients with lower serum levels. Two additional studies were conducted. A single acute dose of 50 mg of phenylpropanolamine produced an increase in maximum urethral closure pressure comparable to the effect recorded following 14 days of therapy with phenylpropanolamine. The mean peak serum level of phenylpropanolamine following the single 50-mg dose was 137 ng/ml (range 72–179 ng/ml). In the second additional study, the daily dose of phenylpropanolamine was increased to 50 mg, t.i.d. This higher dosage regimen produced serum levels of phenylpropanolamine greater than 250 ng/ml. However, the higher dose produced no greater increase in the maximum urethral closure pressure and no greater subjective improvement in incontinence than did the lower dose of phenylpropanolamine (50 mg, b.i.d.).

Norephedrine produced similar effects on urodynamic parameters in patients with slight to mild stress incontinence (Ek et al., 1978a,b; the isomer of norephedrine was not specified). Acute administration of 75–100 mg of norephedrine (PO) increased both the maximum urethral pressure and the maximum urethral closure pressure (Figures 5.11 and 5.12). The bladder pressure was not affected by norephedrine. These effects of norephedrine were reversed by IV administration of phentolamine, demonstrating that the

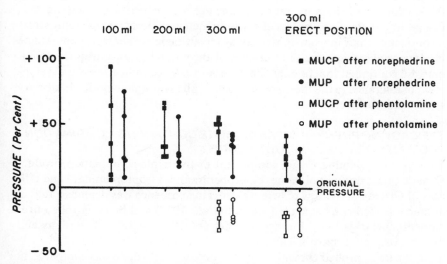

Figure 5.12. Effects of norephedrine and phentolamine on MUP and MUCP. From *Ek et al. (1978a)*.

effects were mediated by actions on α-adrenergic receptors. Similar effects on urodynamic parameters were recorded in women with stress incontinence who took 100 mg of norephedrine (slow-release formulation) b.i.d. for 3 months (Ek et al., 1978b). In subjective evaluation of the therapy with norephedrine, 12/22 patients showed improvement (with two patients becoming continent), 9/22 showed no effect, and placebo was superior to norephedrine in 1/22. The effects of norephedrine were statistically significant ($p <$ .05, Fisher's exact test). Norephedrine was rated as more effective in women with moderate stress incontinence than in women with mild incontinence. Also, norephedrine was more effective in postmenopausal women than in women of reproductive age. In contrast, norephedrine produced no significant effect on urodynamic parameters in women with severe stress incontinence (Obrink & Bunne, 1978). This latter study was an uncontrolled clinical study of 10 women with severe stress incontinence. Norephedrine (100 mg, b.i.d.) was administered for 3 weeks. The results indicate that the efficacy of norephedrine may be a function of the severity of the stress incontinence. On the other hand, Fossberg et al. (1983) systematically compared the efficacy of phenylpropanolamine in women with mild, moderate, and severe stress incontinence. In this placebo-controlled, crossover clinical trial, the efficacy of phenylpropanolamine did not differ between patients with mild, moderate, and severe stress incontinence.

The results of these studies demonstrate that phenylpropanolamine or norephedrine is moderately effective in symptomatic treatment of mild to moderate urinary stress incontinence. The effectiveness of these drugs in patients with severe stress incontinence has not been conclusively investigated. Phenylpropanolamine was less effective in men with postprostatectomy stress incontinence than in women with stress incontinence. Phenylpropanolamine produces only symptomatic treatment of incontinence, and drug treatment must be continued indefinitely. There is no evidence indicating the development of tolerance to the therapeutic effect of phenylpropanolamine in urinary stress incontinence.

EFFICACY OF PHENYLPROPANOLAMINE-CONTAINING COMBINATION PRODUCTS IN STRESS INCONTINENCE

Phenylpropanolamine is one component of the triple-combination product Ornade (phenylpropanolamine, chlorpheniramine, isopropamide). The efficacy of Ornade in therapy of urinary stress incontinence was demonstrated in an uncontrolled clinical study (Stewart et al., 1976) and in a controlled urodynamic investigation (Montague & Stewart, 1979). The study designs and results are summarized in Table 5.22.

In the uncontrolled clinical study, the efficacy of Ornade was compared in women and men with mild to moderate urinary stress incontinence (Stewart et al., 1976). The men were all postprostatectomy patients. Ornade was more effective in women with stress incontinence than in men. The percentages of patients with significant, fair, and no improvement were 59, 8, and 33%, respectively, in women and 27, 9, and 64%, respectively, in men.

Effects of acute administration of Ornade on the urodynamic profile were investigated in women with moderate to marked stress incontinence, and in women with no history of incontinence (Montague & Stewart, 1979). This investigation used a repeated-measures experimental design. Urodynamic profiles were measured before and 1–2 hr after administration of a single Ornade spansule. The experimental design is summarized in Table 5.22, and the results are summarized in Table 5.24. The results were categorized according to the effect of drug treatment on the maximum urethral pressure. The patients were divided into two groups: patients who showed greater than a 20% increase in maximum urethral pressure and patients who showed less than 20% increase. The majority of patients with stress incontinence showed greater than 20% increase in maximum urethral pressure, whereas patients with no urinary incontinence showed less than 20% increase. Furthermore, patients with the greater response to Ornade had low values of maximum urethral pressure in the control condition. These results suggest that the patients with urinary stress incontinence had a low control value for maximum urethral pressure, and that the effect of Ornade was to increase the maximum urethral pressure to a value comparable to that recorded in healthy women in the absence of drug treatment.

EFFICACY OF PHENYLPROPANOLAMINE-CONTAINING PRODUCTS IN OTHER TYPES OF URINARY INCONTINENCE

Although the efficacy of phenylpropanolamine-containing products in urinary incontinence has been most extensively investigated in patients with urinary stress incontinence, urinary incontinence can result from various other

TABLE 5.24. Effects of Ornade on Maximum Urethral Pressure in Healthy Women and Women with Stress Incontinence[a]

Response	Maximum Urethral Pressure			Number of Patients with Stress Incontinence	n
	Control (cm H_2O)	Ornade (cm H_2O)	Percent Increase		
>20% increase	47 (24–68)	73 (42–95)	57 (21–95)	11/12	12
<20% increase	72 (48–86)	73 (48–88)	2 (0–5)	1/6	6

Source: From Montague & Stewart (1979).
[a]Data are mean (range).

pathophysiologic disorders of the urinary system. The efficacy of phenylpropanolamine-containing products in several other types of urinary incontinence has been investigated. The study designs and results are summarized in
Table 5.25. The interpretation of the efficacy of phenylpropanolamine in
these studies is limited for several reasons. In most of these studies, phenylpropanolamine was combined with other drugs and the contribution of
phenylpropanolamine alone was not investigated. In three of the four studies,
the study design was a clinical case management study and double-blind or
placebo-controlled procedures were not used.

Urge incontinence is defined as the involuntary loss of urine associated
with a strong urge to void and is subdivided into motor and sensory urge incontinence. Motor urge incontinence is accompanied by uninhibited detrusor
contractions, whereas sensory urge incontinence is not associated with uninhibited contractions. The efficacies of Lunerin (phenylpropanolamine, brompheniramine) and Rinexin (phenylpropanolamine alone) were compared
in women with sensory urge incontinence (Fossberg et al., 1981) (see also
Table 5.25). The efficacy of drug treatment was assessed subjectively by the
patients keeping daily diaries of micturition frequency and objectively by urodynamic measurements. In addition, the patients were subdivided into
groups of patients with unstable urethras and stable urethras. Stability of the
urethra was diagnosed by urethrocystometry. Both Lunerin and Rinexin produced improvement in sensory urge incontinence as determined from the subjective patient ratings. Furthermore, the drugs were more effective in patients
with unstable urethras. In the combined analysis, it appears that Lunerin was
more effective than Rinexin. However, this may be due to the fact that the
patients who received Lunerin had a higher incidence of unstable urethra. In
contrast, the urodynamic studies did not show any significant effects of drug
treatment on maximum urethral pressure, functional profile length, bladder
compliance, or maximum bladder capacity. The urodynamic studies confirmed the presence of unstable urethra in 21/34 of the patients in the control
condition. Furthermore, drug treatment stabilized the urethra in 14/21
patients.

Incontinence due to an incompetent urethral closure mechanism is a condition that involves continuous leakage of urine, stress incontinence, and an
unstable urethra. The efficacy of Rinexin combined with estriol treatment in
therapy of patients with incompetent urethral closure mechanism was investigated in an uncontrolled clinical management case study (Beisland et al.,
1981) (see also Table 5.25). The results were analyzed by both subjective and
urodynamic methods. The subjective ratings of 14 patients showed that eight
patients became completely continent on the combined drug therapy; subjective improvement was shown in another four patients, whose episodes of incontinence were primarily nocturnal; and the remaining two patients were not

improved by drug therapy. The urodynamic studies confirmed that the urethral function was improved by drug therapy. The maximum urethral pressure was increased in 11 of the 14 patients. The maximum urethral pressures before and during treatment with Rinexin and Klimadurin (estrioli phosphas polymerisat) were 21.6 $\pm$ 10.2 and 31.3 $\pm$ 8.6 cm H_2O, respectively (p < .01). The combined analysis based on both subjective and urodynamic tests is shown in Figure 5.13.

In an uncontrolled clinical trial, Glenning (1984) used phenylpropanolamine to treat eight women whose urinary incontinence was due to very low urethral closure pressure (≤ 30 cm H_2O). Two patients had previously been treated surgically without success; after phenylpropanolamine one of them showed 60% improvement and one showed only minimal improvement. The remaining six patients had not been treated surgically; two received propantheline and imipramine without improvement before virtual complete response to phenylpropanolamine, and four received phenylpropanolamine with excellent response. [Doses and dosing schedule(s) as well as criteria for measuring treatment results were not given.]

Phenylpropanolamine is used also in veterinary medicine for treatment of incontinence. Primary sphincter incompetence, associated with reduced urethral closure pressure, was diagnosed in 11 female and eight male neutered dogs with urinary incontinence (Richter & Ling, 1985). The dogs were given 1.5 mg/kg of phenylpropanolamine orally two or three times daily and were evaluated at least 2 weeks later. After treatment there was a significant increase in maximal urethral closure pressure to within normal range. Urinary incontinence resolved clinically in all but one male and one female dog, and the condition of these two dogs improved considerably.

The efficacy of Eskornade in treatment of diurnal incontinence was assessed in a retrospective study of a large series of children with incontinence (Rees & Ransley, 1980). In this population of 75 children 72 had daytime incontinence (ranging in severity from "giggle incontinence" to complete incontinence), 52 had nocturnal and daytime incontinence, five had anal incontinence secondary to ureterosigmoidostomy surgery, and five had simple nocturnal incontinence. Of the children with diurnal incontinence, 65.6% had incontinence due to incompetent bladder neck. The majority (63%) had been treated unsuccessfully with other drugs. The retrospective analysis demonstrated that 75% of the children showed improvement in incontinence while taking Eskornade. Furthermore, Eskornade decreased incontinence in 82% of the children with bladder neck incompetence.

Under normal circumstances, the smooth muscle of the detrusor of the bladder is under the control of inhibitory reflexes originating in higher brain centers. These inhibitory influences normally prevent spontaneous involuntary contractions of the detrusor. In certain conditions, usually due to neuro-

TABLE 5.25. Efficacy of Phenylpropanolamine-Containing Products in Other Types of Urinary Incontinence[a]

	Drug			Patients			
Tradename	Total Daily Dose of PPA (mg)	Dosing Schedule	Duration of Drug Intake	n	Sex	Age (years)	Diagnosis
Lunerin	100	b.i.d.	3 wk	19	F	16–72	Sensory urge incontinence
Rinexin	100	b.i.d.	2 wk	15	F	7–69	Sensory urge incontinence
Rinexin and Klimadurin[c]	100	b.i.d. q. 4 wk	3–6 mo	14	F	54–94	Incompetent urethral closure mechanism
Rinexin and Klimadurin	100	b.i.d.	4 wk[d]	20	F	49–84	Postmenopausal urethral spincter insufficiency
Eksornade	100–300[e]	b.i.d.–t.i.d.[e]	≥3 months	83[f]	40F,[f] 35M[f]	5–19	Diurnal incontinence
Ornade	NS	NS	NS	128	F	NS	Unstable (neurogenic) bladder (n = 70); other types of incontinence (n = 58)
Ornade	25–50	o.d.	NS	31	16F, 15M	8–40	Refractory enuresis

[a]Abbreviations: NS—not specified; PC—placebo controlled.
[c]Klimadurin—Estroli phosphas polymerisat (Estriol).
[d]Ten patients took 50 mg of phenylpropanolamine PO bid for 4 weeks and 10 patients took 1 mg/day of estriol vaginal suppositories for 4 weeks; these 2 groups switched medication for 4 weeks; combination treatment was given to all 20 patients for 4 weeks.
[e]Dosage was individualized to the patients .
[f]Eight patients were not evaluated due to inadequate follow-up.

TABLE 5.25 Continued

Experimental Design	Results[b]	Reference
Uncontrolled; repeated measures	Subjective improvement 14/19; unstable urethra normalized	Fossberg et al. (1981)
PC; repeated measures	Subjective improvement 8/15; unstable urethra normalized	
Clinical management case study; repeated measures	Subjective response: Good 8/14 Improved 4/14 Unchanged 2/14 Urodynamic response: Improved 11/14	Beisland et al. (1981)
Randomized crossover	Either phenylpropanolamine or estriol alone was effective, but combined treatment was more effective	Beisland et al. (1984)
Retrospective study clinical case management	Subjective response: 75% of patients improved; 82% of patients with bladder neck incontinence improved; 25% of patients not improved	Rees & Ransley (1980)
Retrospective study clinical case management	Unstable bladder: completely inhibited by Ornade 12/70; improved by Ornade 2/70; Urispas[g] was more effective than Ornade	Younglove et al. (1980)
Uncontrolled study	Enuresis stopped in 8/10 patients with urethral instability and 3/6 patients with mixed instability[h]	Penders et al. (1984)

[b]Incidences are number responding per total number.
[g]Urispas—flavoxate.
[h]The remaining 15 patients were treated with propantheline and/or imipramine.

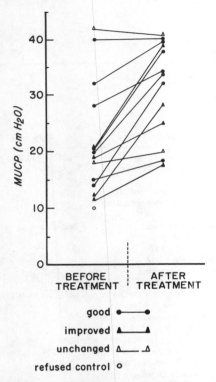

Figure 5.13. Effects of Rinexin® on MUCP in patients with incontinence due to incompetent urethra. From *Beisland et al. (1981)*.

logical damage to the higher brain centers, the detrusor is released from these descending inhibitory influences. The uninhibited contractions of the detrusor can cause a type of urinary incontinence known as the *unstable* (or *neurogenic*) *bladder*. In most cases, the drug of choice for treatment of the neurogenic bladder is a direct-acting antispasmodic drug such as dicyclomine, flavoxate, or oxybutynin (Awad et al., 1979) or an anticholinergic drug (Finkbeiner & Bissada, 1980). However, in selected cases Ornade was completely or partially effective in preventing incontinence due to neurogenic bladder (Younglove et al., 1980) (see also Table 5.25). The mechanism by which phenylpropanolamine-containing products inhibit the neurogenic bladder is unknown. Since Ornade contains an anticholinergic, isopropamide, the effect may be due to anticholinergic effect on the detrusor.

In an uncontrolled study, 31 patients (15 males, 16 females; 8–40 years old) with refractory enuresis underwent simultaneous urethrocystometry for assessment of the vesicosphincter unit as a whole (Penders et al., 1984). Phenylpropanolamine (25-50 mg, Ornade, taken at bedtime) stopped nocturnal enuresis in 8 of 10 patients with diagnosed urethral instability and in 3 of 6 patients with diagnosed mixed (detrusor and urethral) instability. Fifteen patients were treated with propantheline and/or imipramine. There were no adverse side effects related to phenylpropanolamine treatment. The authors noted that Ornade, which is the proposed treatment for urethral instability, stabilized not only the urethra but also the entire vesicosphincter unit. They suggested that phenylpropanolamine be considered as an additional option in the treatment of enuresis.

COMBINED TREATMENT WITH NOREPHEDRINE AND ESTROGENS IN URINARY INCONTINENCE

Since estrogen replacement therapy is effective in treatment of certain types of urinary incontinence, especially in postmenopausal women, the effects of combined therapy with norephedrine and estrogen were investigated to determine whether the two drugs produced additive or synergistic effects (Beisland et al., 1981, 1984; Ek et al., 1980). In a placebo-controlled, crossover study in postmenopausal women with slight to moderate stress incontinence, norephedrine (200 mg/day, PO) combined with estradiol produced greater improvement in both subjective clinical effect and in urodynamic parameters than did estradiol (plus placebo) treatment (Ek et al., 1980). During treatment with norephedrine and estradiol, 8 of 13 women were less incontinent and 5 of 13 women showed no improvement compared to placebo and estradiol. Three women became completely continent during norephedrine and estradiol treatment. The effect of norephedrine was statistically significant ($p < .05$, Fisher's exact test). In the urodynamic study, norephedrine and estradiol produced significant increases in maximum urethral pressure and maximum urethral closure pressure ($p < .05$). However, the magnitude of these effects was similar to the effects recorded when norephedrine alone was given to women with stress incontinence (Ek et al., 1978a,b). Thus the effects were attributed to norephedrine and not to an interaction between norephedrine and estradiol. The combination of norephedrine and estriol was likewise effective in treatment of urinary incontinence due to incompetent urethral closure mechanism (Beisland et al., 1981) (see also Table 5.25 and Figure 5.13).

Beisland et al. (1984) also compared phenylpropanolamine and estriol, separately and combined, in 20 menopausal women with urinary incontinence due to urethral sphincter insufficiency. The study was a randomized, open, comparative crossover trial in which 10 patients took phenylpropanolamine (50 mg PO b.i.d.) and 10 patients took estriol vaginal suppositories

(1 mg/day) for 4 weeks. The groups then switched medication for 4 weeks; finally, all 20 patients took combined treatment for 4 weeks. Both phenylpropanolamine and estriol significantly increased the maximal urethral closure pressure and continence area compared to initial values, but combination treatment was substantially more effective. Phenylpropanolamine was clinically more effective than estriol, but not sufficiently so to obtain complete continence. With combined treatment eight patients became completely continent, nine were considerably improved, and only one remained unchanged.

SIDE EFFECTS OF PHENYLPROPANOLAMINE-CONTAINING PRODUCTS IN TREATMENT OF URINARY INCONTINENCE

The side effects in patients taking phenylpropanolamine-containing products for treatment of urinary incontinence are summarized in Table 5.26. The incidence of side effects was low and the severity of the side effects mild. Similar results were reported for patients taking phenylpropanolamine-containing

TABLE 5.26. Side Effects of Phenylpropanolamine-Containing Products Used in Studies of Efficacy in Urinary Disorders[a]

Tradename: PPA Dose (mg): Reference:	Generic 50 Awad et al. (1978)	Ornade 50 Stewart et al. (1976)[b]	Eskornade 50 Rees & Ransley (1980)[c]	Lunerin or Rinexin[d] 50 Fossberg et al. (1981)
Drowsiness	—	+	14/75	—
Dry mouth, nose	—	3/77	7/75	—
Dizziness	1/20	—	—	+
Headache	1/20	—	—	—
Nosebleeds	—	—	1/75	—
Hypertension	0/20	—	0/75	—
Light-headedness	—	+	—	—
Blurred vision	—	—	2/75	—
Behavioral disturbances	—	—	5/75	—
GI upset	—	—	—	+
Abdominal pain	—	—	1/75	—
Chest tightness	—	—	2/75	—
Rash	—	+	—	—
Fever	—	+	—	—
Total	1/20	9/77	23/75	4/34

[a]Data represent number of patients with side effects per total number of patients. None of these studies used placebo control. Symbol + —side effect present but incidence not reported.
[b]Incidence in females only; incidence in males not reported.
[c]Pediatric patients.
[d]Side effects not reported separately for the two drugs.

decongestant products (Tables 5.9, 5.11, 5.12, 5.13) or appetite-suppressant products (Table 5.20). In one study, behavioral disturbances were reported in five of 75 children given Eskornade for treatment of diurnal incontinence (Rees & Ransley, 1980). Medication was withdrawn because of side effects in eight of 75 patients. In this study, the dose of Eskornade was individualized for each patient. The dose was increased successively until either the child became continent or until side effects developed (the maximum dose allowed was two Eskornade capsules t.i.d., which is three times the recommended daily dose for adults). Because of this dose escalation schedule, and because this was a retrospective study with neither double-blind nor placebo-control procedures, interpretation of the incidence of side effects in this study is limited.

The occurrence of drowsiness and dry mouth in two of the studies with phenylpropanolamine-containing combination products (Rees & Ransley, 1980; Stewart et al., 1976) is consistent with other reports of side effects of these combination products. As mentioned previously, the drowsiness and dry mouth may be responses to the antihistamines and anticholinergic drugs in Ornade and Eskornade.

USE OF PHENYLPROPANOLAMINE FOR CORRECTION OF RETROGRADE EJACULATION

Five case reports and one controlled clinical trial in a single patient have been published demonstrating that phenylpropanolamine reversed retrograde ejaculation. Retrograde ejaculation is a relatively rare cause of infertility. During normal ejaculation, sympathetic reflexes cause contraction of the smooth muscle of the internal urinary sphincter, and this action prevents the ejaculate from entering the urinary bladder. When these sympathetic reflexes are interrupted, retrograde ejaculation occurs. Retrograde ejaculation can occur as the result of surgical or traumatic injury, congenital malformations, neuropathological conditions (especially diabetes mellitus), or side effects of certain drugs. Since the internal urinary sphincter is under the control of the α-adrenergic system, α-adrenergic drugs, including phenylpropanolamine, have been used in pharmacological management of retrograde ejaculation.

Five clinical case reports of successful treatment of retrograde ejaculation with phenylpropanolamine have been reported. In one case (Thiagarajah et al., 1978), the patient was a 27-year-old male with retrograde ejaculation secondary to unilateral orchiectomy and retroperitoneal node dissection. Retrograde ejaculation was corrected by administration of two Ornade spansules 1–2 hr prior to intercourse. Ornade was taken by this schedule for 18 months without conception. On evaluation, the patient's semen volume was

0.15–0.2 ml, with 152–160 million sperm/ml. Approximately 20% of the sperm showed 3+ motility. Homologous insemination was recommended because of the small volume of semen. Homologous insemination of the patient's wife was undertaken during three separate ovulatory cycles. The first cycle was a spontaneous ovulatory cycle, and the second two cycles were induced by administration of clomiphene citrate. The patient ingested two Ornade spansules, and semen was collected by masturbation 2 hr later. The semen volume was 7.0 ml or less, and 3–20 motile sperm per high-powered field were observed microscopically. Pregnancy resulted during the two clomiphene-induced ovulatory cycles. The first pregnancy ended in spontaneous abortion after 8 weeks. The second pregnancy was carried to term and resulted in a normal spontaneous delivery of a healthy baby.

The four other case reports confirm that phenylpropanolamine can reverse retrograde ejaculation. Retrograde ejaculation from undetermined causes was reversed by phenylpropanolamine (50 mg, t.i.d.) in one patient (Kragt & Schellen, 1978). During phenylpropanolamine therapy, the semen volume was 3–5 ml, with 5–30 million sperm/ml. No pregnancy developed during phenylpropanolamine therapy. When phenylpropanolamine treatment was discontinued, retrograde ejaculation reappeared. Similarly, retrograde ejaculation was reversed by administration of one Ornade spansule b.i.d. for 2 months to a man with insulin-dependent diabetes (Stewart & Bergant, 1974) and to a man with physical obstruction of the urethra (Virupannavar & Tomera, 1982). Finally, one case history was published in which retrograde ejaculation was reversed by administration of a phenylpropanolamine-containing decongestant ppoduct in a man with juvenile diabetes (Andaloro & Dube, 1975).

A double-blind, crossover clinical trial of phenylpropanolamine (75 mg, b.i.d.) and three other sympathomimetic amines (dextroamphetamine, 5 mg, q.i.d.; ephedrine, 25 mg, q.i.d.; pseudoephedrine, 60 mg, q.i.d.) was conducted in one patient with oligospermia secondary to bilateral retroperitoneal lymphadenectomy for testicular cancer (Proctor & Howards, 1983). No placebo control was used. Each drug was administered for 4 consecutive days. Semen samples were collected 2 hr after the first dose on day 1 and again on day 4. Each drug treatment was repeated twice. In the absence of drug treatment, there was no anterograde ejaculation. All four drugs produced some anterograde ejaculation with a semen volume of 1–3 ml and an overall mean ($\pm$ standard deviation) sperm count of 2.3 ($\pm$0.7) million sperm/ml. The majority of the sperm were nonmotile and abnormal. The authors noted that there was a larger percentage of nonmotile and abnormal sperm during treatment with phenylpropanolamine than during treatment with the other sympathomimetic amines. Given the limited sample population and high variability of the results, the interpretation of these differences between phenylpropanolamine and the other drugs is questionable. Sperm motility and sperm volume were higher on day 4 than on day 1 of drug treatment. In a second phase of the investigation, the effects of ephedrine with and without chlorpheniramine on semen quality were measured. Addition of the antihistamine did not alter the response to ephedrine. Following the clinical trial, the patient was treated with daily doses of 25 mg of ephedrine (PO, q.i.d.), and conception ensued.

The results of these case reports and the one clinical trial demonstrate that phenylpropanolamine reversed retrograde ejaculation resulting from several causes. The effects were reversed when drug treatment was stopped. In at least one case, the reversal of retrograde ejaculation by phenylpropanolamine was followed by pregnancy and delivery of a normal newborn. Phenylpropanolamine was effective in reversing retrograde ejaculation regardless of whether phenylpropanolamine was given alone or combined with antihistamines.

OVERVIEW OF CLINICAL EFFICACY STUDIES

Phenylpropanolamine has been used extensively as a decongestant and as an appetite suppressant. Phenylpropanolamine's clinical efficacy was demonstrated in uncontrolled case studies conducted as early as the 1930s. In addition, more recent controlled clinical trials and laboratory studies in humans have substantiated the efficacy of phenylpropanolamine.

In terms of the number of published reports, most of the studies investigated the decongestant efficacy of phenylpropanolamine. Phenylpropanolamine, alone or combined with antihistamines and/or anticholinergics, is an effective decongestant. The decongestant efficacy was demonstrated both in healthy volunteers and in patients with various types of congestion (common colds, allergies, rhinitis, sinusitis). Phenylpropanolamine was effective whether administered orally or topically as nose drops. The incidence of side effects in these studies was uniformly low and the side effects reported were mild

Fewer studies of the anorectic efficacy of phenylpropanolamine have been published. Nonetheless, phenylpropanolamine, in association with a low-calorie diet, consistently produces greater weight loss than placebo treatment. In most efficacy studies phenylpropanolamine was taken for 2–8 weeks; in one controlled study phenylpropanolamine was taken for 12 weeks. Patients taking phenylpropanolamine usually lost approximately 1–2 lb/week and patients taking placebo lost approximately 0.5–1 lb/week. These studies are supported by controlled studies showing that phenylpropanolamine reduced appetite and food intake compared to placebo treatment. Phenylpropanolamine was effective either with or without caffeine; however, combination products containing phenylpropanolamine and caffeine are no longer marketed in the United States. No study specifically tested for tolerance to phenylpropanolamine. As with the decongestant studies, side effects associated with phenylpropanolamine were mild and infrequent.

The efficacy of phenylpropanolamine in treatment of various kinds of urinary incontinence was demonstrated by objective laboratory studies and by controlled clinical trials. Finally, phenylpropanolamine was effective in treatment of retrograde ejaculation in several case studies and in one clinical trial.

REFERENCES

Aaronson, A. L., Ehrlich, N. J., Frankel, D. B., Gutman, A. A., & Aaronson, D. W. (1968). Effective oral nasal decongestion. A double-blind, crossover analysis. *Ann Allergy, 26,* 145-150.

Altschuler, S., Conte, A., Sebok, M., Marlin, R. L., & Winick, C. (1982). Three controlled trials of weight loss with phenylpropanolamine. *Internatl J Obes, 6,* 549-556.

Andaloro, V. A., & Dube, A. (1975). Treatment of retrograde ejaculation with brompheniramine. *Urology, 5,* 520-522.

Applebaum, S. M. (1980). Pharmacologic agents in micturitional disorders. *Urology, 16,* 555-568.

Aschan, G. (1974). Decongestion of nasal mucous membranes by oral medication in acute rhinitis. *Acta Otolaryngol, 77,* 433-438.

Aschan, G., & Tham, R. (1974). Objective rhinomanometric clinical testing of an antihistamine (clemastine) combined with adrenergic substance (phenylpropanolamine). *Can J Otolaryngol, 3,* 577-580.

Ashe, G. J. (1968). Oral medications in nasal decongestion. *Ind Med Surg, 37,* 212-214.

Aust, R., Drettner, B., & Falck, B. (1979). Studies of the effect of peroral fenylpropanolamin on the functional size of the human maxillary ostium. *Acta Otolaryngol, 88,* 455-458.

Aviado, D. M., Wnuck, A. L., & De Beer, E. S. (1959). A comparative study of nasal decongestion by sympathomimetic drugs. *Arch Otolaryngol, 69,* 598-605.

Awad, S. A., Downie, J. W., & Kiruluta, H. G. (1978). Alpha-adrenergic agents in urinary disorders of the proximal urethra. Part I. Sphincteric incontinence. *Br J Urol, 50,* 332-335.

Awad, S. A., Downie, J. W., & Kiruluta, H. G. (1979). Pharmacologic treatment of disorders of bladder and urethra: A review. *Can J Surg, 22,* 515-518.

Axelsson, A. (1972). Vasomotor rhinitis treated with Lunerin (Draco), a new sympathomimetic antihistaminic preparation. *Acta Allergol, 27,* 186-194.

Axelsson, A., Jensen, C., Melin, O., Singer, F., & von Sydow, C. (1981). Treatment of acute maxillary sinusitis. *Acta Otolaryngol, 91,* 313-318.

Baptista, R. J., & Beauchemin, R. V. (1981). Treatment of the obese patient: Anorectic drugs. *U.S. Pharmacist,* 41-56.

Beisland, H. O., Fossberg, E., Moer, A., & Sander, S. (1984). Urethral sphincteric insufficiency in postmenopausal females: Treatment with phenylpropanolamine and estriol separately and in combination. *Urol Int, 39,* 211-216.

Beisland, H. O., Fossberg, E., & Sander, S. (1981). Combined treatment with estriol and alpha-adrenergic stimulation in elderly female patients with urinary incontinence. *J Oslo City Hosp, 31,* 39-42.

Bende, M., Andersson, K.-E., Johansson, C.-J., Sjogren, C., & Svensson, G. (1984). Dose-response relationship of a topical nasal decongestant: Phenylpropanolamine. *Acta Otolaryngol (Stockh), 98,* 543-547.

Bende, M., Andersson, K.-E., Johansson, C.-J., Sjogren, C., & Svensson, G. (1985). Vascular effects of phenylpropanolamine on human nasal mucosa. *Rhinology, 23,* 43-48.

Bende, M., & Laurin, L. (1986). Sympathomimetics in nasal allergy. *J Otorhinolaryngol Relat Spec, 48,* 238-242.

Berman, B. A., & Ross, R. N. (1983). Allergic rhinitis. *Cutis, 31,* 458, 460, 464, 470.

Bess, B. E., & Marlin, R. L. (1984). A pilot study of medication and group therapy for obesity in a group of physicians. *Hillside J Clin Psychiatry, 6,* 171-187.

Biaggioni, I., Onrot, J., Parrish, C. K., & Robertson, D. (1986). Marked hypertensive effect of low dose phenylpropanolamine, an over-the-counter appetite suppressant, in subjects with autonomic impairment. Presented at the American Heart Association Meeting, Nov. 17-20, 1986, Dallas, Texas.

Black, N. J. (1937). The control of allergic manifestations by phenylpropanolamine (Propadrine) Hcl. *Lancet, 54,* 101-102.

Blumberg, H., & Morgan, J. P. (1985). Combining anorexiant studies for analysis: A statistical method. In J.P. Morgan, D.V. Kagan, and J.S. Brody (Eds.). *Phenylpropanolamine: Risks, Benefits, and Controversies.* Clinical Pharmacology and Therapeutics Series, Vol. 5. Praeger Scientific, New York (pp. 80-93).

Boyer, W. E. (1938). The clinical use of phenyl-propanol-amine hydrochloride (propadrine) in the treatment of allergic conditions. *J Allergy, 9,* 509-513.

Bradley, M. H., & Raines, J. (1987). Single-blind pilot and double-blind follow-up evaluations of the safety and efficacy of phenylpropanolamine HCl in obese patients with controlled hypertension. *New Engl J Med* (in press).

Bradley, W. E., & Sundin, T. (1982). The physiology and pharmacology of urinary tract dysfunction. *Clin Neuropharmacol, 5,* 131-158.

Bristow, V. G. (1978). Allergic rhinitis. *Med J Aust* (suppl), *2,* 13-17.

Broms, P., Jonson, B., & Lamm, C. J. (1982). Rhinomanometry. II. A system for numerical description of nasal airway resistance. *Acta Otolaryngol, 94,* 157-168.

Broms, P., & Malm, L. (1982). Oral vasoconstrictors in perennial non-allergic rhinitis. *Allergy, 37,* 67-74.

Brooks, C. D., Nelson, A., Parzyck, R., & Maile, M. H. (1981). Protective effect of hydroxyzine and phenylpropanolamine in the challenged allergic nose. *Ann Allergy, 47,* 316-319.

Brummett, R. E. (1983). Treatment of the stuffy nose. *Pharmindex, 25,* 11-16.

Carter, C. H. (1965). Treatment of upper respiratory tract disorders in children: An evaluation of a new pediatric suspension. *Curr Ther Res, 7,* 648-654.

Chait, L. D., Uhlenhuth, E. H., & Johanson, C. E. (1984). Drug preference and mood in humans: Mazindol and phenylpropanolamine. In L.S. Harris (Ed.). *Problems of Drug Dependence, 1983,* NIDA Research Monograph 49: DHHS Publication No. (ADM) 84-1316. Washington, DC (pp 327-328).

Chen, K. K., Wu, C-K., & Henriksen, E. (1929). Relationship between the pharmacological action and the chemical constitution and configuration of the optical isomers of ephedrine and related compounds. *J Pharmacol Exp Ther, 36,* 363-400.

Cohen, B. M. (1975). Physiologic/clinical comparisons of a sustained-release decongestant combination, its components and placebo in patients with allergic rhinitis. *J Asthma Res, 13,* 7-13.

Cohen, B. M. (1978). Clinical correlants of changes in nasal flow/resistance (Rn) measurements. *Allergol Immunopathol, 6,* 217-223.

Collins, M. P., & Church, M. K. (1983). The effect of an anti-allergic, nasal decongestant combination ('Dimotapp') and sodium cromoglycate nose drops on the histamine content of adenoids, middle ear fluid and nasopharyngeal secretions of children with secretory otitis media. *Curr Med Res Opin, 8,* 392-394.

Colton, N. H., Segal, H. I., Steinberg, A., Shechter, F. R., & Pastor, N. (1943). The management of obesity with emphasis on appetite control. *Am J Med Sci, 206,* 75-86.

Cutting, W. C. (1943). The treatment of obesity. *J Clin Endocrinol, 3,* 85-88.

Diokno, A. C. (1983). Practical approach to the management of urinary incontinence in the elderly. *Comp Ther, 9,* 67-75.

Edwards, N., Elcock, H. W., Pyke, R., Griffiths, M. V., & Resouly, A. (1973). An antihistamine-sympathomimetic amine combination in vasomotor rhinitis. *Practitioner, 211,* 220-223.

Ek, A., Andersson, K.-E., & Ulmsten, U. (1978a). The effects of norephedrine and bethanechol on the human urethral closure pressure profile. *Scand J Urol Nephrol, 12,* 97-104.

Ek, A., Andersson, K.-E., Gullberg, B., & Ulmsten, U. (1978b). The effects of long-term treatment with norephedrine on stress incontinence and urethral closure pressure profile. *Scand J Urol Nephrol, 12,* 105-110.

Ek, A., Andersson, K.-E., Gullberg, B., & Ulmsten, U. (1980). Effects of oestradiol and combined norephedrin and oestradiol treatment on female stress incontinence. *Zentralbl Gynaekol, 102,* 839-844.

Erffmeyer, J. E., McKenna, W. R., Lieberman, P. L., Yoo, T. J., & Taylor, W. W. Jr. (1982). Efficacy of phenylephrine-phenylpropanolamine in the treatment of rhinitis. *South Med J, 75,* 562-564.

Fagin, J., Friedman, R., & Fireman, P. (1981). Allergic rhinitis. *Pediatr Clin North Am, 28,* 797-806.

Fazekas, J. F., Ehrmantraut, W. R., & Campbell, K. D. (1959). Comparative effectiveness of phenylpropanolamine and dextro amphetamine on weight reduction. *JAMA, 170,* 1018-1021.

Federal Trade Commission (1967). In the Matter of Alleghany Pharmacal Corp. and Harry Evans, Vincent J. Lynch, and Chester Carity. Docket no. 7176.

Finkbeiner, A. E., & Bissada, N. K. (1980). Drug therapy for lower urinary tract dysfunction. *Urol Clin North Am, 7,* 3-16.

Forquer, B. D., & Linthicum, F. H. (1982). Middle ear effusion in children. A report of treatment in 500 cases. *West J Med, 137,* 370-374.

Forsberg, B., Dalen, A., Lindstrom, O., & Johansson, C. J. (1983). A controlled clinical study of phenylpropanolamine (Rinexin) in acute rhinitis. *Opusc Med, 28,* 39-41.

Fossberg, E., Beisland, H. O., & Sander, S. (1981). Sensory urgency in females: Treatment with phenylpropanolamine. *Eur Urol, 7,* 157-160.

Fossberg, E., Beisland, H. O., & Sander, S. (1982). Urinary incontinence in old age. *Ann Chir Gynaecol, 71,* 228-231.

Fossberg, E., Beisland, H. O., & Lundgren, R. A. (1983). Stress incontinence in females: Treatment with phenylpropanolamine. *Urol Internatl, 38,* 293-299.

Fraser, J. G., Mehta, M., & Fraser, P. A. (1977). The medical treatment of secretory otitis media. *J Laryngol Otol, 91,* 757-765.

Glenning, P. P. (1984). Urodynamics—Is it useful for the gynaecologist? *Aust NZ J Obstet Gynaecol, 24,* 95-97.

Goodman, R. P., Wright, J. T., Jr., Barlascini, C. O., McKenney, J. M., & Lambert, C. M. (1986). The effect of phenylpropanolamine on ambulatory blood pressure. *Clin Pharmacol Ther, 40,* 144-147.

Griboff, S. I., Berman, R., & Silverman, H. I. (1975). A double blind clinical evaluation of a phenylpropanolamine-caffeine-vitamin combination and a placebo in the treatment of exogenous obesity. *Curr Ther Res, 17,* 535-543.

Hamilton, L. H. (1978). Effect of topical decongestants on nasal airway resistance. *Curr Ther Res, 24,* 261-268.

Haugeto, O. K., Schroder, K. E., & Mair, I. W. S. (1981). Secretory otitis media, oral decongestant and antihistamine. *J Otolaryngol, 10,* 359-362.

Heron, T. G. (1972). Double-blind cross-over study of Demazin Chronosules capsules and Eskornade spansules. *S Afr Med J, 46,* 579-581.

Hirsh, L. S. (1939). Controlling appetite in obesity. *J Med Cincinatti, 20,* 84-85.

Hoebel, B. G., Cooper, J., Kamin, M.-C., & Willard, D. (1975a). Appetite suppression by phenylpropanolamine in humans. *Obesity/Bariatric Med, 4,* 192-197.

Hoebel, B. G., Krauss, I. K., Cooper, J., & Willard, D. (1975b). Body weight decreased in humans by phenylpropanolamine taken before meals. *Obesity/Bariatric Med, 4,* 200-206.

Horak, F. (1982). Disophrol syrup versus Rinomar syrup in the treatment of allergic rhinitis in children. *J Int Med Res, 10,* 426-430.

House, M. L. (1981). Obesity control with OTC products. *Pharm Times, 47,* 90-96.

Jackson, R. H., Garrido, R., & Lynes, T. E. (1975). Ru-Tuss in the symptomatic treatment of allergic rhinitis. *Ann Allergy, 35,* 172-174.

Jaffe, G., & Grimshaw, J. J. (1983). Randomized single-blind trial in general practice comparing the efficacy and palatability of two cough linctus preparations, "Pholcolix" and "Actified" Compound, in children with acute cough. *Curr Med Res Opin, 8,* 594-599.

Kalb, S. W. (1942). The effect of amphetamine (Benezedrine) sulphate, propadrine hydrochloride and propadrine hydrochloride in combination with sodium delvinal on the appetite of obese patients. *J Med Soc NJ, 39,* 584-586.

Khan, J. A., Marcus, P., & Cummings, S. W. (1981). *S*-Carboxymethylcysteine in otitis media with effusion. *J Laryngol Otol, 95,* 995-1001.

Kjellman, N.-I. M. (1975). Treatment of children with perennial rhinitis with brompheniramine-maleate and phenylpropanolamine hydrochloride (Lunerin Mite). *Acta Allergol, 30,* 48-57.

Kjellman, N.-I. M., Harder, H., Lindwall, L., & Synnerstad, B. (1978). Longterm treatment with brompheniramine and phenylpropanolamine in recurrent otitis media—a double-blind study. *J Otolaryngol, 7,* 257-261.

Kragt, F., & Schellen, A. (1978). Clinical report about some cases with retrograde ejaculation. *Andrologia, 10,* 381-384.

Krupka, L. R., & Vener, A. M. (1983). Over-the-counter appetite suppressants containing phenylpropanolamine hydrochloride (PPA) and the young adult: Usage and perceived effectiveness. *J Drug Educ, 13,* 141-152.

Lea, P. (1984). A double-blind controlled evaluation of the nasal decongestant effect of Day Nurse in the common cold. *J Int Med Res, 12,* 124-127.

Lofkvist, T., & Svensson, G. (1978). A comparative evaluation of oral decongestants in the treatment of vasomotor rhinitis. *J Int Med Res, 6,* 56-60.

Loth, S., & Bende, M. (1985). The effect of topical phenylpropanolamine on nasal secretion and nasal airway resistance after histamine challenge in man. *Otolaryngol, 10,* 15-19.

McLaurin, J. W., Shipman, W. F., & Rosedale, R. (1961). Oral decongestants. *Laryngoscope, 71,* 54-67.

Meistrup-Larsen, K.-I., Mygind, N., Thomsen, J., Sorensen, H., & Vesterhauge, S. (1978). Oral norephedrine in the treatment of acute otitis media. *Acta Otolaryngol, 86,* 248-250.

Melen, I., Andreasson, L., Ivarsson, A., Jannert, M., & Johansson, C.-J. (1986a). Effects of phenylpropanolamine on ostial and nasal airway resistance in healthy individuals. *Acta Otolaryngol (Stockh), 102,* 99-105.

Melen, I., Friberg, B., Andreasson, L., Ivarsson, A., Jannert, M., & Johansson, C.-J. (1986b). Effects of phenylpropanolamine on ostial and nasal patency in patients treated for chronic maxillary sinusitis. *Acta Otolaryngol (Stockh), 101,* 494-500.

Mercke, U., & Wihl, J.-A. (1973a). Clinical evaluation of an oral combined antihistaminic sympathomimetic preparation. *Acta Allergol, 28,* 108-117.

Mercke, U., & Wihl, J.-A. (1973b). A controlled clinical comparison of Lunerin and Rinomar in allergic rhinitis. *Acta Allergol, 28,* 118-125.

Middleton, R. S. W. (1981). Double blind trial in general practice comparing the efficacy of "Benylin Day and Night" and paracetamol in the treatment of the common cold. *Br J Clin Pract, 35,* 297-300.

Moen, M., & Stein, R. (1982). Urge incontinence. *Ann Chir Gynaecol, 71,* 203-207.

Moller, C., & Bjorksten, B. (1980). Oxatomide in seasonal rhinoconjunctivitis. *Allergy, 35,* 319-322.

Moller, P. (1980). Negative middle ear pressure and hearing thresholds in secretory otitis media. *Scand Audiol, 9,* 171-176.

Montague, D. K., & Stewart, B. H. (1979). Urethral pressure profiles before and after Ornade administration in patients with stress urinary incontinence. *J Urol, 122,* 198-199.

Moran, D. M., Mutchie, K. D., Higbee, M. D., & Paul, L. D. (1982). The use of an antihistamine-decongestant in conjunction with an anti-infective drug in the treatment of acute otitis media. *J Pediatr, 101,* 132-136.

Mullarkey, M. F. (1981). A clinical approach to rhinitis. *Med Clin North Am, 65,* 977-986.

Norlen, L., & Sundin, T. (1982). Influence of the adrenergic nervous system on the lower urinary tract and its clinical implications. *Internatl Rehabil Med, 4,* 37-43.

Obrink, A., & Bunne, G. (1978). The effect of alpha-adrenergic stimulation in stress incontinence. *Scand J Urol Nephrol, 12,* 205-208.

Ouslander, J. G. (1981). Urinary incontinence in the elderly. *West J Med, 135,* 482-491.

Packman, E. W., & London, S. J. (1977). Utility of artificially induced cough as a clinical model for evaluating antitussive drug combinations. *Curr Ther Res Clin Exp, 21,* 855-866.

Parrillo, O. J., & Humoller, F. L. (1966). Clinical evaluation of an antiasthmatic compound. *Nebr State Med J, 51,* 335-337.

Penders, L., de Leval, J., & Petit, R. (1984). Enuresis and urethral instability. *Eur Urol (Switz), 10,* 317-322.

Pentel, P. R., Aaron, C., & Paya, C. (1985). Therapeutic doses of phenylpropanolamine increase supine systolic blood pressure. *Int J Obes, 9,* 115-119.

Pentel, P. R., Asinger, R. W., & Benowitz, N. L. (1985). Propranolol antagonism of phenylpro-panolamine-induced hypertension. *Clin Pharmacol Ther, 37,* 488-494.

Pipkorn, U., & Rundcrantz, H. (1982). The effect of oral decongestants in acute rhinitis as re-lated to variations in body position. *Acta Otolaryngol* (suppl), *386,* 276-278.

Pou, J. W., Quinn, H. J., & Watkins, W. J. (1970). An x-ray evaluation of the symptomatic response to Ru-Tuss tablets in sinusitis. *Curr Ther Res, 12,* 40-46.

Proctor, K. G., & Howards, S. S. (1983). The effect of sympathomimetic drugs on post-lympha-denectomy aspermia. *J Urol, 129,* 837-838.

Randall, J. E., & Hendley, J. O. (1979). A decongestant antihistamine mixture in the prevention of otitis media in children with colds. *Pediatrics, 63,* 483-485.

Rees, D. L. P., & Ransley, P. G. (1980). Eskornade in the treatment of diurnal incontinence in children. *Br J Urol, 52,* 476-479.

Reilly, W. A. (1950). The treatment of obesity in childhood. *Am Pract Dig Treat, 1,* 228-234.

Renvall, U., & Lindqvist, N. (1979). A double-blind clinical study with Monydrin tablets in pa-tients with non-allergic chronic rhinitis. *J Int Med Res, 7,* 235-239.

Renvall, U., & Nilsson, E. (1982). Eustachian tube dysfunction. *Acta Otolaryngol, 94,* 139-143.

Rhea, K. (1971). Treatment of sinusitis associated with atmospheric pollution. *Clin Med, 78,* 28-29.

Richter, K. P., & Ling, G. V. (1985). Clinical response and urethral pressure profile changes after phenylpropanolamine in dogs with primary sphincter incompetence. *J Am Vet Med Assoc, 187,* 605-611.

Robinson, J. M. (1982). The lower urinary tract. *Br J Clin Pharmacol, 13,* 761-773.

Saunte, C., & Johansson, S.-A. (1978). Clinical trial with Lunerin Mixture and Lunerin Mite in children with secretory otitis media. *J Int Med Res, 6,* 50-55.

Schnore, S. K., Sangster, J. F., Gerace, T. M., & Bass, M. J. (1986). Are antihistamine-decon-gestants of value in the treatment of acute otitis media in children? *J Fam Pract, 22,* 39-43.

Sebok, M. (1985). A double-blinded, placebo-controlled, clinical study of the efficacy of a phenylpropanolamine/caffeine combination product as an aid to weight loss in adults. *Curr Ther Res, 37,* 701-708.

Silverman, H. I. (1963). Phenylpropanolamine—misused? Or simply abused? *Am J Pharm, 135,* 45-54.

Silverstone, T. (1982). Psychopharmacology of hunger and food intake in humans. *Pharmacol Ther, 19,* 417-434.

Sorri, M., Sipila, P., Palva, A., & Karma, P. (1982). Can secretory otitis media be prevented by oral decongestants. *Acta Otolaryngol* (suppl), *386,* 115-116.

Stewart, B. H., & Bergant, J. A. (1974). Correction of retrograde ejaculation by sympathomi-metic medication: Preliminary report. *Fertil Steril, 25,* 1073-1074.

Stewart, B. H., Banowsky, L. H., & Montague, D. K. (1976). Stress incontinence: Conservative therapy with sympathomimetic drugs. *J Urol, 115,* 558-559.

Stockton, A. B., Pace, P. T., & Tainter, M. L. (1931). Some clinical actions and therapeutic uses of racemic synephrine. *J Pharmacol Exp Therap, 41,* 11-20.

Tainter, M. L. (1944). Actions of benzedrine and propadrine in the control of obesity. *J Nutr, 27,* 89-105.

Thiagarajah, S., Vaughan, E. D., & Kitchin, J. D. (1978). Retrograde ejaculation: Successful pregnancy following combined sympathomimetic medication and insemination. *Fertil Steril, 30,* 96-97.

Thomsen, J., Mygind, N., Meistrup-Larsen, K. I., Sorensen, H., & Vesterhauge, S. (1979). Oral decongestant in acute otitis media. *Internatl J Pediatr Otorhinolaryngol, 1,* 103-108.

Virupannavar, C., & Tomera, F. (1982). An unusual case of retrograde ejaculation and a brief review of management. *Fertil Steril, 37,* 275-276.

Weintraub, M. (1985). Phenylpropanolamine as an anorexiant agent in weight control: A review of published and unpublished studies. In J. P. Morgan, D. V. Kagan, and J. S. Brody (Eds.). *Phenylpropanolamine: Risks, Benefits, and Controversies.* Clinical Pharmacology and Therapeutics Series, Vol. 5. Praeger Scientific, New York (pp. 53-79).

Weintraub, M., Ginsberg, G., Stein, E. C., Sundaresan, P. R., Schuster, B., O'Connor, P., & Byrne, L. M. (1986). Phenylpropanolamine OROS (Acutrim) vs. placebo in combination with caloric restriction and physician-managed behavior modification. *Clin Pharmacol Ther, 39,* 501-509.

Wenger, A. P., & Lapsa, P. (1970). Three-way measurement of an oral nasal decongestant. *Clin Med, 77,* 15-18.

Williams, R. H., Daughaday, W. H., Rogers, W. F., Asper, S. P., & Towery, B. T. (1948). Obesity and its treatment with particular reference to the use of anoxerigenic compounds. *Ann Int Med, 29,* 510-532.

Williams, M. E., & Pannill, F. C. (1982). Urinary incontinence in the elderly. *Ann Int Med, 97,* 895-907.

Winter, C. A., & Flataker, L. (1954). Antitussive compounds: Testing methods and results. *J Pharmacol Exp Ther, 112,* 99-108.

Wright, D. (1981). Sinusitis acute and chronic. *Practitioner, 225,* 1555-1564.

Younglove, R. H., Newman, R. L., & Wall, L. A. (1980). Medical management of the unstable bladder. *J Reprod Med, 24,* 215-218.

AUTHOR INDEX

Note: Numbers in *italics* indicate pages on which the complete reference appears.

405

SUBJECT INDEX